Idiopathic Pulmonary Fibrosis

*Edited by Salim Surani
and Venkat Rajasurya*

Published in London, United Kingdom

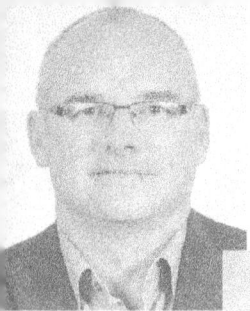
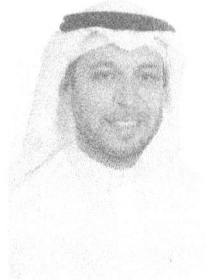
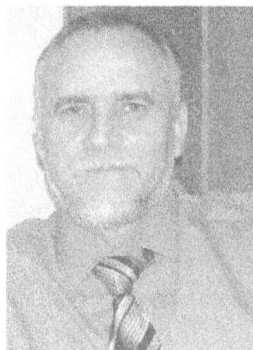
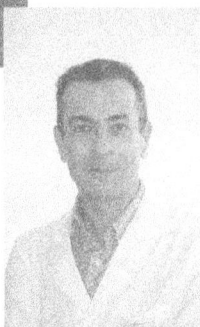
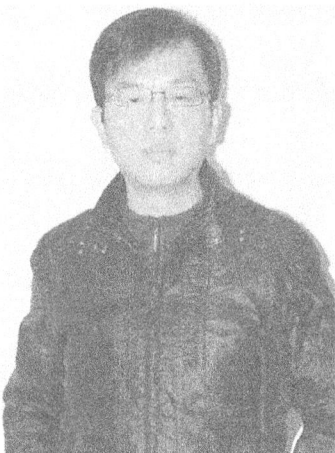
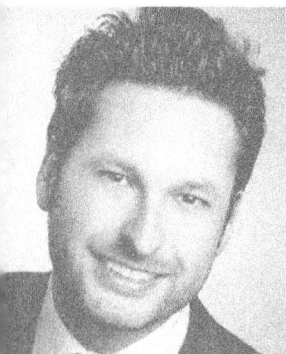
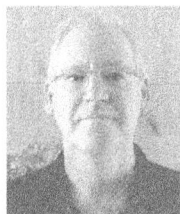

IntechOpen

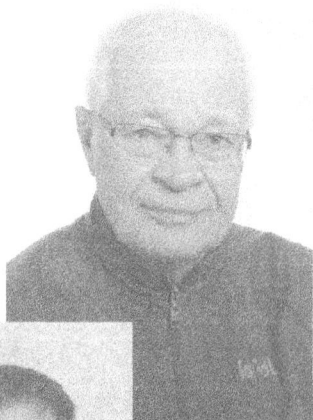
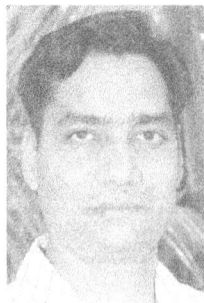
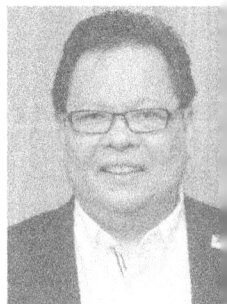
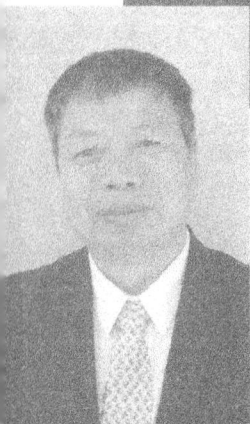
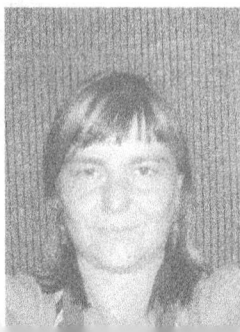
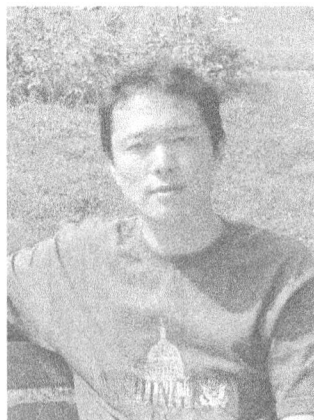

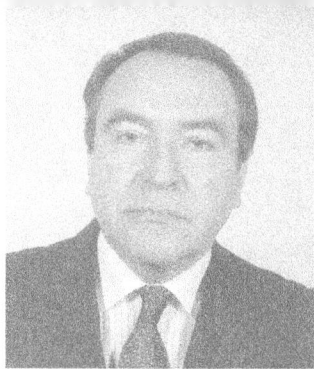

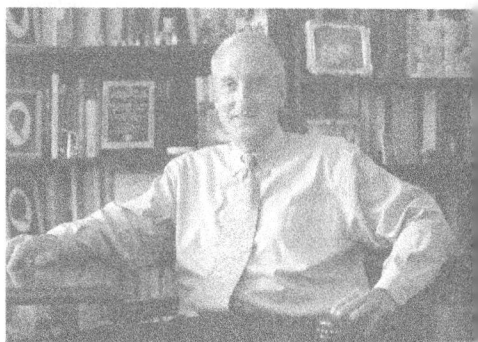

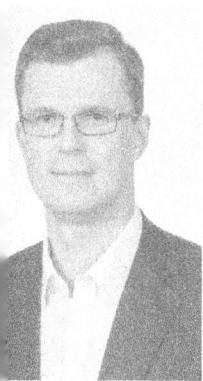

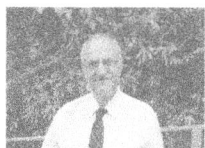

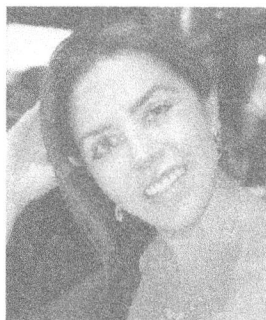

Supporting open minds since 2005

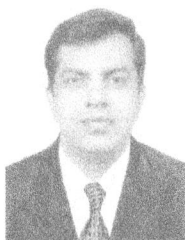

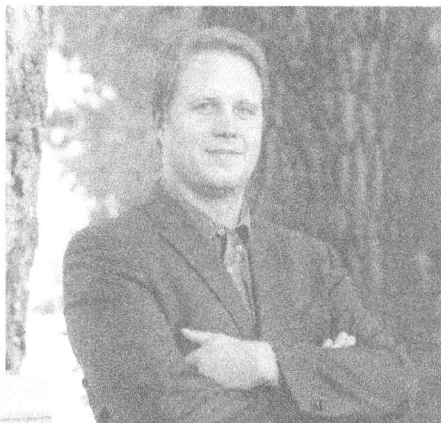

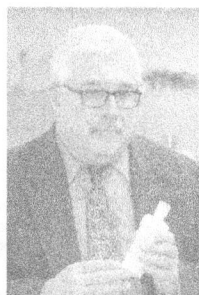

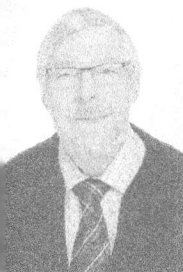

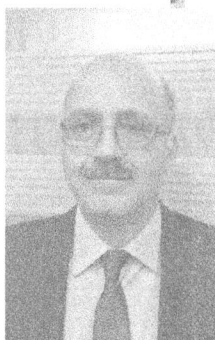

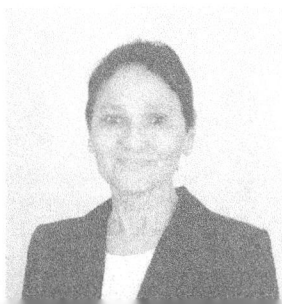

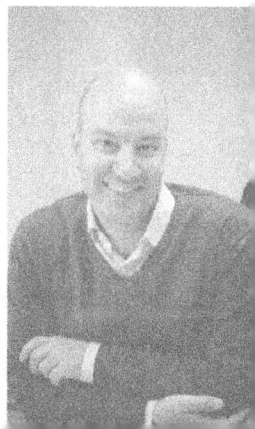

Idiopathic Pulmonary Fibrosis
http://dx.doi.org/10.5772/intechopen.87624
Edited by Salim Surani and Venkat Rajasurya

Contributors

Sanja Stankovic, Mihailo Stjepanovic, Milika Asanin, Nitesh Kumar Jain, Thoyaja Koritala, Anwar Khedr, Hisham Ahmed Mushtaq, Amos Lal, Simon Zec, Syed Anjum Khan, Rahul Kashyap, Aysun Tekin, Shikha Jain, Ramesh Adhikari, Aishwarya Reddy Korsapati, Mool Chand, Vishwanath Pattan, Vikas Bansal, Ali Rabaan, Hasnain Bawaadam, Aman Sethi, Lavanya Dondapati, Raghavendra Tirupathi, Ibtisam Rauf, Mack Sheraton, Maureen Muigai, David Rokser, Chetna Dengri, Kovid Trivedi, Samir Gautam, Brian Bartlett, April Lanz, Sumeet Yadav, Greta Zoesch, Stephanie Welle, M.S. Chandramouli, Salim Surani, Anupam Sule, Jama Abbas, Mohamed Hassan, Adham Mohsen, Amit Munshi Sharma, Mikael Mir, Lia Nandi, Hariprasad Reddy Korsapati, Sachin M. Patil, Pahnwat T. Taweesedt, Kejal Gandhi, Reena Shah, Ruben A. Peredo, Moiz Ehtesham, Anupama Tiwari, Rose Sneha George, Ladan Panahi, George Udeani, Andrew Scott Tenpas, Theresa Ofili, Elizabeth Marie Aguilar, Sarah Burchard, Alexandra Ruth Ritenour, April Jacob Chennat, Nehal Ahmed, Chairat Atphaisit, Crystal Chi, Jesus Cruz III, Monica D. Deleon, Samantha Lee, Zack Mayo, Mackenzie Mcbeth, Mariel Morales, Jennifer N. Nwosu, Kelly Palacios, Jaycob M. Pena, Nitza Vara, Humayun Anjum, Ryan Goetz, Thomas S. Kaleekal

Notice
Statements and opinions expressed in the chapters are these of the individual contributors and not necessarily those of the editors or publisher. No responsibility is accepted for the accuracy of information contained in the published chapters. The publisher assumes no responsibility for any damage or injury to persons or property arising out of the use of any materials, instructions, methods or ideas contained in the book.

First published in London, United Kingdom, 2022 by IntechOpen
IntechOpen is the global imprint of INTECHOPEN LIMITED, registered in England and Wales, registration number: 11086078, 5 Princes Gate Court, London, SW7 2QJ, United Kingdom
Printed in Croatia

British Library Cataloguing-in-Publication Data
A catalogue record for this book is available from the British Library

Additional hard and PDF copies can be obtained from orders@intechopen.com

Idiopathic Pulmonary Fibrosis
Edited by Salim Surani and Venkat Rajasurya
p. cm.
Print ISBN 978-1-83969-239-0
Online ISBN 978-1-83969-240-6
eBook (PDF) ISBN 978-1-83969-241-3

We are IntechOpen,
the world's leading publisher of
Open Access books
Built by scientists, for scientists

6,000+
Open access books available

148,000+
International authors and editors

185M+
Downloads

Our authors are among the

156
Countries delivered to

Top 1%
most cited scientists

12.2%
Contributors from top 500 universities

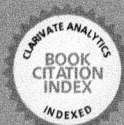

Interested in publishing with us?
Contact book.department@intechopen.com

Numbers displayed above are based on latest data collected.
For more information visit www.intechopen.com

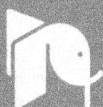

Meet the editor

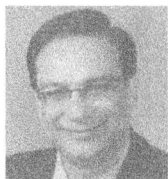

Dr. Salim Surani serves as Adjunct Clinical Professor of Medicine, Department of Pulmonary, Critical Care & Sleep Medicine, Texas A&M University, as well as Clinical Professor of Pharmacology, Texas A&M University–Kingsville. In addition, he serves as a voluntary professor at the University of Houston, Texas, and a research collaborator at Mayo Clinic, Minnesota. He has served as the program director for the Pulmonary Fellowship Program at Bay Area Medical Center, Corpus Christi, Texas. He completed a fellowship in Pulmonary Medicine at Baylor College of Medicine, Houston, Texas. Dr. Surani obtained a master's degree in Public Health and Epidemiology from Yale University, Connecticut, and a master's degree in Health Management from the University of Texas, Dallas. Dr. Surani is on the board of trustees and has served as secretary for the CHEST Foundation. He is also on the membership committee of the American College of Chest Physicians. He has also served as a chair of practice operations for the network of the American College of Chest Physicians. He serves on the award committee for ACCP and the American Academy of Sleep Medicine (AASM). He is an editor in chief, editorial board member, and reviewer for several peer-reviewed journals. He has served as a steering committee member for the executive committee of networks of the American College of Chest Physicians. Dr. Surani has authored more than 300 articles in journals and has written several books and book chapters. He has been involved in teaching residents for more than two decades. He has received faculty of the year awards numerous times. He has established himself as a master clinician who has trained significant numbers of practicing primary care, internal medicine, and emergency physicians in the Coastal Bend region of the United States. He has served as an independent grant reviewer for the Government of Australia, the Government of Singapore, as well as the European Nation via Rannis. Dr. Surani has established several ICU-intensivist models in the region and has served in every possible leadership role in the hospital system. He also helped start an emergency medicine residency program. He also started a pulmonary critical care fellowship with the American Osteopathic Association (AOA) and successfully led the program with no citations. He then converted the program into a pulmonary medicine fellowship program when the Accreditation Council for Graduate Medical Education (ACGME) and AOA merged, leading to its accreditation. He has served as a speaker at several regional, national, and international scientific conferences. His areas of expertise include critical care, sleep medicine, ICU infections, and practice operations. Dr. Surani serves as a resident health expert for KIII-TV, Texas (an affiliate of ABC News). He has also served on committees for several national organizations and has received several community and teaching awards, including the Health Care Hero award and humanitarian awards by the American College of Physicians, the American College of Chest Physicians, and the Texas Medical Association. Dr. Surani is highly regarded among his peers and is very well respected as a mentor, clinician, and humanitarian.

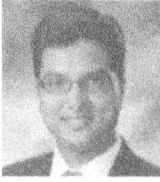

Dr. Venkat Rajasurya currently works as an attending pulmonary critical care physician at MultiCare Health System, Tacoma, Washington. He previously worked as an attending physician in the Novant Health system in North Carolina and has worked as a clinical assistant professor at the Southern Illinois University program in Decatur, Illinois for 4 years, and served as director of multiple clinical and leadership committees at Decatur Memorial Hospital, Decatur, Illinois. Dr. Rajasurya completed his fellowship in Pulmonary Critical Care at Cook County/ Rush University Hospital, Chicago, Illinois. He served as the medical advisor for the Illinois Society of Respiratory Care for three years. He has played a key role in the training and education of medical and pharmacy residents as well as physician assistants throughout his career. He has served as a co-investigator for several clinical trials at MultiCare Institute for Research & Innovation, Tacoma, Washington, and Southeastern Research Center, Winston Salem, North Carolina. Dr. Rajasurya has authored and reviewed articles and serves as an editorial board member for peer-reviewed journals. He has given oral presentations at several national and international conferences. His areas of interest include obstructive airway diseases, interstitial lung diseases, lung cancer, sepsis, critical care management of acute conditions, and resident education. He is an active member of the American College of Chest Physicians and was awarded FCCP for his excellence, dedication, and leadership in chest medicine. He is also actively involved in the Society of Critical Care Medicine and the American Thoracic Society. In addition to multiple teaching and research awards throughout his career, he was awarded the prestigious Gold Doc Award by the Arnold P. Gold Foundation for humanism in medicine.

Contents

Preface

Idiopathic pulmonary fibrosis (IPF) is the most common and important type of idiopathic interstitial pneumonia, characterized by chronic, progressive fibrosing interstitial pneumonia of unknown etiology with a high fatality rate. The incidence and prevalence of the disease increase with age. Worldwide, IPF affects more than 3 million people. In the United States and Europe, the reported incidence of IPF is 2.8–9.3 per 100,000 per year and the prevalence is 18–495 cases per 100,000 adults depending on the age of the cohort. Regional variance has been seen, suggesting that environmental factors play a role.

Over the past decades, we have seen tremendous advancement in the diagnosis and treatment of IPF, which has led to a better understanding of the disease's epidemiology, diagnostics, and optimal treatment modalities. There has been a big push to decrease the time to diagnosis from symptom onset, as it can take one to two years. The pathogenesis of the disease is complex and it is important to rule out several other diseases that can lead to pulmonary fibrosis. The hallmark of IPF is the usual interstitial pneumonia (UIP) pattern seen on high-resolution computed tomography (HRCT) and histology. The diagnosis requires a multidisciplinary team approach, and several guidelines have been published in recent years to help clinicians diagnose this disease in a timely manner.

Recent guidelines have updated the diagnostic modalities and have accepted transbronchial cryobiopsy as an acceptable alternative to surgical biopsy. Moreover, progressive pulmonary fibrosis has now been defined as having two of the following three criteria: physiological progression, radiological progression, and worsening symptoms.

Two antifibrotic drugs are now available, which are not curative but have shown to significantly slow down the decline in lung function associated with IPF. Some recent guidelines have given a conditional recommendation to nintedanib, while more research is suggested for pirfenidone (which was the first to make its way into IPF treatment).

This book describes the epidemiology and diagnosis of IPF in detail. There has been a significant advancement in biomarkers and thus we have included a chapter on biomarkers in IPF. In the area of therapeutics, the book discusses pharmacological management as well as exacerbation of IPF. IPF is a complex disease and gastro-esophageal reflux (GERD) has been shown to play a role. As such, there is a chapter addressing the role of GERD in IPF. The book ends with a discussion of pulmonary involvement in Sjogren's disease. Lung transplant remains the cornerstone of management of IPF and despite treatment with antifibrotic agents, most patients with this disease will progress to advanced end-stage lung disease.

We hope this book will update clinicians' knowledge and aid them in taking care of patients with IPF.

Salim Surani, MD, MPH, MSHM, FACP, FAASM, FCCM, FCCP
Adj. Clinical Professor of Medicine and Pharmacology,
Texas A&M University,
Texas, USA

Venkat Rajasurya
Multicare Health System,
Tacoma, WA, USA

Section 1

Epidemiology

Chapter 1

Epidemiology of Idiopathic Pulmonary Fibrosis

Sachin M. Patil

Abstract

Idiopathic pulmonary fibrosis (IPF) is a type of interstitial lung disease (ILD) classified under idiopathic fibrotic disorders of the lung. It is the most common type of ILD presenting clinically in the seventh decade of life, almost always at the later stage of illness, attributed to its earlier nonspecific presentation. The term IPF is used when no specific cause for pulmonary fibrosis is identified. Initially described in 1944, recent advances in lung biopsy and pathology have described the disease in detail. This led to further classification of ILD. Also, there have been multiple recent studies indicative of an increased incidence. However, accurate epidemiological data for IPF is minimal, with some being contradictory. Inconsistency in the case definition criteria and methodology has resulted in epidemiological inaccuracy when used to detect patients in the study population. To avoid inaccuracy American Thoracic Society collaborated with the European, Japanese, and Latin American Thoracic Society to arrive at a consensus resulting in 2010 IPF evidence-based guidelines. Notable epidemiological differences are observed in the European, American, and Asian countries. Some countries have set up national registries to collect essential patient data for future studies and comparison with other countries. In this topic, we try to glean over the epidemiology of IPF.

Keywords: Epidemiology, Idiopathic, Interstitial, Fibrosis, Lung, Disease

1. Introduction

IPF is a rare pulmonary disease affecting patients often in their sixth or the seventh decade of life. The disease course is progressive, causing permanent damage to the pulmonary tissue resulting in restrictive lung disease and hypoxia. Pharmacological therapeutic options are sparse and limited to new medications such as nintedanib and pirfenidone [1]. Without lung transplantation, IPF is lethal, and the patient dies from acute pulmonary failure in two to four years on average [1]. Lung transplantation has altered the disease course and improved longevity. As it is a rare disease, an accurate, consistent epidemiological methodology needs to be followed for data collection to measure the incidence and prevalence of IPF [1]. The consensus evidence-based guidelines in 2011 guide how to arrive at a diagnosis after ruling out other ILD causes and the need for multidisciplinary specialist's input.

2. Predisposing risk factors

2.1 Age and gender

As the patient's age increases, the IPF incidence increases with a more significant occurrence in men than women as per epidemiological studies [2]. The mean age at which diagnosis was established was 66 years. On average, most patients diagnosed with IPF lie between the age of 40 to 70 years [3]. Occurrence in younger patients (< 40 years) is rare. In most studies, men accounted for most cases except for a Norwegian study which disclosed a higher prevalence in females [4]. A recent study with an IPF score algorithm was generated using logistic regression to measure the exact incidence and prevalence values of 14.6/100,000 person-years and 58.7/100,000 person-years. The IPF score algorithm had a positive predictive value (PPV) of 83.3% [1].

The Gender-Age-Physiology (GAP) index calculated to predict IPF mortality by dividing the IPF into three stages GAP one, two, and three did not anticipate a decline in pulmonary function based on the severity of the GAP index [5]. IPF disproportionately affecting 71% of males was observed in a recent retrospective cohort study [6]. Age-adjusted males were strongly linked to an increased risk (40%) for lung transplantation or death [6]. In males, the cough was associated with dyspnea due to smoking-related airway disease, whereas in females, it was due to acid reflux disease. A lower diffusion capacity than predicted for age, senility, dry or productive cough with phlegm correlated with a decreased survival in males free of transplant compared to females. This may be due to excessive male exposure to risk factors in the environment, such as cigarette or occupational smoke particulate material and sex hormones [6]. Sex hormones modulate the immune system with a humoral immune response augmentation by estrogen and androgens, suppressing the cell-mediated and humoral immune response [7].

Age is a substantial independent predictor of IPF [8]. Aging lung undergoes anatomical and physiological changes predisposing it to IPF. The elderly may have abnormal recruitment of protective mesenchymal cells and fibrocytes in response to acute lung injury [9]. Increased endoplasmic reticulum oxidative stress, unfolded protein response lead to apoptosis of type 2 alveolar epithelial cells increasing susceptibility to IPF in the elderly [10]. Immune changes are seen in adaptive than in innate immunity. Adaptive immunity changes affect the T lymphocytes more than the B lymphocytes. There is a decrease in differentiation, antibody affinity, and interaction with T cells & B cells. There is a decline in naïve T cells (with short telomere and restricted repertoire), transition to Th2 response phenotype, an abnormal increase in memory, and effector cells with large CD28 deficient CD8 endstage clonal population [11, 12]. The T cell response leads to an inadequate vaccination and abnormal viral response [13, 14]. Many IPF patients have a shorter telomere with no detectable mutation in telomerase [15]. The elderly with a short telomere on exposure to susceptible environmental exposure may trigger apoptosis resulting in fibrosis. Old lungs may provide the appropriate local milieu for gammaherpesvirus or any other virus to cause fibrosis [9]. Smoking promotes epigenetic changes in deoxyribonucleic acid methylation, histone modifications, and microribonucleic acid [16].

Increased mortality in IPF is associated with a consecutive increase in oxygen desaturation episodes during a six-minute walk test. Males during their disease course experienced frequent faster desaturation events than females. In contrast to males, the disease progression rate is slower, in females contributing to survival differences. This may contribute to but does not entirely inform more remarkable female survival in IPF. Even in fibrotic diseases, females have lesser fibrosis than males, possibly due to sex hormone exposure [17]. Most females at their diagnosis of IPF are in a postmenopausal state with diminished estrogen levels. The precise role of hormonal imbalance on the fibrotic process needs clarification with further studies.

2.2 Smoking

Smoking is a practice of burning raw or refined tobacco plant leaves and breathing in the resulting smoke for taste. Smoking is an ancient frequent recreational drug use still in practice. Tobacco smoke contains multiple active chemicals which are either absorbed in the mucosa or delivered to the lungs. Tobacco smoke exposure results in multiple lung diseases such as chronic obstructive pulmonary disease (COPD) and lung cancer. Tobacco smoke contains numerous chemicals exerting various delirious cellular effects on multiple organs affecting their metabolic function. As a primary intermediary, the lung faces the brunt of tobacco smoke exposure in active and passive smokers. Tobacco smoke exposure contains acrolein, benzene, benzopyrene, acetaldehyde, formaldehyde, carbon monoxide, 1,3-butadiene, and tobacco-specific nitrosamines with human toxicity potential. Additionally, the long-term effects of flavors and additives used in cigarettes on tobacco smoke and lung are unknown. Another issue is the lack of regulation regarding performance standards for ingredients used in making cigarettes [18].

Smoking has been included as a potential etiologic agent recently over the last few decades due to its significant prevalence among the IPF patient population [19]. However, the association was proposed as early as 1969, which independently increases the significant risk of IPF disease [20]. Another disease that shares the pathological features of COPD and IPF, known as combined pulmonary fibrosis and emphysema (CPFE), is seen predominantly in male smokers. Smoking may also enhance the systemic immune response to numerous environmental etiological agents, increasing the IPF risk by 60% in smokers [21]. The cytological effect of smoking in IPF can be direct or indirect, impacting the clinical course and survival. The evidence for a direct effect of smoking causing pulmonary fibrosis is minimal [22]. Tobacco use prevalence in IPF patients ranges from 41–83%, the range attributed to the definition criteria used in various studies [3, 23]. Alveoli is the main target of the IPF, resulting in diminished diffusion capacity for carbon monoxide. Alveolar wall fibrosis seen in smokers is due to cigarette smoke exposure, and there is an increase in fibrosis based on the duration and intensity of exposure [24]. Increased oxidative stress in current and ex-smokers may promote IPF disease progression [25]. IPF is also known as senescence disease due to its occurrence in tobacco smoke exposure patients' in an age-dependent style [26].

Smoking results in a small airway inflammatory cell recruitment comprising neutrophils, macrophages, and langerhans cells, resulting in severe immune and other lung cell defects. However, only a few patients end up having clinically significant diffuse lung disease. Probably only a minority of patients progress into a vicious inflammation cycle resulting in IPF due to constant environmental stimuli and lapse of anti-inflammatory mechanisms [23]. A brief outline of the IPF pathogenesis is explained in **Figure 1** [19]. Persistent cigarette smoke exposure (CSE) leads to a predominant M2 macrophage activation in the lung. In contrast to the M1 Phenotype, the M2 macrophages are ineffective in host defense, inadequately clear noxious agents, and increase fibrotic mediators synthesis.

This results in a vicious, inflammatory cascade causing an increased expression of transforming growth factor α 1 (TGF α 1), epidermal growth factor (EGF), and mixed metalloproteinase (MMP) expression on epithelial cells leading to an epithelial to mesenchymal transition of the epithelial cells. This increases the pulmonary myofibroblasts, which are relatively resistant to apoptosis, have a lower activation threshold, augmented profibrotic response, and are activated by apoptosis debris.

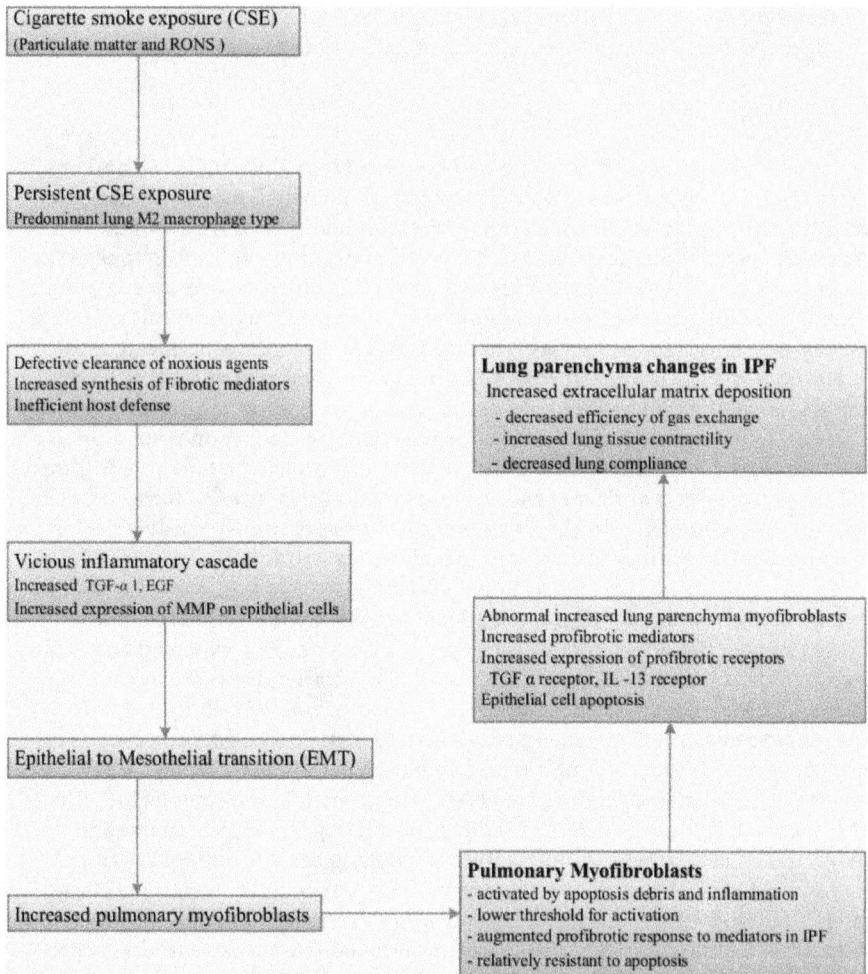

Figure 1.
Pathogenesis of idiopathic pulmonary fibrosis. RONS, reactive oxygen and nitrogen species; TGF, transforming growth factor; EGF, epidermal growth factor; MMP, matrix metalloproteinase; IL, interleukin.

This leads to an abnormal increase in lung parenchyma myofibroblasts, profibrotic mediators, profibrotic receptor expression, and epithelial cell apoptosis. Finally, the lung parenchyma changes kick in with increased extracellular matrix (ECM) deposition making it difficult for gas exchange. The thick ECM increases lung contractility and decreases lung compliance.

Telomere dysfunction noted in the epithelial precursor cells simulating senescence can be seen sporadically and in patients with genetic abnormalities [27]. In IPF, the primary cell type affected is the alveolar epithelial precursor cell. The Wnt and the Notch signal pathways are essential in sustaining and separating the precursor cells (epithelial and mesenchymal). Defective functioning of these pathways results in pneumocyte loss followed by significant inflammation during defective attempts at repair due to molecular signals' release [27]. Smoking causes a decrease in histone acetylation and methylation, resulting in the antifibrotic cyclooxygenase-2 gene and interferon-gamma inducible protein suppression [19].

In an earlier study comparing survival disparities and smoking status in IPF patients, smokers had lower survival than nonsmokers [27]. Lifetime nonsmokers had a better outcome than prior smokers and the combination of all smokers, including active and ex-smokers. This survival disparity suggests that smoking results in a decrement of IPF patient's survival. Current smokers had better survival than former smokers due to a healthy smoker effect [27]. The reasoning for this effect is that a smoker with the advanced symptomatic disease will quit smoking for health benefits. In a recent study analyzing differences in severity adjusted survival among active and prior smokers, active smokers' minimal survival benefit diminished on adding age to the model [28]. The healthy smoker effect was absent in this study. The earlier study's survival disparity was not apparent after a composite physiologic index (calculated from the pulmonary function tests) was added to the severity adjustment [27].

Current smokers are younger than ex-smokers and nonsmokers, explaining the more prolonged survival seen in these patients [28]. Smoking-associated comorbidities were frequent in current smokers with more pack-years of smoking than ex-smokers [28]. The frequent comorbidities associated with smoking include cardiovascular disease (CVD), coronary artery disease, hypertension, cerebrovascular disease, diabetes, and heart failure may affect IPF mortality. Females had a higher incidence of asthma and diabetes than males, while active smokers had a higher incidence of COPD and lung cancer than nonsmokers. In the recent study, only a diagnosis of CVD, COPD at any time, and insulin use at the time of diagnosis resulted in a poor survival on severity adjustment analysis [28]. Smoking prevention is an important cause to decrease mortality and morbidity in the western and third world.

2.3 Environmental factors

Occupational disclosure to surrounding elements contributes around 26% population attributable fraction (PAF) of total cases of IPF [29]. This suggests that IPF is a heterogeneous disease. Exposure to environmental agents occurs during the occupation, residence in a specific area, and recreational activities. The exposure may be due to a single agent or multiple agents, which is difficult to quantify. Recently air pollution has been recognized as a critical etiology and an exacerbating factor for IPF [30]. In comparison to the population size exposed to these agents, only a few develop IPF. IPF occurs more so in individuals with genetic susceptibilities exposed to these environmental agents. There are three factors essential in the pathogenesis of IPF; one is the environmental agent exposure, the second is the duration of exposure, while the third is the host response to the persistent exposure controlled by genetic susceptibility. Persistent environmental agent exposure results in a biochemical reaction (in most cases oxidative stress) followed by an insistent immune response to the agent, causing lung fibrosis [31]. As IPF is a rare disease, case–control studies are best suited for it. They come with many challenges regarding data collection as they are subjected to multiple factors that dilute the study's purpose. These factors include disease misclassification (pneumoconiosis classified as IPF), exposure misclassification (recall bias), and variable susceptibility to fibrogenic agents(dose and duration of exposure along with genetic susceptibilities) [31]. Adequate clinical significance is denied to occupational and environmental history when clinical information is obtained from the patients. Pulmonary tissue biopsy analysis in IPF patients with Particle induced X-ray emission revealed a high content of silicon, magnesium, titanium, and high surface silicon to a sulfur ratio [32, 33]. Elementary analysis of hilar and mediastinal lymph nodes using fluorescent x-ray analysis disclosed high nickel content and a minimum silicon elevation [34]. Over the last two to three decades, multiple case–control investigations have identified various environmental agents suspected to be a causative factor for

IPF [35]. These include metal dust (brass, aluminum, arsenic, cadmium, copper, molybdenum, tungsten, cobalt, uranium, vanadium, lead, and steel), raising birds, farming, wood dust, hairdressing, stone cutting/polishing, and organic dust from livestock & vegetation.

A southern European case–control study found two occupations with an increased prospect of having IPF, which increased with the exposure duration. One group included the farmers, veterinarians, gardeners, and the other group included metallurgical and steel industry workers [36]. A self-reported exposure history correlated with the increased risk, and the authors evaluated the history with a job-exposure matrix (JEM). Although an American multicenter study identified multiple jobs related to an increased risk of IPF, the multivariate regression model revealed the strongest link between raising birds and exposure to vegetable or animal dust [37]. Three occupations in the United States of America (USA), namely metal mining, wood building (mobile homes), and structured metal fabricated products, had an increased IPF mortality risk based on the mortality data [38]. A Korean study on dust exposure divulged its impact on IPF patient's prognosis. Patients with exposure had an earlier IPF diagnosis, prolonged symptom duration at diagnosis, and increased mortality than those with no exposure [39].

Organic dust involves farming, gardening, animal husbandry, poultry farming, carpentry, and pesticides. Animal husbandry is an agriculture branch related to animal rearing for food and other products with significant exposure to animal feeds, products, and waste. A multicenter case–control study done in Egypt was the first to reveal an increased IPF risk in females than males [40]. Females were at a higher risk while working in poultry farming, farming with organic dust, and occupational pesticide exposure. Males carried an increased risk in carpentry, chemical, and petrochemical industries occupations. Both sexes had an increased risk with cat or bird exposure. IPF risk was minimal in sales and clerical jobs [40]. A Belgian multidisciplinary team studied 244 IPF patients, divided them based on prior exposure to molds or birds, and simultaneously compared them to chronic hypersensitivity pneumonitis patients. Patients exposed to birds or molds were associated with a decreased fatality than unexposed patients [41].

Mineral and metal dust exposure are well known to increase the IPF risk. A British study done in a major engineering company evaluated IPF mortality in employees exposed to occupational metal exposure. It revealed a strong association between IPF fatality and metal exposure strength and duration [42]. A multicenter Japanese study disclosed that patients with clerical occupations had a lower risk of IPF than patients with prior metal exposure [43]. Hilar lymph nodes histopathological analysis in IPF patients compared to controls revealed excess aluminum and silicon related to an increased risk of IPF [44]. Two smaller South Korean case–control studies revealed an increased IPF risk with exposure to stone, sand, silica, and metal dust [45, 46]. Asbestos occupational exposure results in asbestosis are well established; however, the effects of mild to moderate exposure on IPF are unclear. A study comparing United Kingdom (UK) asbestos imports per year to IPF mortality for any relationship was done. The overall asbestos exposure outcome was not addressed in this study. Linear regression models revealed a significant positive linear association between imports and IPF mortality, suggesting an association between IPF mortality and asbestos exposure [47]. UK is undergoing a national study by the name IPF Job Exposure study (IPF-JES) to evaluate the IPF risk associated with occupational asbestos exposure.

Wood dust exposure during carpentry and woodworks is related to a higher IPF risk and follows a dose–response association in UK based case–control study [48]. A Swedish multicenter case–control study on occupational exposure revealed a higher IPF risk in males with birch dust and hardwood dust exposure and no increased risk with metal exposure [49]. A similar increased association was observed in an Italian case series and an Egyptian multicenter case–control study [40, 50]. Air pollutants present in the environment may have an important role apart from smoking in IPF incidence. An Italian study evaluated the relationship between IPF occurrence in patients persistently exposed to ambient air pollutants (nitrogen dioxide, particulate matter [aerodynamic diameter less than 10 μm], and ozone) [30]. Final results were not adjusted for smoking which was a limitation of this study. An increment in nitrogen dioxide concentration resulted in a significant IPF incidence rate increase with no association observed with ozone and particulate matter. IPF acute exacerbation risk is higher in patients exposed to nitrogen dioxide and ozone in the prior six weeks [51]. Conflicting results of studies on lung function decline on ambient particulate matter (APM) exposure have been observed. One study revealed an accelerated lung function decrement in patients exposed to APM with an aerodynamic diameter of less than 10 μm, and no relationship was noted with APM with an aerodynamic diameter of less than 2.5 μm [52]. No association with a lung function decrease rate and ambient air pollutant exposure was identified in a 25 patient prospective group study [53]. A large French cohort study evaluated the effect of air pollutants on IPF disease outcomes [54]. Patients exposed to ozone had a higher risk of IPF acute exacerbations, whereas those exposed to APM with an aerodynamic diameter of less than 10 or 2.5 μm had increased mortality. In conclusion, APM exposure regularly can play a role in pathophysiology and may affect IPF disease progression.

A 2019 meta-analysis reviewed the literature and case–control studies. The following exposures (metal dust, silica, wood dust & vapor, gas, dust, or fumes) were significant statistically [29]. The pooled odds ratio for agricultural work was elevated with no significance. A recent South Korean meta-analysis revealed a statistically significant association with pesticide, metal, and wood dust exposure. No significance was observed with stone or sand dust and textile dust exposure. Agricultural workers and woodworkers had a significant increase in IPF risk statistically, whereas no significance was seen in textile workers [55]. In this Japanese study, consumption of fish rich in polyunsaturated fatty acids had a significantly lower odds ratio with regards to IPF, and it may have a suppressive effect on lung fibrosis [56]. A decline in IPF rate is achievable if environmental exposure is modified. It is a demanding process to obtain a detailed exposure history as it is subject to recall bias, difficulty in quantifying heterogeneous exposure intensity and its cumulative variation [57]. Also, it is difficult to identify a specific exposure effect when multiple are in play. For obtaining accurate epidemiological data, a standard operational definition for occupational and environmental history needs to be arrived at based on consensus so that it is easier to compare multiple studies (case–control and cohort) precisely to understand the IPF occurrence. If occupational and environmental exposure results in IPF, implementing measures to alter the exposure or improve the occupational environment may decrease IPF risk, and prevention may become a public health issue.

2.4 GERD (gastroesophageal reflux disease)

Gastroesophageal disease is a suspected risk factor for IPF development and progression currently under intense debate [58, 59]. The prevalence of pulmonary fibrosis was statistically significant in veterans with GERD history compared to healthy controls [60]. GERD incidence in IPF is higher than the average population and ranges from 8–87%. The variation is due to the methods used in diagnosis, diagnosis definition used and the types of data collected [61–63]. The greater incidence could be due to the common risk factors such as smoking and aging [64].

The gastroesophageal abnormalities seen in IPF patients include transient lower esophageal sphincter (LES) relaxations, decreased upper esophageal sphincter tone, and significantly greater proximal esophageal acid exposure cumulatively [65]. The decreased lung compliance in IPF due to fibrosis creates a negative intrapleural pressure which on transmission to the intrathoracic area decreases the LES tone resulting in reflux [66]. In animal models, the burden of proof is most substantial for GERD associated with IPF [67]. Chronic microaspiration insults may lead to pulmonary parenchyma damage attracting persistent inflammation resulting in fibrotic remodeling [68, 69]. Tracheal pepsin is a predictable indicator of aspiration [70]. The presence of bile salts and pepsin in bronchoalveolar lavage (BAL) suggests both acidic and nonacidic refluxate as risk factors for IPF disease [71]. BAL pepsin levels in post-transplant IPF patients were higher than in other chronic lung diseases [72].

PPI (Proton pump inhibitors) used in GERD are a reactive oxygen species scavenger, stimulate antioxidant production, decrease pro-inflammatory cytokines, inhibit profibrotic molecule expression, and decelerate pulmonary epithelial cell apoptosis [73]. Multiple studies and metanalysis have reviewed the use of PPI in IPF patients for GERD. Initial studies revealed PPI use was associated with fewer acute exacerbations, lower hospitalization rates, lesser radiological fibrosis score, stable or improved lung function, and more extended transplant-free survival [59, 74–76]. GERD symptoms and pathophysiology are well addressed by LARS (Laparoscopic antireflux surgery) as it restores the gastroesophageal junction anatomy and controls both acidic and nonacidic reflux [65]. IPF patients post-LARS had a nonsignificant decline in acute exacerbations, hospitalization related to pulmonary issues, and death than the nonsurgical group in a small group of 72 patients [77]. A pooled analysis on the antacid treatment effect on disease progression in IPF placebo patients included in the pirfenidone trials revealed no improved outcomes [78]. Instead, advanced IPF patients on antacid therapy had a greater risk of pulmonary and nonpulmonary infections. PPI use in IPF patients has given mixed results in studies, possibly due to their inability to correct the GERD anatomy. PPI can only alter the gastric refluxate's pH, making it more alkaline with no acidic and nonacidic microaspiration prevention [65]. A meta-analysis and systematic review evaluated the efficacy and safety of GERD therapy in IPF [79]. It revealed a significant decline in acute exacerbations, mortality related to IPF, and improved transplant-free survival. GERD pharmacological therapy did not result in all-cause mortality reduction. Another meta-analysis via systematic review analyzed the GERD and IPF association, and it revealed a possible association confounded by smoking [80].

In a post-hoc data evaluation of the INPULSIS trials, IPF acute exacerbations frequently occurred on antacid therapy than those not on it [81]. PPI use results in alkaline gastric pH, which loses its bactericidal effect and increases respiratory infections on aspiration [69]. The clinical data available does not agree with a GERD and IPF relationship [82]. In most patients, refluxes are silent with the absence of any symptoms, and the best way to diagnose them is via esophageal MII-pH or high-resolution manometry. Alternatively, bronchoscopy with BAL presence of pepsin and bile salts can be used in IPF [69]. During meta-analysis, a lack of clarity with GERD diagnostic definitions was identified. It was difficult to pinpoint which criteria were used to select the patient and how many met them [78]. The heterogeneous methods used have made it difficult to assess the association. Meta-analysis always encounters various issues with case–control studies and requires accurate interpretation of the association, however small it may be [83]. More extensive randomized trials are needed to study the effect of LARS in IPF patients. Future prospective studies would be better suited to accurately evaluate the evidence and analyze the PPI effect on the IPF clinical course.

2.5 Viral infections

The role of viral infections in IPF pathogenesis is unclear. It could either be an initiator of IPF or could exacerbate a preexisting disease based on the type of viral infection. Immunosenescence predisposes old lungs to viral infections due to T cell inefficiency. Lack of improved outcomes on the treatment of IPF with immunosup-pressants indicates the need for an intact immune system to control the disease process [84]. IPF therapy with antiviral medications has improved pulmonary function [85, 86]. Herpesvirus deoxyribonucleic acid (DNA) was recovered in 97% of IPF subjects compared to 36% of controls. This supports the idea of a herpes virus causing chronic antigenic stimulation in lung tissue [85]. Multiple animal models have supported a virus as an etiology for IPF. Experimental horse infection with an equine gammaherpesvirus resulted in pulmonary fibrosis [87]. Murine infection with a *Murine herpesvirus 68* (MHV 68) two to 10 weeks before introduc-ing a fibrotic insult accelerated lung fibrosis even in the presence of a weaker insult [88]. MHV68 pulmonary installation in an old mouse leads to pulmonary fibrosis due to the upregulation of TGF β, which was absent in the younger mice [89]. MHV 68 can cause lung fibrosis after a stem cell transplant in animal models [90]. MHV 68 infection after a fibrotic lung insult can result in fibrosis [91]. MHV 68 in interferon-gamma deficient mice causes pulmonary fibrosis [92].

Serological evidence against herpes virus was detected in IPF patients, including *Epstein–Barr virus* (EBV), *Cytomegalovirus* (CMV), *Herpes simplex virus 1*. CMV antibodies were present in 80% of patients with IPF compared to 30% of control subjects [93]. EBV antibodies were recovered in 60% of IPF patients versus 22% and control in another study [94]. EBV DNA presence in the lung relates with arterial sclerosis and an increase in pulmonary hypertension suggestive of an influence in pulmonary hypertension development [95]. 96% of IPF lungs were positive for EBV DNA versus 71% of controls [96]. 9 out of 29 IPF patients had viral latent membrane protein in the epithelial cells compared to none in control. 61% of IPF patients with a lung biopsy revealed the productive EBV rearrangement of DNA [97]. *Herpes saimiri* DNA was detected in the regenerating epithelium in all IPF patient lung biopsy compared to none in control [98]. *Herpes saimiri* causes infection in 7% of humans, and this infection rate is suggestive of it as an etiologi-cal agent for infrequent sporadic IPF [99]. MHV 68 has high homology to *Herpes saimiri*. In sporadic IPF cases, two or more herpesviruses were detected in the lung than a single herpesvirus identified in the familial IPF cases. In the familial IPF cases, the virus was either CMV or *Human herpesvirus 8* (HHV 8) [85]. At-risk family members of IPF patients revealed the presence of epithelial dysfunction and fibrotic remodeling. Biopsy specimens revealed herpesvirus antigen elucidation in alveolar epithelial cells, and a cell-free BAL sample revealed herpesvirus DNA.

Adenovirus gene product E1A upregulates TGF-beta and stimulates epithelial cells to express mesenchymal markers [100]. Administration of adenovirus into the airway resulted in an acute inflammatory lung response followed by fibrosis in a dose-dependent manner [101]. In IPF patients, serology has not revealed significant adenovirus antibodies compared to controls. A Japanese study revealed *hepatitis C* (HCV) antibodies in 28% of IPF patients compared to 3.6% of a controlled cohort [102]. IPF incidence in HCV patients was greater at ten years and 20 years after the infection [103]. In another study involving 62 IPF patients, serology revealed HCV antibodies' presence in only one patient, indicating no increased prevalence [104]. *Torque-Teno Virus* (TTV) single-stranded DNA virus was the most frequent one identified in IPF patients with acute exacerbation [105]. Although it was detected in 36.4% of IPF patients, about 50% died in four years [106]. TTV DNA titer reflects the host's immunosuppressive state due to treatment [107]. Experimental *Human Boca virus subtype one* infection in human cell culture lines causes respiratory disease and can persist in the lung causing chronic lung disease triggering fibrogenesis [108]. *Human Boca virus* was isolated from BAL in 2 patients in Germany who presented with acute usual interstitial pneumonia due to human bocavirus infection [109].

Two studies evaluated the presence of viral infection in acute IPF exacerbation. In the first study, most cases of acute exacerbation did not have any viral infections. Only TTV was identified in a substantially small number of cases [105]. In the second study, viruses were detected on the nasopharyngeal swabs in 60% of acute IPF exacerbation cases than 43.3% of stable patients. In this study, none of the patients were on any corticosteroids or antimicrobials. In acute cases, the inflammatory cytokines were elevated than in stable IPF and controls [110]. A meta-analysis of retrospective studies disclosed that chronic infection with CMV, EBV, HHV 7 & 8 substantially increased the risk of IPF without acute exacerbation of IPF. HHV 6 was not related to any significant risk of IPF. A nonsignificant greater risk of IPF was seen in younger patients with viral infections [111]. Viral infections predispose aged lungs to fibrosis, either by reactivating the infection or via latency promoting epithelial to mesenchymal transition. Latent infections alter the local milieu by increasing profibrotic mediators but cannot cause fibrosis by themselves and need another local lung insult. Latent viral infection is ineffective in causing acute exacerbations in animal models. The viral ability to increase exacerbations involves lytic replication in animal models not observed in all human patients [99]. CMV and Influenza are unable to use this mechanism to cause exacerbations.

2.6 Bacterial infections

Bacterial infections are suspected to be a cause for acute IPF exacerbations. In mouse lung fibrosis models, *Streptococcus pneumoniae* initiated pulmonary fibrosis via its pore creating cytotoxin pneumolysin, which was preventable by treatment with clarithromycin or amoxicillin at 24 hours or 48 hours [112]. The evaluation of IPF patient lung microbiome reveals staphylococcus and streptococcus species' presence in significant numbers during the disease progression [113]. The bacterial load in IPF patients BAL was larger than controls and the species in abundance were *Haemophilus*, *Streptococcus*, *Neisseria*, and *Veillonella* [114]. In murine models, *Pseudomonas aeruginosa* infection did not lead to augmentation of bleomycin-induced fibrosis [91].

2.7 Geographical and racial factors

To better understand the etiology of IPF, it is ideal for identifying geographical areas with more significant cases and evaluate the involved triggers. A study from Spain analyzed the IPF cases location and consistently highly polluted areas to recognize any risk factors [115]. Locations associated with the higher prevalence of IPF cases correlated maximally with the APM 2.5 μm exposure than other risk factors. Patients in such areas may need screening for IPF to identify these cases early in the disease course. A Japanese study identified substantial ethnic differences regarding the IPF disease course [116]. These studies are essential as they reveal the genetic trait polymorphisms associated with IPF. The incidence of IPF in males is 2.7 times higher than in females in Japan, possibly due to more male smokers than females. Males also have higher mortality than females, with a mortality ratio of 2.68 compared to that of 1.59 in the USA [117]. Clinical data on ethnic disparities with regards to IPF mortality are limited. Acute IPF exacerbation accounts for most deaths in IPF patients, and cardiac disease is a less frequent cause than in

Western countries. The variable used in the prognostification of IPF, such as age and gender, did not perform well in Japanese [118]. The GAP system fared poorly, and no substantial survival differences were noted in different IPF stages. Most Japanese carry single nucleotide polymorphisms (SNPs) rs2736100 in intron 2 of the TERT (Telomerase reverse transcriptase) gene, codes for the telomerase reverse transcriptase.

A retrospective study reviewed the ethnic and racial disparities in USA IPF outcomes using Organ Procurement and Transplantation Network data from 1995 to 2003 [119]. Black and Hispanic patients tended to be female and younger at diagnosis than whites. More significant medical comorbidities (hypertension, diabetes mellitus, and poor performance) were observed in Black and Hispanic patients. Whites had more private insurance, college education and lived in better neighborhood areas. The age-adjusted mortality rate and risk of having double lung transplantation were higher in Blacks and Hispanics. The poor mortality was partly attributed to the poor lung function when they were listed for lung transplantation. Race might be a proxy marker for the genetic makeup producing a specific phenotype [119]. Another retrospective study done in the USA evaluated the ethnic and racial differences based on National Center for Health Statistics data from 1989 to 2007 [120]. Among the IPF total census, 87.2% were Whites,5.4% Hispanics, 5% Blacks, and others 2.2%. As mentioned in the prior study, Blacks and Hispanics were younger at diagnosis and death. When age and gender were controlled, the race was a significant predictor for IPF death with a similar IPF risk in all races. Hispanics were at an increased death risk from IPF than Whites and Blacks. Blacks had a higher risk of death from pulmonary hypertension and lung cancer than Whites and Hispanic patients. Hispanics were more likely to be coded with IPF than Whites and Blacks. The differences mentioned above are due to blacks dying at an early age and less likely to smoke than Whites. Access to health care has been inadequate due to the lack of medical insurance in Blacks.

2.8 Genetic factors

Familial causes of IPF constitute less than 5% of all cases, with at least two family members being affected [121]. The diagnostic criteria used to identify cases are similar to the one used for sporadic cases. Familial inheritance is via an autosomal dominant pattern with partial penetrance [122]. In 15% of familial cases, the cause is gene mutations encoding the ribonucleic acid (RNA)(TERC) or protein component (TERT) of the telomerase enzyme [123, 124]. Another 25% have sporadic or familial IPF with no telomerase RNA component (TERC) or telomerase reverse transcriptase (TERT) mutation but have circulating leucocyte telomere shortening [125]. A substantial congregation of familial cases was observed in the Finnish population [126]. ELMOD2, a gene on chromosome 4q31, has been identified as a susceptible gene for familial IPF [127]. A significant familial association has been detected with surfactant protein C and A2 gene mutation [121, 128]. Sporadic mutations of surfactant protein C gene are rarely associated with IPF [129]. A Mucin 5B (MUC5B) gene polymorphism of the promoter (rs35705950) is substantially associated with familial and sporadic IPF [130]. MUC5B promoter polymorphism presence can be used for IPF prediction and prognostification; however, it is not seen in 40% of cases [131, 132]. New loci (FAM13A, DSP, OBFC1, ATP11A, DPP9) and prior associations (TERT, MUC5B, TERC) were confirmed by a genome-wide association study in White patients. The newer loci were essential in immune defenses, DNA repair, and cell adhesion [133]. Peripheral blood markers may be used to identify a protein signature made up of MMP 1, MMP 7, MMP 8, Insulin-like growth factor-binding protein 1(IGFBP1) & tumor necrosis factor receptor superfamily member 1A (TNFRSA1F), which was able to differentiate IPF patients from healthy controls with a specificity of 98.1% and sensitivity of 98.6% [134]. Higher plasma concentrations of MMP 7, vascular cell adhesion molecule 1 (VCAM-1), IL-8, Intercellular Adhesion Molecule 1 (ICAM-1), and S100 calcium-binding protein A12 (S100A12) predict poor survival in IPF patients [135]. The gene microarray expression process can help in understanding the pathophysiology and therapeutic target candidates [136]. Currently, no genetic factors are associated with sporadic IPF in a consistent pattern.

3. Vital statistics and measures to improve them

Epidemiologic studies carried out before 2013 are highly heterogeneous in their methods and cannot be compared [137]. Even with this heterogeneity, the incidence shows a gradual increase across the world [138]. The IPF incidence has increased in all studies except for two quality studies, one each from Denmark and USA [139, 140]. When all studies are considered, the IPF incidence ranges from 0.22 to 93.7 per 100,000 per year. After removing underreported, South American and Asian studies, the incidence was 2.8 to 9.3 per 100,000 per year for the USA and European studies together [138]. In Europe, the higher rates were observed in the UK, while Scandinavia and Southern Europe revealed lower rates [4, 139, 141–143]. In the USA, using the narrow criteria, the incidence rates were lower at an incidence of 5–8 per 100,000 per year [38, 144, 145]. Incidence rates in South America were at 0.4 to 1.2 per 100,000 per year [146, 147]. East Asia studies based on insurance claims indicate an incidence rate of IPF at 1.2–3.8 per 100,000 per year [148, 149]. In contrast, in Japan, the mortality statistics suggest a greater incidence rate and an adjusted mortality rate of 10.26 per 100,000 [150]. Age-adjusted mortality has accelerated from 3.2 per 100,000 in 1979 to 7.57 per 100,000 from 1999 to 2003 in USA [38, 151]. In the UK, age-adjusted mortality has increased from 2.54 per 100 000 (1968–2008) to 5.5.10 per 100 000 (2005–2008) [141]. In Brazil, mortality had risen from 0.65 per 100 000 in 1996 to 1.21 per 100 000 in 2010 [146].

Overall, increased incidence rates are observed in the UK, European, South American, and East Asian epidemiological studies [141, 146–148, 152, 153]. USA mortality rates have declined as in Denmark after reaching a plateau [2, 139, 154]. Younger patients have a more prolonged median survival due to earlier treatment of recognized comorbidities and avoiding the use of ineffective treatment such as immunosuppressants and corticosteroids [117]. IPF diagnosis and treatment are getting more specific, and widespread acceptance of IPF international guidelines will improve accurate, comparable IPF clinical data [155]. National IPF registries from different countries will yield valuable data on IPF epidemiology. In general, the current IPF epidemiological data does not have substantial consistency.

The ideal sample should be large to validate the clinical diagnosis by medical records review [138]. Uncertainty of diagnosis can be avoided by using internationally accepted guidelines and consolidate its use in all studies. Other things to be considered are liberal use of imaging techniques, avoid broad diagnostic codes to identify IPF, and reinforce clinical guidelines in practicing physicians [138]. IPF score algorithm improved the positive predictive value by incorporating the IPF risk factors to identify fewer false-positive cases accurately [1]. The increasing prevalence can be attributed to the IPF patients living longer than ten years before [117]. Prevalence is affected by disease definition, guidelines used for diagnosis, the difference in methodology, and health care systems. Gender differences are due to smoking habit variations and occupational exposure. Incidence is influenced by diagnostic improvements, population age, availability of drugs, and improved health care. Mortality is affected by clinical recognition of IPF and diagnostic coding [155]. Insurance databases reveal an underrepresentation of lower socioeconomic strata and non-White patients, impacting the overall incidence and prevalence [1]. Care should be ascertained during medical record review for confirmation as they can be inaccurate. Using medicare beneficiary data excludes younger IPF patients, which a national IPF registry can avoid [117].

4. Conclusion

IPF datasets currently overestimate the prevalence, whereas the questionnaire studies underestimate it. Obtaining the correct epidemiological data is essential in identifying IPF clinical course and prognosis. Initiation and maintenance of a national registry with appropriate epidemiology data collection is an excellent beginning. An attempt should be garnered towards using algorithms or other tools in epidemiological studies to establish their efficacy. Epidemiological studies should attempt to use a similar case definition standardized across multiple countries to compare effectively and decrease the heterogeneity. As the IPF incidence increases, it has become a substantial public health concern. Future studies need to stress clinical epidemiology, pathophysiology & diagnostic biomarkers for an accurate understanding of epigenetic mechanisms and their pathways to provide a clue about future therapeutic targets. Clinical research into the epigenetic processes, disease pathophysiology, and diagnostic procedures needs to be encouraged and supported to improve life quality, prolong survival, and ultimately find a cure.

Acknowledgements

"None, No external funding was received in preparation of this manuscript."

Conflict of interest

"The author declares no conflict of interest."

Notes/thanks/other declarations

"A special thanks to the editor for allowing me to author this manuscript."

Acronyms and abbreviations

IPF	Idiopathic pulmonary fibrosis
ILD	Interstitial lung disease
PPV	Positive predictive value
GAP	Gender-Age-Physiology
COPD	Chronic obstructive pulmonary disease
CPFE	Combined pulmonary fibrosis and emphysema
CSE	Cigarette smoke exposure
TGF	Transforming growth factor
EGF	Epidermal growth factor
MMP	Mixed metalloproteinases

ECM	Extracellular matrix
CVD	Cardiovascular disease
PAF	Population attributable fraction
JEM	Job-exposure matrix
USA	United States of America
IPF-JES	IPF-Job Exposure study.
UK	United Kingdom
APM	Ambient particulate matter
GERD	Gastroesophageal reflux disease
LES	Lower esophageal sphincter
BAL	Bronchoalveolar lavage
PPI	Proton pump inhibitor
LARS	Laparoscopic antireflux surgery
DNA	Deoxyribonucleic acid
MHV	Murine herpesvirus
EBV	Epstein–Barr virus
CMV	Cytomegalovirus
HHV	Human herpesvirus
HCV	Hepatitis C virus
TTV	Torque-Teno virus
SNP	Single nucleotide polymorphism
TERT	Telomerase reverse transcriptase
RNA	Ribonucleic acid
TERC	Telomerase RNA component
MUC5B	Mucin5b
FAM13A	Family with sequence similarity 13, Member A
DSP	Desmoplakin
OBFC1	Oligosaccharide-binding fold-containing Protein 1
ATP11A	ATPase Phospholipid Transporting 11A
DPP9	Dipeptidyl Peptidase 9
IGFBP	Insulin-like growth factor-binding protein
TNFRSA1F	Tumor necrosis factor receptor superfamily member 1A
VCAM	Vascular cell adhesion molecule
IL	Interleukin
ICAM	Intercellular adhesion molecule
S100A12	S100 calcium-binding protein A12

Author details

Sachin M. Patil
University of Missouri, Columbia, MO, USA

*Address all correspondence to: drssmp1@gmail.com

IntechOpen

References

[1] Esposito DB, Lanes S, Donneyong M, Holick CN, Lasky JA, Lederer D, et al. Idiopathic Pulmonary Fibrosis in United States Automated Claims. Incidence, Prevalence, and Algorithm Validation. Am J Respir Crit Care Med. 2015;192(10):1200-1207.

[2] Coultas DB, Zumwalt RE, Black WC, Sobonya RE. The epidemiology of interstitial lung diseases. Am J Respir Crit Care Med. 1994;150(4):967-972.

[3] American Thoracic Society. Idiopathic pulmonary fibrosis: diagnosis and treatment. International consensus statement. American Thoracic Society (ATS), and the European Respiratory Society (ERS). Am J Respir Crit Care Med. 2000;161(2 Pt 1):646-664.

[4] von Plessen C, Grinde O, Gulsvik A. Incidence and prevalence of cryptogenic fibrosing alveolitis in a Norwegian community. Respir Med. 2003;97(4): 428-435.

[5] Salisbury ML, Xia M, Zhou Y, Murray S, Tayob N, Brown KK, et al. Idiopathic Pulmonary Fibrosis: Gender-Age-Physiology Index Stage for Predicting Future Lung Function Decline. Chest. 2016;149(2):491-498.

[6] Zaman T, Moua T, Vittinghoff E, Ryu JH, Collard HR, Lee JS. Differences in Clinical Characteristics and Outcomes Between Men and Women With Idiopathic Pulmonary Fibrosis: A Multicenter Retrospective Cohort Study. Chest. 2020;158(1):245-251.

[7] McGee SP, Zhang H, Karmaus W, Sabo-Attwood T. Influence of sex and disease severity on gene expression profiles in individuals with idiopathic pulmonary fibrosis. Int J Mol Epidemiol Genet. 2014;5(2):71-86.

[8] Fell CD, Martinez FJ, Liu LX, Murray S, Han MK, Kazerooni EA, et al. Clinical predictors of a diagnosis of idiopathic pulmonary fibrosis. Am J Respir Crit Care Med. 2010;181(8): 832-837.

[9] Naik PK, Moore BB. Viral infection and aging as cofactors for the development of pulmonary fibrosis. Expert Rev Respir Med. 2010;4(6): 759-771.

[10] Salminen A, Kaarniranta K. ER stress and hormetic regulation of the aging process. Ageing Res Rev. 2010;9(3):211-217.

[11] Aw D, Silva AB, Palmer DB. Immunosenescence: emerging challenges for an ageing population. Immunology. 2007;120(4):435-446.

[12] Goronzy JJ, Lee WW, Weyand CM. Aging and T-cell diversity. Exp Gerontol. 2007;42(5):400-406.

[13] Goronzy JJ, Fulbright JW, Crowson CS, Poland GA, O'Fallon WM, Weyand CM. Value of immunological markers in predicting responsiveness to influenza vaccination in elderly individuals. J Virol. 2001;75(24): 12182-12187.

[14] Khan N, Hislop A, Gudgeon N, Cobbold M, Khanna R, Nayak L, et al. Herpesvirus-specific CD8 T cell immunity in old age: cytomegalovirus impairs the response to a coresident EBV infection. J Immunol. 2004;173(12): 7481-7489.

[15] Alder JK, Chen JJ, Lancaster L, Danoff S, Su SC, Cogan JD, et al. Short telomeres are a risk factor for idiopathic pulmonary fibrosis. Proc Natl Acad Sci U S A. 2008;105(35):13051-13056.

[16] Yang IV, Schwartz DA. Epigenetics of idiopathic pulmonary fibrosis. Transl Res. 2015;165(1):48-60.

[17] Han MK, Murray S, Fell CD, Flaherty KR, Toews GB, Myers J, et al. Sex differences in physiological progression of idiopathic pulmonary fibrosis. Eur Respir J. 2008;31(6): 1183-1188.

[18] Hecht SS. Research opportunities related to establishing standards for tobacco products under the Family Smoking Prevention and Tobacco Control Act. Nicotine Tob Res. 2012;14(1):18-28.

[19] Oh CK, Murray LA, Molfino NA. Smoking and idiopathic pulmonary fibrosis. Pulm Med. 2012;2012:808260.

[20] Rao RN, Goodman LR, Tomashefski JF, Jr. Smoking-related interstitial lung disease. Ann Diagn Pathol. 2008;12(6):445-457.

[21] Baumgartner KB, Samet JM, Stidley CA, Colby TV, Waldron JA. Cigarette smoking: a risk factor for idiopathic pulmonary fibrosis. Am J Respir Crit Care Med. 1997;155(1): 242-248.

[22] Katzenstein AL, Mukhopadhyay S, Zanardi C, Dexter E. Clinically occult interstitial fibrosis in smokers: classification and significance of a surprisingly common finding in lobectomy specimens. Hum Pathol. 2010;41(3):316-325.

[23] Vassallo R, Ryu JH. Smoking-related interstitial lung diseases. Clin Chest Med. 2012;33(1):165-178.

[24] Franks TJ, Galvin JR. Smoking-Related "Interstitial" Lung Disease. Arch Pathol Lab Med. 2015;139(8):974-977.

[25] MacNee W. Pulmonary and systemic oxidant/antioxidant imbalance in chronic obstructive pulmonary disease. Proc Am Thorac Soc. 2005;2(1):50-60.

[26] Selman M, Rojas M, Mora AL, Pardo A. Aging and interstitial lung diseases: unraveling an old forgotten player in the pathogenesis of lung fibrosis. Semin Respir Crit Care Med. 2010;31(5):607-617.

[27] Antoniou KM, Hansell DM, Rubens MB, Marten K, Desai SR, Siafakas NM, et al. Idiopathic pulmonary fibrosis: outcome in relation to smoking status. Am J Respir Crit Care Med. 2008;177(2):190-194.

[28] Karkkainen M, Kettunen HP, Nurmi H, Selander T, Purokivi M, Kaarteenaho R. Effect of smoking and comorbidities on survival in idiopathic pulmonary fibrosis. Respir Res. 2017;18(1):160.

[29] Blanc PD, Annesi-Maesano I, Balmes JR, Cummings KJ, Fishwick D, Miedinger D, et al. The Occupational Burden of Nonmalignant Respiratory Diseases. An Official American Thoracic Society and European Respiratory Society Statement. Am J Respir Crit Care Med. 2019;199(11):1312-1334.

[30] Conti S, Harari S, Caminati A, Zanobetti A, Schwartz JD, Bertazzi PA, et al. The association between air pollution and the incidence of idiopathic pulmonary fibrosis in Northern Italy. Eur Respir J. 2018;51(1).

[31] Taskar VS, Coultas DB. Is idiopathic pulmonary fibrosis an environmental disease? Proc Am Thorac Soc. 2006;3(4):293-298.

[32] Inoue M. [Quantitative and qualitative analyses of inorganic dusts in idiopathic interstitial pneumonia (IIP)]. Hokkaido Igaku Zasshi. 1986;61(5): 745-754.

[33] Monso E, Tura JM, Marsal M, Morell F, Pujadas J, Morera J. Mineralogical microanalysis of idiopathic pulmonary fibrosis. Arch Environ Health. 1990;45(3):185-188.

[34] Hashimoto H, Tajima H, Mizoguchi I, Iwai K. [Elemental analysis

of hilar and mediastinal lymph nodes in idiopathic pulmonary fibrosis]. Nihon Kyobu Shikkan Gakkai Zasshi. 1992;30(12):2061-2068.

[35] Raghu G, Collard HR, Egan JJ, Martinez FJ, Behr J, Brown KK, et al. An official ATS/ERS/JRS/ALAT statement: idiopathic pulmonary fibrosis: evidence-based guidelines for diagnosis and management. Am J Respir Crit Care Med. 2011;183(6):788-824.

[36] Paolocci G, Folletti I, Toren K, Ekstrom M, Dell'Omo M, Muzi G, et al. Occupational risk factors for idiopathic pulmonary fibrosis in Southern Europe: a case-control study. BMC Pulm Med. 2018;18(1):75.

[37] Baumgartner KB, Samet JM, Coultas DB, Stidley CA, Hunt WC, Colby TV, et al. Occupational and environmental risk factors for idiopathic pulmonary fibrosis: a multicenter case-control study. Collaborating Centers. Am J Epidemiol. 2000;152(4): 307-315.

[38] Pinheiro GA, Antao VC, Wood JM, Wassell JT. Occupational risks for idiopathic pulmonary fibrosis mortality in the United States. Int J Occup Environ Health. 2008;14(2):117-123.

[39] Lee SH, Kim DS, Kim YW, Chung MP, Uh ST, Park CS, et al. Association between occupational dust exposure and prognosis of idiopathic pulmonary fibrosis: a Korean national survey. Chest. 2015;147(2):465-474.

[40] Awadalla NJ, Hegazy A, Elmetwally RA, Wahby I. Occupational and environmental risk factors for idiopathic pulmonary fibrosis in Egypt: a multicenter case-control study. Int J Occup Environ Med. 2012;3(3):107-116.

[41] De Sadeleer LJ, Verleden SE, De Dycker E, Yserbyt J, Verschakelen JA, Verbeken EK, et al. Clinical behaviour of patients exposed to organic dust and

diagnosed with idiopathic pulmonary fibrosis. Respirology. 2018;23(12): 1160-1165.

[42] Hubbard R, Cooper M, Antoniak M, Venn A, Khan S, Johnston I, et al. Risk of cryptogenic fibrosing alveolitis in metal workers. Lancet. 2000;355(9202): 466-467.

[43] Miyake Y, Sasaki S, Yokoyama T, Chida K, Azuma A, Suda T, et al. Occupational and environmental factors and idiopathic pulmonary fibrosis in Japan. Ann Occup Hyg. 2005;49(3): 259-265.

[44] Kitamura H, Ichinose S, Hosoya T, Ando T, Ikushima S, Oritsu M, et al. Inhalation of inorganic particles as a risk factor for idiopathic pulmonary fibrosis--elemental microanalysis of pulmonary lymph nodes obtained at autopsy cases. Pathol Res Pract. 2007;203(8):575-585.

[45] Koo JW, Myong JP, Yoon HK, Rhee CK, Kim Y, Kim JS, et al. Occupational exposure and idiopathic pulmonary fibrosis: a multicentre case-control study in Korea. Int J Tuberc Lung Dis. 2017;21(1):107-112.

[46] Kim SY, Kang DM, Lee HK, Kim KH, Choi J. Occupational and Environmental Risk Factors for Chronic Fibrosing idiopathic Interstitial Pneumonia in South Korea. J Occup Environ Med. 2017;59(11):e221-e2e6.

[47] Barber CM, Wiggans RE, Young C, Fishwick D. UK asbestos imports and mortality due to idiopathic pulmonary fibrosis. Occup Med (Lond). 2016;66(2):106-111.

[48] Hubbard R, Lewis S, Richards K, Johnston I, Britton J. Occupational exposure to metal or wood dust and aetiology of cryptogenic fibrosing alveolitis. Lancet. 1996;347(8997): 284-289.

[49] Gustafson T, Dahlman-Hoglund A, Nilsson K, Strom K, Tornling G, Toren K. Occupational exposure and severe pulmonary fibrosis. Respir Med. 2007;101(10):2207-2212.

[50] Ricco M. Lung fibrosis and exposure to wood dusts: Two case reports and review of the literature. Med Pr. 2015;66(5):739-747.

[51] Johannson KA, Vittinghoff E, Lee K, Balmes JR, Ji W, Kaplan GG, et al. Acute exacerbation of idiopathic pulmonary fibrosis associated with air pollution exposure. Eur Respir J. 2014;43(4): 1124-1131.

[52] Winterbottom CJ, Shah RJ, Patterson KC, Kreider ME, Panettieri RA, Jr., Rivera-Lebron B, et al. Exposure to Ambient Particulate Matter Is Associated With Accelerated Functional Decline in Idiopathic Pulmonary Fibrosis. Chest. 2018;153(5): 1221-1228.

[53] Johannson KA, Vittinghoff E, Morisset J, Wolters PJ, Noth EM, Balmes JR, et al. Air Pollution Exposure Is Associated With Lower Lung Function, but Not Changes in Lung Function, in Patients With Idiopathic Pulmonary Fibrosis. Chest. 2018;154(1): 119-125.

[54] Sese L, Nunes H, Cottin V, Sanyal S, Didier M, Carton Z, et al. Role of atmospheric pollution on the natural history of idiopathic pulmonary fibrosis. Thorax. 2018;73(2):145-150.

[55] Park Y, Ahn C, Kim TH. Occupational and environmental risk factors of idiopathic pulmonary fibrosis: a systematic review and meta-analyses. Sci Rep. 2021;11(1):4318.

[56] Iwai K, Mori T, Yamada N, Yamaguchi M, Hosoda Y. Idiopathic pulmonary fibrosis. Epidemiologic approaches to occupational exposure. Am J Respir Crit Care Med. 1994;150(3): 670-675.

[57] Trethewey SP, Walters GI. The Role of Occupational and Environmental Exposures in the Pathogenesis of Idiopathic Pulmonary Fibrosis: A Narrative Literature Review. Medicina (Kaunas). 2018;54(6).

[58] Lee JS, Ryu JH, Elicker BM, Lydell CP, Jones KD, Wolters PJ, et al. Gastroesophageal reflux therapy is associated with longer survival in patients with idiopathic pulmonary fibrosis. Am J Respir Crit Care Med. 2011;184(12):1390-1394.

[59] Lee JS, Song JW, Wolters PJ, Elicker BM, King TE, Jr., Kim DS, et al. Bronchoalveolar lavage pepsin in acute exacerbation of idiopathic pulmonary fibrosis. Eur Respir J. 2012;39(2): 352-358.

[60] el-Serag HB, Sonnenberg A. Comorbid occurrence of laryngeal or pulmonary disease with esophagitis in United States military veterans. Gastroenterology. 1997;113(3):755-760.

[61] Raghu G, Freudenberger TD, Yang S, Curtis JR, Spada C, Hayes J, et al. High prevalence of abnormal acid gastro-oesophageal reflux in idiopathic pulmonary fibrosis. Eur Respir J. 2006;27(1):136-142.

[62] Tobin RW, Pope CE, 2nd, Pellegrini CA, Emond MJ, Sillery J, Raghu G. Increased prevalence of gastroesophageal reflux in patients with idiopathic pulmonary fibrosis. Am J Respir Crit Care Med. 1998;158(6): 1804-1808.

[63] Behr J, Kreuter M, Hoeper MM, Wirtz H, Klotsche J, Koschel D, et al. Management of patients with idiopathic pulmonary fibrosis in clinical practice: the INSIGHTS-IPF registry. Eur Respir J. 2015;46(1):186-196.

[64] Sonnenberg A. Effects of environment and lifestyle on gastroesophageal reflux disease. Dig Dis. 2011;29(2):229-234.

[65] Allaix ME, Rebecchi F, Morino M, Schlottmann F, Patti MG. Gastroesophageal Reflux and Idiopathic Pulmonary Fibrosis. World J Surg. 2017;41(7):1691-1697.

[66] Gibson GJ, Pride NB. Pulmonary mechanics in fibrosing alveolitis: the effects of lung shrinkage. Am Rev Respir Dis. 1977;116(4):637-647.

[67] Lee JS. The Role of Gastroesophageal Reflux and Microaspiration in Idiopathic Pulmonary Fibrosis. Clin Pulm Med. 2014;21(2):81-85.

[68] Raghu G, Meyer KC. Silent gastro-oesophageal reflux and microaspiration in IPF: mounting evidence for anti-reflux therapy? Eur Respir J. 2012;39(2): 242-245.

[69] Ghisa M, Marinelli C, Savarino V, Savarino E. Idiopathic pulmonary fibrosis and GERD: links and risks. Ther Clin Risk Manag. 2019;15:1081-1093.

[70] Krishnan U, Mitchell JD, Messina I, Day AS, Bohane TD. Assay of tracheal pepsin as a marker of reflux aspiration. J Pediatr Gastroenterol Nutr. 2002;35(3):303-308.

[71] Savarino E, Carbone R, Marabotto E, Furnari M, Sconfienza L, Ghio M, et al. Gastro-oesophageal reflux and gastric aspiration in idiopathic pulmonary fibrosis patients. Eur Respir J. 2013;42(5):1322-1331.

[72] Davis CS, Mendez BM, Flint DV, Pelletiere K, Lowery E, Ramirez L, et al. Pepsin concentrations are elevated in the bronchoalveolar lavage fluid of patients with idiopathic pulmonary fibrosis after lung transplantation. J Surg Res. 2013;185(2):e101-e108.

[73] Ghebre Y, Raghu G. Proton pump inhibitors in IPF: beyond mere suppression of gastric acidity. QJM. 2016;109(9):577-579.

[74] Ghebremariam YT, Cooke JP, Gerhart W, Griego C, Brower JB, Doyle-Eisele M, et al. Pleiotropic effect of the proton pump inhibitor esomeprazole leading to suppression of lung inflammation and fibrosis. J Transl Med. 2015;13:249.

[75] Raghu G, Yang ST, Spada C, Hayes J, Pellegrini CA. Sole treatment of acid gastroesophageal reflux in idiopathic pulmonary fibrosis: a case series. Chest. 2006;129(3):794-800.

[76] Lee JS, Collard HR, Anstrom KJ, Martinez FJ, Noth I, Roberts RS, et al. Anti-acid treatment and disease progression in idiopathic pulmonary fibrosis: an analysis of data from three randomised controlled trials. Lancet Respir Med. 2013;1(5):369-376.

[77] Raghu G, Pellegrini CA, Yow E, Flaherty KR, Meyer K, Noth I, et al. Laparoscopic anti-reflux surgery for the treatment of idiopathic pulmonary fibrosis (WRAP-IPF): a multicentre, randomised, controlled phase 2 trial. Lancet Respir Med. 2018;6(9):707-714.

[78] Kreuter M, Wuyts W, Renzoni E, Koschel D, Maher TM, Kolb M, et al. Antacid therapy and disease outcomes in idiopathic pulmonary fibrosis: a pooled analysis. Lancet Respir Med. 2016;4(5):381-389.

[79] Fidler L, Sitzer N, Shapera S, Shah PS. Treatment of Gastroesophageal Reflux in Patients With Idiopathic Pulmonary Fibrosis: A Systematic Review and Meta-Analysis. Chest. 2018;153(6):1405-1415.

[80] Bedard Methot D, Leblanc E, Lacasse Y. Meta-analysis of Gastroesophageal Reflux Disease and Idiopathic Pulmonary Fibrosis. Chest. 2019;155(1):33-43.

[81] Costabel U, Behr J, Crestani B, Stansen W, Schlenker-Herceg R, Stowasser S, et al. Anti-acid therapy in

idiopathic pulmonary fibrosis: insights from the INPULSIS(R) trials. Respir Res. 2018;19(1):167.

[82] Corrao S, Natoli G, Argano C, Scichilone N. Gastroesophageal Reflux Disease and Idiopathic Pulmonary Fibrosis: No Data for Supporting a Relationship After a Systematic Review. Chest. 2019;156(1):190-192.

[83] Kahrilas IJ, Kahrilas PJ. Reflux Disease and Idiopathic Lung Fibrosis: Association Does Not Imply Causation. Chest. 2019;155(1):5-6.

[84] Idiopathic Pulmonary Fibrosis Clinical Research N, Raghu G, Anstrom KJ, King TE, Jr., Lasky JA, Martinez FJ. Prednisone, azathioprine, and N-acetylcysteine for pulmonary fibrosis. N Engl J Med. 2012;366(21): 1968-1977.

[85] Tang YW, Johnson JE, Browning PJ, Cruz-Gervis RA, Davis A, Graham BS, et al. Herpesvirus DNA is consistently detected in lungs of patients with idiopathic pulmonary fibrosis. J Clin Microbiol. 2003;41(6):2633-2640.

[86] Egan JJ, Adamali HI, Lok SS, Stewart JP, Woodcock AA. Ganciclovir antiviral therapy in advanced idiopathic pulmonary fibrosis: an open pilot study. Pulm Med. 2011;2011:240805.

[87] Williams KJ, Robinson NE, Lim A, Brandenberger C, Maes R, Behan A, et al. Experimental induction of pulmonary fibrosis in horses with the gammaherpesvirus equine herpesvirus 5. PLoS One. 2013;8(10):e77754.

[88] Vannella KM, Luckhardt TR, Wilke CA, van Dyk LF, Toews GB, Moore BB. Latent herpesvirus infection augments experimental pulmonary fibrosis. Am J Respir Crit Care Med. 2010;181(5):465-477.

[89] Naik PN, Horowitz JC, Moore TA, Wilke CA, Toews GB, Moore BB. Pulmonary fibrosis induced by gamma-herpesvirus in aged mice is associated with increased fibroblast responsiveness to transforming growth factor-beta. J Gerontol A Biol Sci Med Sci. 2012;67(7):714-725.

[90] Coomes SM, Farmen S, Wilke CA, Laouar Y, Moore BB. Severe gammaherpesvirus-induced pneumonitis and fibrosis in syngeneic bone marrow transplant mice is related to effects of transforming growth factor-beta. Am J Pathol. 2011;179(5):2382-2396.

[91] Ashley SL, Jegal Y, Moore TA, van Dyk LF, Laouar Y, Moore BB. gamma-Herpes virus-68, but not Pseudomonas aeruginosa or influenza A (H1N1), exacerbates established murine lung fibrosis. Am J Physiol Lung Cell Mol Physiol. 2014;307(3):L219-L230.

[92] Ebrahimi B, Dutia BM, Brownstein DG, Nash AA. Murine gammaherpesvirus-68 infection causes multi-organ fibrosis and alters leukocyte trafficking in interferon-gamma receptor knockout mice. Am J Pathol. 2001;158(6):2117-2125.

[93] Yonemaru M, Kasuga I, Kusumoto H, Kunisawa A, Kiyokawa H, Kuwabara S, et al. Elevation of antibodies to cytomegalovirus and other herpes viruses in pulmonary fibrosis. Eur Respir J. 1997;10(9):2040-2045.

[94] Manika K, Alexiou-Daniel S, Papakosta D, Papa A, Kontakiotis T, Patakas D, et al. Epstein-Barr virus DNA in bronchoalveolar lavage fluid from patients with idiopathic pulmonary fibrosis. Sarcoidosis Vasc Diffuse Lung Dis. 2007;24(2):134-140.

[95] Calabrese F, Kipar A, Lunardi F, Balestro E, Perissinotto E, Rossi E, et al. Herpes virus infection is associated with vascular remodeling and pulmonary hypertension in idiopathic pulmonary fibrosis. PLoS One. 2013;8(2):e55715.

[96] Tsukamoto K, Hayakawa H, Sato A, Chida K, Nakamura H, Miura K. Involvement of Epstein-Barr virus latent membrane protein 1 in disease progression in patients with idiopathic pulmonary fibrosis. Thorax. 2000;55(11):958-961.

[97] Kelly BG, Lok SS, Hasleton PS, Egan JJ, Stewart JP. A rearranged form of Epstein-Barr virus DNA is associated with idiopathic pulmonary fibrosis. Am J Respir Crit Care Med. 2002;166(4): 510-513.

[98] Folcik VA, Garofalo M, Coleman J, Donegan JJ, Rabbani E, Suster S, et al. Idiopathic pulmonary fibrosis is strongly associated with productive infection by herpesvirus saimiri. Mod Pathol. 2014;27(6):851-862.

[99] Moore BB, Moore TA. Viruses in Idiopathic Pulmonary Fibrosis. Etiology and Exacerbation. Ann Am Thorac Soc. 2015;12 Suppl 2:S186-92.

[100] Hayashi S, Hogg JC. Adenovirus infections and lung disease. Curr Opin Pharmacol. 2007;7(3):237-243.

[101] Zhou Q, Chen T, Bozkanat M, Ibe JC, Christman JW, Raj JU, et al. Intratracheal instillation of high dose adenoviral vectors is sufficient to induce lung injury and fibrosis in mice. PLoS One. 2014;9(12):e116142.

[102] Ueda T, Ohta K, Suzuki N, Yamaguchi M, Hirai K, Horiuchi T, et al. Idiopathic pulmonary fibrosis and high prevalence of serum antibodies to hepatitis C virus. Am Rev Respir Dis. 1992;146(1):266-268.

[103] Arase Y, Suzuki F, Suzuki Y, Akuta N, Kobayashi M, Kawamura Y, et al. Hepatitis C virus enhances incidence of idiopathic pulmonary fibrosis. World J Gastroenterol. 2008;14(38):5880-5886.

[104] Irving WL, Day S, Johnston ID. Idiopathic pulmonary fibrosis and

hepatitis C virus infection. Am Rev Respir Dis. 1993;148(6 Pt 1):1683-1684.

[105] Wootton SC, Kim DS, Kondoh Y, Chen E, Lee JS, Song JW, et al. Viral infection in acute exacerbation of idiopathic pulmonary fibrosis. Am J Respir Crit Care Med. 2011;183(12): 1698-1702.

[106] Bando M, Ohno S, Oshikawa K, Takahashi M, Okamoto H, Sugiyama Y. Infection of TT virus in patients with idiopathic pulmonary fibrosis. Respir Med. 2001;95(12):935-942.

[107] Bando M, Nakayama M, Takahashi M, Hosono T, Mato N, Yamasawa H, et al. Serum torque teno virus DNA titer in idiopathic pulmonary fibrosis patients with acute respiratory worsening. Intern Med. 2015;54(9): 1015-1019.

[108] Khalfaoui S, Eichhorn V, Karagiannidis C, Bayh I, Brockmann M, Pieper M, et al. Lung Infection by Human Bocavirus Induces the Release of Profibrotic Mediator Cytokines In Vivo and In Vitro. PLoS One. 2016;11(1): e0147010.

[109] Windisch W, Schildgen V, Malecki M, Lenz J, Brockmann M, Karagiannidis C, et al. Detection of HBoV DNA in idiopathic lung fibrosis, Cologne, Germany. J Clin Virol. 2013;58(1):325-327.

[110] Weng D, Chen XQ, Qiu H, Zhang Y, Li QH, Zhao MM, et al. The Role of Infection in Acute Exacerbation of Idiopathic Pulmonary Fibrosis. Mediators Inflamm. 2019;2019:5160694.

[111] Sheng G, Chen P, Wei Y, Yue H, Chu J, Zhao J, et al. Viral Infection Increases the Risk of Idiopathic Pulmonary Fibrosis: A Meta-Analysis. Chest. 2020;157(5):1175-1187.

[112] Knippenberg S, Ueberberg B, Maus R, Bohling J, Ding N, Tort

Tarres M, et al. Streptococcus pneumoniae triggers progression of pulmonary fibrosis through pneumolysin. Thorax. 2015;70(7): 636-646.

[113] Han MK, Zhou Y, Murray S, Tayob N, Noth I, Lama VN, et al. Lung microbiome and disease progression in idiopathic pulmonary fibrosis: an analysis of the COMET study. Lancet Respir Med. 2014;2(7):548-556.

[114] Molyneaux PL, Cox MJ, Willis-Owen SA, Mallia P, Russell KE, Russell AM, et al. The role of bacteria in the pathogenesis and progression of idiopathic pulmonary fibrosis. Am J Respir Crit Care Med. 2014;190(8): 906-913.

[115] Shull JG, Pay MT, Lara Compte C, Olid M, Bermudo G, Portillo K, et al. Mapping IPF helps identify geographic regions at higher risk for disease development and potential triggers. Respirology. 2021;26(4):352-359.

[116] Saito S, Lasky JA, Hagiwara K, Kondoh Y. Ethnic differences in idiopathic pulmonary fibrosis: The Japanese perspective. Respir Investig. 2018;56(5):375-383.

[117] Raghu G, Chen SY, Yeh WS, Maroni B, Li Q, Lee YC, et al. Idiopathic pulmonary fibrosis in US Medicare beneficiaries aged 65 years and older: incidence, prevalence, and survival, 2001-11. Lancet Respir Med. 2014;2(7): 566-572.

[118] Kondoh Y, Taniguchi H, Kataoka K, Furukawa T, Ando M, Murotani K, et al. Disease severity staging system for idiopathic pulmonary fibrosis in Japan. Respirology. 2017;22(8):1609-1614.

[119] Lederer DJ, Arcasoy SM, Barr RG, Wilt JS, Bagiella E, D'Ovidio F, et al. Racial and ethnic disparities in idiopathic pulmonary fibrosis: A UNOS/OPTN database analysis. Am J Transplant. 2006;6(10):2436-2442.

[120] Swigris JJ, Olson AL, Huie TJ, Fernandez-Perez ER, Solomon J, Sprunger D, et al. Ethnic and racial differences in the presence of idiopathic pulmonary fibrosis at death. Respir Med. 2012;106(4):588-593.

[121] Wang Y, Kuan PJ, Xing C, Cronkhite JT, Torres F, Rosenblatt RL, et al. Genetic defects in surfactant protein A2 are associated with pulmonary fibrosis and lung cancer. Am J Hum Genet. 2009;84(1):52-59.

[122] Marshall RP, Puddicombe A, Cookson WO, Laurent GJ. Adult familial cryptogenic fibrosing alveolitis in the United Kingdom. Thorax. 2000;55(2): 143-146.

[123] Armanios MY, Chen JJ, Cogan JD, Alder JK, Ingersoll RG, Markin C, et al. Telomerase mutations in families with idiopathic pulmonary fibrosis. N Engl J Med. 2007;356(13):1317-1326.

[124] Tsakiri KD, Cronkhite JT, Kuan PJ, Xing C, Raghu G, Weissler JC, et al. Adult-onset pulmonary fibrosis caused by mutations in telomerase. Proc Natl Acad Sci U S A. 2007;104(18):7552-7557.

[125] Cronkhite JT, Xing C, Raghu G, Chin KM, Torres F, Rosenblatt RL, et al. Telomere shortening in familial and sporadic pulmonary fibrosis. Am J Respir Crit Care Med. 2008;178(7): 729-737.

[126] Allam JS, Limper AH. Idiopathic pulmonary fibrosis: is it a familial disease? Curr Opin Pulm Med. 2006;12(5):312-317.

[127] Hodgson U, Pulkkinen V, Dixon M, Peyrard-Janvid M, Rehn M, Lahermo P, et al. ELMOD2 is a candidate gene for familial idiopathic pulmonary fibrosis. Am J Hum Genet. 2006;79(1):149-154.

[128] Thomas AQ, Lane K, Phillips J, 3rd, Prince M, Markin C, Speer M, et al. Heterozygosity for a surfactant protein

C gene mutation associated with usual interstitial pneumonitis and cellular nonspecific interstitial pneumonitis in one kindred. Am J Respir Crit Care Med. 2002;165(9):1322-1328.

[129] Rickard CM, Roberts BL, Foote J, McGrail MR. Intensive care research coordinators: who are they and what do they do? Results of a binational survey. Dimens Crit Care Nurs. 2006;25(5): 234-242.

[130] Seibold MA, Wise AL, Speer MC, Steele MP, Brown KK, Loyd JE, et al. A common MUC5B promoter polymorphism and pulmonary fibrosis. N Engl J Med. 2011;364(16):1503-1512.

[131] Hunninghake GM, Hatabu H, Okajima Y, Gao W, Dupuis J, Latourelle JC, et al. MUC5B promoter polymorphism and interstitial lung abnormalities. N Engl J Med. 2013;368(23):2192-2200.

[132] Peljto AL, Zhang Y, Fingerlin TE, Ma SF, Garcia JG, Richards TJ, et al. Association between the MUC5B promoter polymorphism and survival in patients with idiopathic pulmonary fibrosis. JAMA. 2013;309(21):2232-2239.

[133] Fingerlin TE, Murphy E, Zhang W, Peljto AL, Brown KK, Steele MP, et al. Genome-wide association study identifies multiple susceptibility loci for pulmonary fibrosis. Nat Genet. 2013;45(6):613-620.

[134] Ostrowski LE, Yin W, Rogers TD, Busalacchi KB, Chua M, O'Neal WK, et al. Conditional deletion of dnaic1 in a murine model of primary ciliary dyskinesia causes chronic rhinosinusitis. Am J Respir Cell Mol Biol. 2010;43(1): 55-63.

[135] Sime PJ, Xing Z, Graham FL, Csaky KG, Gauldie J. Adenovector-mediated gene transfer of active transforming growth factor-beta1 induces prolonged severe fibrosis in rat lung. J Clin Invest. 1997;100(4):768-776.

[136] Zuo F, Kaminski N, Eugui E, Allard J, Yakhini Z, Ben-Dor A, et al. Gene expression analysis reveals matrilysin as a key regulator of pulmonary fibrosis in mice and humans. Proc Natl Acad Sci U S A. 2002;99(9): 6292-6297.

[137] Nalysnyk L, Cid-Ruzafa J, Rotella P, Esser D. Incidence and prevalence of idiopathic pulmonary fibrosis: review of the literature. Eur Respir Rev. 2012;21(126):355-361.

[138] Hutchinson J, Fogarty A, Hubbard R, McKeever T. Global incidence and mortality of idiopathic pulmonary fibrosis: a systematic review. Eur Respir J. 2015;46(3):795-806.

[139] Kornum JB, Christensen S, Grijota M, Pedersen L, Wogelius P, Beiderbeck A, et al. The incidence of interstitial lung disease 1995-2005: a Danish nationwide population-based study. BMC Pulm Med. 2008;8:24.

[140] Fernandez Perez ER, Daniels CE, Schroeder DR, St Sauver J, Hartman TE, Bartholmai BJ, et al. Incidence, prevalence, and clinical course of idiopathic pulmonary fibrosis: a population-based study. Chest. 2010;137(1):129-137.

[141] Navaratnam V, Fleming KM, West J, Smith CJ, Jenkins RG, Fogarty A, et al. The rising incidence of idiopathic pulmonary fibrosis in the U.K. Thorax. 2011;66(6):462-467.

[142] Karakatsani A, Papakosta D, Rapti A, Antoniou KM, Dimadi M, Markopoulou A, et al. Epidemiology of interstitial lung diseases in Greece. Respir Med. 2009;103(8):1122-1129.

[143] Xaubet A, Ancochea J, Morell F, Rodriguez-Arias JM, Villena V, Blanquer R, et al. Report on the incidence of interstitial lung diseases in Spain. Sarcoidosis Vasc Diffuse Lung Dis. 2004;21(1):64-70.

[144] Raghu G, Weycker D, Edelsberg J, Bradford WZ, Oster G. Incidence and prevalence of idiopathic pulmonary fibrosis. Am J Respir Crit Care Med. 2006;174(7):810-816.

[145] Olson AL, Swigris JJ, Lezotte DC, Norris JM, Wilson CG, Brown KK. Mortality from pulmonary fibrosis increased in the United States from 1992 to 2003. Am J Respir Crit Care Med. 2007;176(3):277-284.

[146] Costa CHD, Accar J, Torres GR, Silva VL, Barros NP, Graça NP. Incidence And Mortality Of Interstitial Pulmonary Fibrosis In Brazil. A42 INTERSTITIAL LUNG DISEASE: EPIDEMIOLOGY, EVALUATION AND PATHOGENESIS. p. A1458-A.

[147] Fortuna FP, Perin C, Cunha L, Moreira JdS, Rubin AS. Mortality caused by idiopathic pulmonary fibrosis in the State of Rio Grande do Sul (Brazil). Jornal de Pneumologia. 2003;29(3): 121-124.

[148] Lai CC, Wang CY, Lu HM, Chen L, Teng NC, Yan YH, et al. Idiopathic pulmonary fibrosis in Taiwan - a population-based study. Respir Med. 2012;106(11):1566-1574.

[149] Mok Y, Jee SH, Danoff SK. Incidence And Mortality Of Idiopathic Pulmonary Fibrosis In South Korea. A42 INTERSTITIAL LUNG DISEASE: EPIDEMIOLOGY, EVALUATION AND PATHOGENESIS. p. A1460-A.

[150] Munakata M, Asakawa M, Hamma Y, Kawakami Y. [Present status of idiopathic interstitial pneumonia--from epidemiology to etiology]. Nihon Kyobu Shikkan Gakkai Zasshi. 1994;32 Suppl:187-92.

[151] Mannino DM, Etzel RA, Parrish RG. Pulmonary fibrosis deaths in the United States, 1979-1991. An analysis of multiple-cause mortality data. Am J Respir Crit Care Med. 1996;153(5):1548-1552.

[152] Gribbin J, Hubbard RB, Le Jeune I, Smith CJ, West J, Tata LJ. Incidence and mortality of idiopathic pulmonary fibrosis and sarcoidosis in the UK. Thorax. 2006;61(11):980-985.

[153] Kolek V. Epidemiology of cryptogenic fibrosing alveolitis in Moravia and Silesia. Acta Univ Palacki Olomuc Fac Med. 1994;137:49-50.

[154] Hubbard R, Johnston I, Coultas DB, Britton J. Mortality rates from cryptogenic fibrosing alveolitis in seven countries. Thorax. 1996;51(7): 711-716.

[155] Kaunisto J, Salomaa ER, Hodgson U, Kaarteenaho R, Myllarniemi M. Idiopathic pulmonary fibrosis--a systematic review on methodology for the collection of epidemiological data. BMC Pulm Med. 2013;13:53.

Section 2

Diagnosis

Chapter 2

Biomarkers in Idiopathic Pulmonary Fibrosis

Sanja Stankovic, Mihailo Stjepanovic and Milika Asanin

Abstract

Numerous published papers are investigating the utility of biomarkers in Idiopathic Pulmonary Fibrosis (IPF) diagnosis, treatment, and outcome prediction. This chapter will summarize our current knowledge about biomarkers associated with alveolar epithelial cell damage and dysfunction (Krebs von den Lungen, surfactant proteins, the mucin MUC5B, CA 15-3, CA 125, CA 19-9, defensins, Clara cell protein (CC16), telomere shortening), biomarkers associated with fibrogenesis, fibroproliferation and extracellular matrix (ECM) remodeling (MMPs and their inhibitors, osteopontin, periostin, insulin-like growth factors, fibulin-1, heat shock protein 47, lysyl oxidase-like 2, circulating fibroblasts, extracellular matrix neoepitopes) and biomarkers related to immune dysfunction and inflammation (C-C chemokine ligand-18, C-C chemokine 2, YKL-40, C-X-C motif chemokine 13, S100A4, S100A8/9, S100A12, autoantibodies to heat shock protein 72, toll-like receptor 3, soluble receptor for advanced glycosylated end products, endothelial damage (vascular endothelial growth factor, interleukin 8, endothelin 1). The future directions in incorporating IPF biomarkers into clinical practice will be reviewed.

Keywords: idiopathic pulmonary fibrosis, biomarkers, extracellular matrix, remodeling and fibroproliferation, alveolar epithelial cell dysfunction, immune dysfunction diagnosis, prognosis

1. Introduction

Idiopathic pulmonary fibrosis (IPF) is a chronic fibrotic lung disease of unknown etiology, progressive and irreversible interstitial lung disease (ILD). IPF is the most common form of idiopathic interstitial pneumonia. It affects around 3 million people worldwide [1]. The increasing count of IPF cases is evident. The prognosis for patients with IPF is poor, with a median survival of 3–5 years if untreated [1]. IPF generally affects adults over 50 years, mainly in their sixth or seventh decade, but the earlier onset was noted in familial IPF. According to the epidemiological data, the incidence rates in Europe and North America are between 2.8 and 19 cases per 100,000 people per year [2]. The number of cases older than 65 years of age is about 400 per 100,000. The IPF has a prevalence of 8.2 cases per 100,000 and belongs to the rare diseases group [3]. The first IPF manifestation is shortness of breath (up to 85% of cases), chronic non-productive cough (up to 75%), tiredness, loss of appetite, and progressive exertional dyspnea, followed by an impaired quality of life [4]. More rarely, it can be an acute exacerbation (AE), acute episodes of sudden, rapid worsening of the disease of dyspnea over just a few weeks, and a consequent significant increase in mortality risk [5].

The pathogenesis of IPF is not completely understood. For many years, IPF was principally an inflammatory disease, given the increase in inflammatory cells in the lungs. Dramatic advances in the understanding of IPF pathogenesis mechanisms over the past decade were based on proteomics data. It discovered proteins in terms of prognosis, diagnosis, and IPF progression. Today, we think about IPF as an epithelial-driven disease. IPF originates from unknown microinjuries resulting from recurrent exposures of the lung epithelium to stimuli or predisposition, followed by initiation of alveolar epithelial cells (AECs) dysfunction, fibroblast recruitment, and proliferation and progression of fibrosis through fibroblast differentiation, myofibroblasts proliferation, and accumulation of extracellular matrix and remodeling [6].

Usually, pulmonary function tests reveal reduced total lung capacity, low carbon monoxide diffusing capacity, and arterial hypoxemia. Although the course of the disease is variable, IPF has a poor prognosis, mortality is high, and reported median survival is from 2.5 to 5 years from the time of diagnosis [7, 8].

The most frequent cause of death is respiratory failure. Although there is no identified cause for the IPF, men are more frequently affected than women. Genetic and environmental factors may contribute to the development or worsen the prognosis of IPF. A history of smoking increases the risk of developing IPF. Occupational and environmental risk factors for IPF are agricultural exposure, dusts from metal, asbestos, wood, chemicals, air pollution, etc. Although IPF is a disease that is limited to the lungs, numerous comorbidities have been increasingly recognized in patients with IPF, such as cardiovascular, pulmonary hypertension and ischemic heart disease, gastroesophageal reflux, lung cancer, chronic obstructive pulmonary disease/pulmonary emphysema, depression, sleep apnea, and diabetes [9].

Diagnosis of IPF is challenging because the initial symptoms are vague, nonspecific, often mild, and may be attributed to advancing age or other diseases. Frequently the diagnosis is complex, requiring a multidisciplinary evaluation as recommended by international guidelines. The diagnosis of IPF continues to be a diagnosis of exclusion of other known causes for pulmonary fibrosis. High-resolution computed tomography (HRCT) plays a central role in the diagnosis of IPF. The presence of the HRCT pattern of usual interstitial pneumonitis is the hallmark of IPF diagnosis. In the case of the inconsistent pattern of UIP, significant inter-observer variability, surgical lung biopsy is necessary despite possible complications: triggering of the pneumothorax, pulmonary collapse, etc. Specific combinations of HRCT patterns and histopathology patterns in patients subjected to lung tissue sampling (transbronchial lung cryobiopsy or surgical lung biopsy) are an important part of the diagnosis.

In summary, the required criteria for diagnosing IPF is the combination of exclusion of known causes of ILD and presence of UIP pattern on chest HRCT or exclusion of known causes of ILD and specific HRCT/histology combinations. In the case of atypical HRCT presentation, lung biopsy is recommended. However, not all patients are eligible due to age and comorbidity limits. The average time from the symptoms' onset to the correct diagnosis is approximately 1.5 years [10–12].

Current guidelines also support the use of clinical, radiological, and physiologic evaluations to estimate IPF disease severity and predict disease progression [12]. These include quality of life questionnaires and quantitation of IPF exacerbation frequency; serial measurements of forced vital capacity (FVC), diffusing capacity for the lungs for carbon monoxide (DLCO), and 6-min walk test (6MWT) distances; and sequential HRCT scans when indicated. Composite scoring systems such as the Composite-Physiologic Index (CPI) and Gender Age Physiology (GAP) index, which incorporate demographic and physiological data, may represent more accurate prognostic models [13, 14].

IPF patients usually respond poorly to therapy. The treatment is based on the use of antifibrotic drugs (nintedanib or pirfenidone), which slow down the disease progression, but they do not significantly improve the survival of these patients. Lung transplantation is the only treatment option that increases survival in IPF. Early intervention may help improve clinical outcomes [15].

2. Biomarkers

A growing body of knowledge highlights IPF diagnosis, and providing accurate prognostic information is difficult using the currently available clinical, radiological, and physiologic findings. Furthermore, pulmonary function tests, clinical assessments, and imaging are very good for some cases, but not good for others. For example, lung biopsy is often not feasible in an elderly population with co-morbidities, etc. [16].

With the development of new treatments for IPF, it is critical to identify patients at an earlier stage of disease and rapidly identify those patients who will progress to worse clinical outcomes. That's why there has been an emergence of molecular biomarkers. Compared to today's diagnostic methods, an optimal biomarker for discriminating patients with IPF from healthy subjects or non-IPF patients should be less invasive, more rapid, and reproducible, easier to obtain from patients.

At the same time, we are the witnesses that non-invasive biomarkers can provide very important information for the clinical assessment of patients. Although considerable advances have been made in the last decade in revealing IPF pathogenesis, this is not the case with IPF biomarkers. Similar to the previous guidelines, current existing guidelines such as 2021 German Respiratory Society (DGP), 2018 American Thoracic Society (ATS), European Respiratory Society (ERS), Japanese Respiratory Society (JRS), American Latin Thoracic Association (ALAT) guidelines strongly recommend not to measure any serum biomarker for IPF diagnosis and distinguishing IPF from other interstitial lung diseases in patients with newly detected ILD of apparently unknown cause who are clinically suspected of having IPF. Also, no guidelines on prognostic biomarkers are available [12, 17–20].

Although there is no molecular biomarker in widespread clinical use for IPF, advancements in this field have been achieved; a growing body of literatures indicates a fascinating field of IPF biomarkers has reported changes in the level of various biomarkers in IPF patients, which implies the potential to become a new tool for clinical practice of IPF.

IPF biomarkers include:

a. predisposition biomarkers for identification of patients at risk for developing IPF

b. diagnostic biomarkers for identification of IPF patients and differentiation of IPF patients from healthy controls or patients with other ILD or another lung disease

c. prognostic biomarkers for staging disease severity, monitoring disease progression, herald worsening of IPF or the onset of an acute exacerbation or more accurate prediction of mortality

d. therapeutic biomarkers that are a reliable measure of efficacy and safety during treatment

e. biomarkers used as a surrogate endpoint in clinical trials helping predict clinical benefit based on epidemiologic/therapeutic/pathophysiologic evidence [21–23].

It is very well known that the ideal biomarker should be noninvasive, easily measured by a single, readily available test, to have high sensitivity/specificity, to be reproducible, accurate, widely available, and cost/effective [24].

Before considering the clinical implementation of the biomarker candidate, it must be evaluated critically with respect to key analytical and clinical characteristics. Criteria to be satisfied for definitive clinical implementation of biomarker related to the test such as adequate assays for its measurement, its predictive value defined in specific clinical contexts, optimal cut-off(s), and known timing of measurement (release kinetics) [25, 26].

Biomarkers should be measured from body fluids or tissues (serum, urine, exhaled breath condensates bronchoalveolar lavage fluid (BALF) transbronchial biopsy, surgical lung biopsy, etc.) with a recommendation to use easily obtainable body fluids or tissues. Although airway biomarkers could be obtained non-invasively via exhaled breath, is simple to collect and unlimited in quantity, most studies used bronchoscopy to obtain these biomarkers via BALF [27].

Additionally, incremental marker value should be examined, and the data about the effect on patient management and outcome and cost-effectiveness should be available. Also, validation across sexes, ages, ethnicities, and disease severity to assure generalizability is very welcome.

This chapter will summarize our current knowledge about IPF biomarkers associated with alveolar epithelial cell damage and dysfunction, biomarkers related to extracellular matrix remodeling and fibroproliferation, as well as biomarkers related to immune dysfunction.

3. Markers of alveolar epithelial cell damage and dysfunction

Markers that belong to this group are the most studied biomarkers and offer the most convincing data. The increase in serum levels of these markers can be attributed to an increase in the production of these proteins by regenerating alveolar type II cells and/or to an enhanced permeability following the destruction of the alveolar-capillary barrier [28].

3.1 Krebs von den Lungen-6 (KL-6) antigen

Krebs von den Lungen-6 (KL-6) antigen is a high molecular weight glycoprotein belonging to the group of human transmembrane mucins, expressed on type II pneumocytes, bronchial epithelium, as well as in glandular epithelium, including breast and pancreatic epithelium [22].

It was originally studied as a potential tumor marker in adenocarcinoma, whereas today's research is mainly based on KL-6 as a diagnostic and prognostic biomarker in ILD [22]. It shows marked inter-individual variability in serum levels.

Although few studies have revealed the KL-6 role as a diagnostic marker for IPF and found a higher value of KL-6 in patients IPF compared to controls. KL-6 was approved in Japan more than twenty years ago as a diagnostic biomarker in ILD [29].

Serum concentrations of KL-6 depend on the polymorphism of the MUC1 gene encoding its synthesis, which accounts for the different values in people of different ethnicities [29]. For these reasons, validation in the non-Asian population is necessary for this biomarker to be internationally used in patients with IPF [30].

However, KL-6 has been mostly studied as a prognostic biomarker. KL-6 values are predominantly increased in ILD, characterized by damage to AECs and progressive thinning of the interstitium, including IPF. A serum cut-off value of ≥ 1000 U/ml is associated with a poorer prognosis of patients with ILD and a higher risk of death [30].

KL-6 fluctuations in the follow-up of IPF patients have also been reported to be potentially useful in predicting functional disease progression [31]. Few studies examined the prognostic significance of serial measurements of KL-6 levels in IPF. Sokai et al. [32] found that serial measurements of serum KL-6 may provide additional prognostic information than physiological parameters in patients with IPF. Wakamatsu et al. [33] found that patients with both initial serum KL-6 values <1000 U/mL and no serial increase in KL-6 had more favorable prognoses than those with serial increases in KL-6 or initial serum KL-6 values ≥ 1000 U/mL. Bennett et al. [34] revealed that higher KL-6 levels in BALF are related to the more severe and extended disease.

As previously discussed, the course of IPF varies widely, and some patients experiencing acute exacerbations of IPF, but the risk factors contributing to AE are unclear. It was noticed that basal values of KL-6 are significantly higher in patients who develop AE compared to patients with stable IPF [30]. Qui et al. [35], in systematic review and meta-analysis, investigated the risk factors for AE in IPF patients. The meta-analysis included seven articles involving 14 risk factors for AE in IPF patients, and poor pulmonary function, mechanical procedures, higher serum KL-6, and secondary pulmonary hypertension were associated with increased risks of AE in IPF patients.

Meta-analysis of 10 studies in IPF found that KL-6 had the strongest association with diagnosis of lung fibrosis compared with the three other examined markers (SP-D, SP-A, and MMP7) until for prognostic studies (decline in forced vital capacity and/or mortality) in IPF, KL-6 showed significant prognostic value [36].

Recently published systematic review and meta-analysis [37] was evaluated the robustness of available evidence for the use of KL-6 measurements in blood to predict prognosis in IPF patients. Twenty-six studies were included in the systematic review, and 14 studies were mainly performed on Asian patients in meta-analysis. The meta-analysis found that IPF patients with increased KL-6 concentrations had a significantly increased risk of developing AE, but the relation of KL-6 concentrations with mortality was not found.

3.2 Mucin 5B

Secreted mucins are the most abundant glycoprotein component of mucus. Secreted mucins (MUC2, MUC5AC, MUC5B, MUC6–8, and MUC19) are secreted into the extracellular space [38] MUC5B is among the major best-described, secreted gel-forming mucins. The main tissues expression of MUC 5B is; respiratory tract, submandibular glands, endocervix. Mucin 5B is one of the main components of respiratory secretions, and it participates in defense of the respiratory system from infections [39, 40]. However, the accumulation of this gel-forming glycoprotein further contributes to impaired gas exchange and complicates the clinical features of IPF patients [41]. The over-expression of mucin 5B in a study in mice showed a negative effect on mucociliary clearance, so inhaled harmful substances remain in the airways longer and initiate damage, and consequently tissue repair with fibrotic changes [42].

In 2011, a genome-wide linkage study identified a locus on chromosome 11 that was significantly associated with IPF risk. A common single nucleotide polymorphism (SNP) (rs35705950) in the promoter of the gene encoding for Mucin 5B (MUC5B) is associated with an increased risk for IPF [43, 44]. Meta-analysis of Zhu et al. [45] revealed a strong association between the MUC5B promoter rs35705950 polymorphism and the risk of IPF, and confirmed that the minor T allele is significantly associated with an increased risk of IPF compared.

The same polymorphism has been associated with higher concentrations of MUC5B and its distribution, predominantly in the epithelial cells of small airways [46]. Mutations in this gene are not the only cause of increased mucin expression. Recent data indicate that increased DNA methylation is also associated with increased MUC5B expression [47]. This association has not been clarified yet and is certainly a topic for future research.

It was also shown that mucin 5B could be a good prognostic marker. Namely, the mutation in the promoter region of the MUC5B gene is associated with a lower risk of lethal outcome [48]. It has not yet been found how the same mutation leads simultaneously to an increased risk of disease. Yet, it is associated with a better prognosis and a higher degree of survival.

3.3 Oncomarkers

Certain similarities between IPF and lung cancer have already been identified. Both diseases primarily affect the lower parts of the lung lobes; risk factors such as smoking, exposure to harmful substances in the living and work environment, viral infections, and others are also common. There are also certain similarities in pathogenetic mechanisms, such as genetic and epigenetic changes, dysfunctions at the molecular and cellular levels, and activation of certain signaling pathways [49]. All the above indicates the possibility of using certain tumor markers in IPF when assessing the severity of the disease and predicting the outcome [50].

Carbohydrate antigen 19-9 (CA 19-9) is a marker of epithelial damage, widely used as a serum tumor marker of carcinoma of the pancreas and digestive system [51]. An increase in the concentration of this marker has been observed in patients with IPF, but the significance of determining it is still speculative.

Another widely used tumor marker that indicates the severity of the disease in IPF is CA 15-3. This glycoprotein, or the most significant tumor marker of breast cancer, is elevated in patients with pulmonary fibrosis. It is useful in predicting the severity of the disease, and after lung transplantation, there is a decrease in its concentration [50].

Carcinoembryonic antigen (CEA), a glycoprotein used as a serum tumor marker of colon, rectum, stomach, pancreas, lung, and breast cancer, also stands out as a useful marker in IPF [52]. The values of this analyte are elevated in IPF and are associated with the severity of the disease [52].

Yin and Lloyd [53] recently identified MUC16 as a transmembrane mucin corresponding to the CA125 antigen, long known as a marker for ovarian cancer. Recently, CA125 was identified as a serum biomarker for disease progression and death in IPF patients.

In the analysis from the PROFILE study, examining 123 serum proteins in IPF patients, Maher et al. [54] singled out primarily CA19-9, CA125, and SP-D as three markers with the greatest potential for routine use in clinical practice. Although these three biomarkers are all secreted in small amounts by the pulmonary epithelium in states of health, SP-D being secreted by alveolar type 2 cells and CA19-9 and CA-125 by the bronchial epithelium, they are secreted abundantly by the metaplastic epithelium of IPF patients. Mahler et al. [54] indicate that the potential of these parameters is reflected precisely in their ability to distinguish patients from healthy people (SP-D) reliably, predict disease progression (CA 19-9), and dynamically reflect disease progression and overall mortality (CA 125) [54]. By examining the concentrations of CA19-9 in the final stage of IPF, Balestro et al. [55] got results consistent with previous research. Namely, most patients at this stage of the disease had CA19-9 values above the threshold (37kU/L). As confirmed by the results of several studies on different populations, CA19-9 is a reliable marker of disease progression [50, 54, 55].

The direct mechanisms of the increase in the concentration of tumor markers in idiopathic pulmonary fibrosis remain unclear. Nevertheless, research results are consistent in that these already widely used markers are useful in assessing the severity and progression of IPF [49, 50]. The great potential of these molecules is reflected, among other things, in the fact that they are already in routine use, as well as that there are commercial tests for their determination, unlike many of the aforementioned potential markers of the IPF.

3.4 Surfactant proteins

Surfactant proteins are lipoprotein complexes synthesized and then secreted exclusively by alveolar epithelial cells, bronchial epithelial cells, as well as Clara cells [56]. They are encoded by SFTPA, SFTPB, SFTPC, and SFTPD genes [57]. Their role is to reduce surface tension in the alveoli and prevent their collapse [58].

Surfactant proteins themselves, as well as mutations in the genes encoding these proteins, have been described as potential biomarkers in IPF [22]. Mutations in the genes for surfactant proteins (SP) C and A2 have been associated with the development of oxidative stress and damage to the endoplasmic reticulum, but an additional profibrotic stimulus is necessary to induce the development of pulmonary fibrosis [59–61].

However, SP-A and SP-D are the most studied surfactants in IPF, as well as surfactants studied for the longest time. The mechanisms by which SP-A and SP-D from pneumocytes enter the circulation are hyperplasia of AECs and thus increased synthesis of these proteins, and loss of AEC integrity i.e., increased permeability of the basement membrane of the pulmonary epithelium to the interstitium [58].

In the serum of patients with IPF, there was a significant increase in the concentration of SP-A and D, while in contrast, their concentration in BAL was lower compared to healthy, control subjects [58]. In addition, an increase in SP-D has been found in patients with acute exacerbations of the disease [62]. This surfactant protein may be useful in detecting patients who are more prone to disease progression and poorer outcomes [54]. There is evidence that SP-D is a biomarker that can be used for differential diagnosis of interstitial lung disease, as its level is higher in IPF than in other ILDs [63].

Wang et al. [64], in a meta-analysis of 21 articles, evaluated the use of serum SP-A and SP-D for differential diagnosis and prognosis of IPF. Serum SP-A levels were significantly higher in patients with IPF than in patients with non-IPF ILD. In the AE of IPF, serum SP-A/D was higher than those in the stable stage.

Studies, therefore, show that these proteins, as well as KL-6 and matrix metalloproteinase-7 (MMP-7), are predictive markers; however, in some studies, only SP-A and SP-D are independent predictors of mortality [65]. In addition, SP-D has proved to be a more sensitive marker than SP-A, with a sensitivity of 77% (SP-A sensitivity is 33%). However, these markers are not specific to IPF, but their increase is also observed in other interstitial lung diseases. Also, a study conducted in South Korea has shown that the application of these biomarkers in IPF, combined with clinical parameters, does not significantly contribute to the assessment of outcome compared to the application of clinical parameters alone. However, if KL-6 is included in the assessment, the contribution of biomarkers to clinical parameters becomes significant [65].

Compared with SP-A and SP-D in the serum of patients with IPF, the data for SP-B are limited. SP-B is a component of pulmonary surfactant, produced by alveolar epithelial cells, which is synthesized as a preproprotein [66]. The maturation process of this protein involves primarily the removal of the signal peptide, followed by the glycosylation of the C-terminal region, and finally, the cleavage of the N- and C-terminal propeptides [67]. Mature surfactant protein B is hydrophobic and strongly associated with phospholipids rich in surfactants. At the same time, its precursors, proSP-B, and C-proSP-B are more hydrophilic so that they can be found in the supernatant of bronchoalveolar lavage [68]. In healthy subjects, concentrations of both mature and SP-B precursors are almost undetectable in serum [69]. The study of Khan et al. [68] has been studied SP-B precursor, C-pro-SP-B, as a new biomarker in serum of patients with different chronic lung diseases, including ILDs. The highest C-proSP-B levels were detected in the serum IPF patients. In a multivariate analysis, C-proSP-B levels were able to discriminate IPF patients from patients with all other pulmonary diseases ($p < 0.0001$). SP-B pre-proteins might serve as a biomarker in pulmonary diseases with alveolar or interstitial damage in IPF.

3.5 Clara cell secretory protein (CC16)

Clara cells are exocrine bronchiolar cells with several different physiological functions, including a protective and regenerative role, as well as a role in maintaining pulmonary homeostasis [70]. These cells' protective and regulatory function is achieved through the secretion of various surfactants, glycosaminoglycans, enzymes, and other proteins [70]. In addition, these cells are involved in the biotransformation of many harmful substances that enter the lungs through the inhaled air [71].

CC16 is a 16 kDa homodimeric secretory protein of Clara cells with anti-inflammatory and antioxidant properties and has been studied as a potential therapeutic agent in various lung diseases [70]. It is encoded by the SCGB1A1 gene. Low serum CC16 values are associated with decreased lung function in children, accelerated decline in lung function in adults, and an increased risk of death, primarily in lung cancer [72].

In contrast, significantly high values of CC16 have been observed in the serum and bronchoalveolar lavage of patients with IPF [72]. Also, CC16 values are high in other interstitial lung diseases, such as sarcoidosis, although the values are significantly higher in IPF [72]. It is assumed that the activation of Clara cells after the alveolar epithelium damage leads to elevated serum concentrations of CC16. However, the exact role of CC16 in the alveolar repair process has not been thoroughly tested [70]. Although CC16 is a potential biomarker in various lung diseases, further studies are needed since CC16 values do not correlate with disease severity; there are no reference values, nor can it be used independently in diagnostics since it is a non-specific marker [70].

3.6 Telomeres

Telomeres are repetitive nucleotide sequences at the ends of chromosomes, whose role is to protect chromosomes from degradation [73]. As DNA polymerase cannot completely replicate the DNA strand, wherein a sequence of about 50 nucleotides is lost during each replication, the importance of telomeres is reflected in the fact that during replication, these non-coding parts of chromosomes are lost. The loss of telomere parts is compensated by the telomerase enzyme, which incorporates guanine-rich sequences at the ends of chromosomes during cell replication. However telomeres become shorter during repeated replications, resulting in cell aging and apoptosis [74].

It has been found that approximately one-third of patients with familial IPF have shortened telomeres, and/or mutations in the gene encoding telomerases [75]. When examining telomere length in peripheral blood leukocytes in patients with IPF, it was found that 40% of patients with familial IPF and a quarter of patients with sporadic IPF have shortened telomeres, below the 10th percentile [76]. In a 2014 cohort study involving over three hundred patients with IPF, it was found that telomere length in peripheral blood leukocytes was an independent predictor of mortality [77]. It was also found that telomere shortening in peripheral blood leukocytes as a surrogate marker for telomere mutations, so telomere length in peripheral blood may be examined in the family of a carrier of these mutations, instead of carrying out genetic analysis, which would indicate a risk factor for familial IPF [78].

3.7 αvβ6 integrin

Integrins are receptors found on the surface of cells, and they have a role in their binding to the extracellular matrix, in the interconnection of cells, and their migration, proliferation, and innate immune response [79]. Structurally they are heterodimers, made of different α and β subunits, and the αvβ6 integrin itself consists of αv and β6 subunits. The β6 subunit is expressed only in epithelial cells, so the whole integrin is present only. This integrin is extremely important for the pathogenesis of IPF, as it can activate transforming growth factor beta (TGF-β), which is involved in the interaction of lung epithelial cells and fibroblasts [80]. In patients with IPF, higher concentrations of this integrin have been found in lung tissue [81]. Also, higher concentrations of integrin are associated with a poorer prognosis [82].

4. Markers of fibrogenesis and extracellular matrix remodeling

4.1 Matrix metalloproteinases (MMP)

Matrix metalloproteinases (MMP) are zinc-dependent proteases, which degrade the extracellular matrix. They can modulate the proliferation, migration, and apoptosis of smooth muscle cells, endothelial cells, and some types of immune system cells. So far, 23 members of this family have been discovered, encoded by 24 genes, where two genes serve to encode the same matrix metalloproteinase - MMP-23 [83]. Under physiological conditions, the activity of these enzymes, collectively called matrixins, is regulated at the level of transcription, activation of their inactive zymogen precursors, interaction with extracellular matrix components, and finally inhibition by endogenous inhibitors [84]. Matrixins are divided into seven categories: collagenases, gelatinases, stromelysins, membrane-type MMP, matrilysins, metalloelastases, and other types of matrixins [85].

Although MMPs are expected to prevent fibrotic changes due to their many functions and role in ECM degradation, these enzymes can have both a profibrotic and an antifibrotic role [85]. More details on members of the MMP-7 and MMP-1 matrix families, specifically elevated in the serum of patients with IPF, will be provided below.

4.1.1 MMP-7 (matrilysine)

This metalloproteinase is expressed in alveolar epithelial cells, phagocytes, and fibrocytes. An increase in MMP-7 levels has been observed in patients with IPF, and this enzyme has been confirmed as a biomarker of IPF [86]. The expression of this matrixin in the lung epithelium in IPF is further increased by osteopontin, a marker that will be discussed later [87]. Two SNPs have been identified in the promoter of the MMP-7 gene, which causes increased transcription, and are associated with the development of idiopathic pulmonary fibrosis [88]. In addition, as an enzyme that effectively removes tissue pathway factor inhibitor (TPFI), MMP-7 creates a procoagulant environment in the alveolar space, which has been observed in many fibrotic diseases, including IPF. Although this enzyme is also involved in the regeneration of lung epithelium after damage, in studies in mice lacking the MMP-7 gene, it was not possible to induce pulmonary fibrosis (PF) with bleomycin, suggesting that this metalloproteinase nevertheless promotes the development of PF [89]. This fact singles out MMP-7 as a potential new therapeutic target.

White et al. study tested the differentiation of IPF from a heterogeneous comparator group that included various other ILDs [63]. In another study, the serum MMP7 levels of IPF patients were compared to a group of patients with other ILD. Serum MMP7 values had a median sensitivity, specificity, accuracy, and diagnostic odds ratio of 71.7, 64.4, 68.4, and 4.7%, respectively [90]. MMP7 indicates a correct IPF diagnosis in more than half of the patients, suggesting an incorrect classification in about one-third of patients. Based on these data, the diagnostic value of these serum biomarkers is currently considered insufficient to support clinical use [17].

The Bosentan Use in Interstitial Lung Disease (BUILD)-3 trial that assessed potential prognostic capabilities of few biomarkers showed that MMP-7 is higher than healthy controls. Baseline MMP-7 levels were good predictors of worsening and could predict changes in FVC as early as month 4. MMP-7 shows the potential to be a reliable predictor of lung function decline and disease progression [91].

Despite the promising data regarding MMP-7 as a prognostic biomarker of IPF, it is not included in clinical practice due to the lack of reproducible, uniform cut-off values in different studies. There are major discrepancies between different studies about collection matrices; for example, EDTA collection tubes suppress MMP activity while PBMC layers are sometimes [10% of cases) contaminated by neutrophils, therefore significantly affecting predictive cut-off thresholds [92].

4.1.2 MMP-1 (collagenase type I)

This type of matrixin degrades the extracellular matrix collagen; it is not expressed in healthy tissue but during physiological and pathophysiological processes [87]. Along with MMP-7, MMP-1 is the most studied matrixin in IPF. The combination of these two matrixins in the diagnosis of IPF has a positive predictive value of up to 91% (for concentrations of MMP-7 > 2.6 ng/mL and MMP-1 > 8.9 ng/mL). Additionally, elevated values of these two MMPs can reliably distinguish IPF from other ILDs [86].

4.2 Osteopontin

Osteopontin (OPN) is an acidic phosphorylated glycoprotein secreted by various cells, including osteoclasts, activated T-lymphocytes, and activated macrophages [93]. Osteopontin is a multifunctional cytokine involved in various biological processes, including cell adhesion, chemotaxis, and reparative processes [87]. In this regard, the biological role of osteopontin in the pathogenesis of cardiovascular diseases, diabetes, glomerulonephritis, and several types of cancer is suggested [93, 94].

The function of osteopontin in the occurrence of pulmonary fibrosis was tested in experimental mouse models, where the role in promoting the migration, adhesion, and proliferation of fibroblasts in the bleomycin-induced pulmonary fibrosis was demonstrated [93, 94]. In addition, analysis of lung biopsy samples of patients with IPF showed that osteopontin is a cytokine with the highest expression [93].

Osteopontin serum values are significantly higher in AE of IPF, compared to values in stable IPF, which is associated with a poorer prognosis [87, 95]. Although OPN is increased in serum and BALF of IPF patients [96], it is not specific in differentiating IPF from other ILDs [93].

The studies did not show the correlation between OPN concentration and SP-A and KL-6 concentrations, which can be explained by the different origins of these markers. Serum values of KL-6 and SP-A better reflect a later phase of the fibrosis process, i.e., the remodeling phase [93]. Although OPN values are highest in patients with IPF, no significant differences were observed compared to the values in patients with other ILD subtypes, indicating the limited use of this biomarker in differential diagnosis [94].

4.3 Periostin

Periostin is an extracellular matrix protein from the fascicline family, and it is involved in the pathogenesis of various diseases accompanied by increased levels of inflammation and fibrosis [97]. Studies have shown that periostin is a protein that is highly expressed in the lungs of patients with IPF [97, 98]. The highest level of periostin expression in the lungs is in fibroblasts, in the areas of active fibrosis [97]. Stimulation of periostin synthesis in fibroblasts is influenced by various factors, including TGF-β and IL-4/IL-13 [98]. Experimental mouse models have shown that suppression of the periostin gene or administration of neutralizing antibodies protects to a large extent against bleomycin-induced pulmonary fibrosis [99]. Also, periostin acts in cooperation with inflammatory cytokines, such as TNF-α, by activating NF-κB, which is accompanied by the production of inflammatory cytokines and chemokines, leading further to the development of pulmonary fibrosis [97].

All this indicates the importance of the biological role of periostin in the pathogenesis of PF. However, elevated serum levels of periostin are also observed in other inflammatory diseases, which is why there is a need to develop a test that will enable greater diagnostic specificity [98]. There is a test designed to determine specifically periostin monomers, which is a better diagnostic marker compared to total periostin [98]. In addition, both total and monomeric periostin are better predictive markers of short-term deterioration of IPF compared to conventional markers KL-6, SP-D, and LDH [98]. The potential role of periostin in the treatment of patients with IPF should also be noted since experimental mouse models have shown that suppression of periostin expression or administration of neutralizing antibodies may result in improvement in the fibroproliferative phase [99].

4.4 Lysyl oxidase 2-like protein (LOXL2)

Lysyl oxidase (LOX) and lysyl oxidase-like proteins (LOXL) represent a group of enzymes with important roles in extracellular matrix remodeling, including covalent binding of elastin and collagen [100]. The LOXL proteins promote collagen accumulation and deposition, participating in ECM stabilization. In addition to the enzymatic function, LOX also has a function in regulating the transcription of elastin and collagen III genes [101].

Four LOX isoenzymes (LOX1-LOX4) encoded by genes located on different chromosomes have been identified [101]. Changes in LOX expression, i.e., increased LOX activity, have been associated with the mechanisms of fibrotic changes in certain lung, liver, and kidney diseases [101]. Increased LOX expression was observed in experimental mouse models in bleomycin-induced pulmonary fibrosis [101].

Also, elevated serum concentrations of LOXL2 in patients with IPF have been associated with a higher risk of disease progression but cannot be correlated with disease severity [101, 102]. Given its role in the pathogenesis of pulmonary fibrosis, the applicability of LOXL2 as a potential therapeutic target was examined. However, the study of the use of a monoclonal anti-LOXL2 antibody (simtuzumab) in the treatment of patients with IPF was discontinued in the second phase of the clinical trials due to the lack of efficiency [101]. One of the potential reasons for failure is the impossibility of adequate penetration into the lung tissue, but there were not enough data for a complete evaluation [101]. In any case, further testing of the diagnostic, predictive and prognostic value of LOXL2 as a biomarker in IPF is necessary.

4.5 Insulin-like growth factors and their binding proteins

IGFs are hormones or growth factors primarily synthesized in the liver. For the most part, they are bound to some of their binding proteins (IGF-BP), which modulate their effects and bioavailability [103]. The IGF binding protein family consists of six members, which also originate primarily from the liver. IGF and IGF-BP are synthesized locally in many tissues to achieve their autocrine and paracrine effects, respectively [104].

Studies have shown a significant increase in circulating concentrations of these binding proteins in newly diagnosed IPF patients. In contrast, in those patients who started using antifibrotic drugs, lower levels of GFBP-2 were found than in patients who do not receive this type of therapy [105]. IGFBP-2 values do not return to the levels of healthy subjects, even with the use of antifibrotic therapy [105].

As IGFs are very strong growth factors, their significant increase in the process of fibrosis, and even lung fibrosis, is expected. However, Guiot et al. [105] found a decrease in the concentration of these analytes in the serum of IPF patients. These surprising results can be explained in several ways. It is possible that IGF-BP, by binding to the extracellular matrix in the lungs with fibrotic changes, locally releases IGF and thus enables its effects in such an environment. On the other hand, an increase in the concentration of binding proteins to insulin-like growth factors means that these factors bind to a greater extent, thus reducing their effectiveness, which can also have a protective role in IPF [106–108].

4.6 Fibulin 1

Fibulin 1 (Fbln1) is a secretory glycoprotein with a significant role in embryonic morphogenesis and alveolar septal formation [109]. Four isoforms of this protein (Fbln1a/b/c/d) have been isolated, differing from each other in C-terminal sequences [110]. However, the identification of individual variants is difficult due to the unavailability of antibodies specific to certain isoforms [111]. Fbln1 has an important role in tissue repair and has been associated with several different respiratory diseases [111]. The importance of the Fbln1c form in the pathogenesis of various respiratory diseases is especially emphasized, which is achieved through the stimulation of fibroblast proliferation and remodeling of the extracellular matrix [110, 111]. Experimental mouse models have shown that the inhibition of Fbln1c expression reduces the proliferation of smooth muscle cells and fibroblasts and collagen deposition around the small airways [111]. In addition, mouse models have shown a significant role of Fbln1c in chronic inflammation, where the inhibition of Fbln1c expression reduces the influx of inflammatory cells into the bronchoalveolar lavage and the synthesis of cytokines and chemokines in the lungs [111]. Accordingly, Fbln1 is mentioned as a potential biomarker and therapeutic target in respiratory and other diseases involving inflammation and remodeling [111].

Elevated values of Fbln1 in the serum and lungs of patients with IPF compared to healthy subjects suggest a role of Fbln1 in the pathogenesis of this disease [109]. High values of Fbln1 in the lungs are a consequence of increased production in smooth muscle cells and fibroblasts; apart from that, under the influence of TGF-β, exogenously synthesized Fbln1 is incorporated into the extracellular matrix [111]. The high serum concentration of Fbln1 correlates with decreased lung function and is associated with acute exacerbation of the disease [109, 112]. Fbln1 values are higher in patients with IPF compared to other ILDs. Still, they are in correlation with pulmonary function in other types of disease, suggesting that Fbln1 may be a predictive marker of disease progression in other ILDs, such as idiopathic nonspecific pneumonia [109].

4.7 Neoepitopes

Excessive deposition of the extracellular matrix is critical to the pathogenesis of IPF. Collagen is the main component of the extracellular matrix, whose synthesis and degradation take place in a balanced way in healthy lungs, while in IPF, this balance is disturbed [113, 114]. During synthesis, the procollagen is cleaved, and during the degradation of collagen molecules, MMPs cut parts of this molecule, which reveals different neoepitopes in all these processes [115].

Peptides formed during synthesis and newly formed neoepitopes are released into the circulation and detected in the blood. Studies have shown that serum concentrations of neoepitopes of collagen synthesis PRO-C3 and PRO-C6 (collagen type 3 and type 6) are higher in patients with IPF compared to healthy subjects of the same age. Their elevated concentration is associated with IPF progression [115]. The concentration of collagen degradation markers (C1M, C3M, C6M, and CRPM) is also elevated in IPF. Longitudinal changes in serum concentrations of these neoepitopes follow the progression of fibrosis and can predict mortality in individuals with IPF in three months [116]. Biomarkers of collagen synthesis and degradation have the potential to improve clinical trials in IPF, prognostic evaluation, and make decisions on therapy [115].

4.8 Heat shock protein 47 (HSP47)

HSP47 is a protein necessary for the synthesis and secretion of collagen molecules. Increased expression of HSP40 is closely related to excessive production and accumulation of collagen, so these data indicate a significant role of this molecule in fibrotic processes and its correlation with the activity of such diseases. It has been shown that a significant increase in the concentration of HSP47 occurs during the acute exacerbation of the disease, compared to the stable form of IPF. Additionally, this biomarker has been found to be superior to better known and studied markers of pulmonary fibrosis, such as KL-6 and SP-A and D [117]. It was assumed that, as HSP47 concentrations in the exacerbation phase of the disease are higher than during stable disease, this distinction would also exist between patients with a stable form of the disease and healthy subjects. However, these assumptions have been refuted in the research conducted [117, 118].

The precise role of HSP47 in the pathogenesis of IPF has not been determined, but this molecule is likely responsible for the additional effect of pirfenidone in the inhibition of fibrotic processes. In addition to direct suppression of type I collagen expression, it is possible that pirfenidone partially achieves its anti-fibrotic effect by suppressing the expression of HSP47 depending on TGF-β1 [119].

4.9 Circulating fibroblasts and fibrocytes

The lungs are characteristic of IPF patients in the regions of the so-called fibroblast foci, where ECM production is most active. In these foci, the predominant cells are myofibroblasts, where under the effect of various cell mediators, the proliferation of these cells takes place, with the inhibition of their apoptosis [120]. Myofibroblasts are cells that phenotypically correspond to the stage between fibroblasts and smooth muscle cells [121].

There are two hypotheses on the origin of myofibroblasts: traditional – that they are formed from fibroblasts after their activation by inflammatory stimuli and more recent – that they are formed by differentiation of alveolar epithelial cells [122].

Fibrocytes are cells originating from the monocytic lineage. In case of tissue damage, migrate to the site of damage attracted by chemotactic factors and then differentiate into fibroblast-like cells. They are present in the circulation and can produce ECM. Fibrocytes express different markers, and these are primarily CD45 leukocyte markers and type I collagen. During its differentiation, it has been found that CD45 expression gradually decreases while type I collagen expression remains unchanged. It has also been found that their differentiation is accelerated under the effect of TGF- β [123]. Although they have a protective role in the process of tissue remodeling and damage repair, it is considered that fibrocytes are involved in the progression of pulmonary fibrosis. Studies show that in the blood of IPF patients, an increased number of circulating fibrocytes is associated with a poor disease outcome [124, 125]. It has been found that, compared to healthy subjects, in patients with IPF, there is a significantly higher number of circulating fibrocytes, identified precisely as CD45+, collagen type I+ cells. In addition, in patients with AE of the disease, these cells are present in ten times greater numbers than in the case with a stable state [125].

5. Markers of immune system dysfunction and inflammation

Although IPF is primarily not an inflammatory disorder, inflammatory and immune-mediated pathways are activated in IPF patient's lungs.

5.1 CC chemokine ligand 18 (CCL18)

CC chemokine ligand 18 (CCL18) is a protein secreted by myeloid lineage cells: monocytes, macrophages, and dendritic cells. In patients with idiopathic pulmonary fibrosis, alveolar macrophages produce large amounts of CCL18 [126, 127]. Th2 cytokines lead to alternative activation of alveolar macrophages, which thus activated have a role in tissue and fibrosis healing [128, 129]. Alternatively, activated macrophages produce CCL18, which leads to increased collagen production by pulmonary fibroblasts, and collagen then stimulates alveolar macrophages to produce CCL18 by a positive feedback loop. In this way, the process of fibrosis is continuously maintained [126].

Increased serum concentrations of CCL18 in IPF are negatively correlated with pulmonary function tests and associated with disease progression [126, 127]. In a prospective study of 72 patients, significantly higher mortality was observed in the group of patients with a CCL 18 concentration above 150 ng/mL [130]. It was also found that pirfenidone used in the treatment of IPF significantly reduces the expression of CCL18 in macrophages [130].

Data obtained from meta-analysis Elhai et al. showed that CCL18 has a significant prognostic value [36]. Based on previous research, it can be concluded that CCL18 is a good prognostic marker in IPF.

In a posthoc analysis of phase 3 ASCEND and CAPACITY trials [131], concentrations of IPF biomarkers in IPF patients who received pirfenidone 2403 mg/day or placebo were investigated, and their associations with changes in FVC and disease progression over one year. CCL18 was consistently prognostic for absolute change in percentage of FVC% and was the most consistent predictor of disease progression across IPF cohorts.

5.2 CC chemokine ligand 2 (CCL2)

CC chemokine ligand 2 (CCL2) is one of the chemokines involved in the recruitment of mononuclear phagocytes, thereby promoting inflammation and the development of tissue fibrosis [132]. Additionally, the recruitment of fibrocytes into the lungs most likely occurs because of interactions between chemokine ligands (including CCL-2) and their receptors [133]. More than 20 years ago, it was established that significantly higher serum concentrations of this chemoattractant are present in patients with idiopathic pulmonary fibrosis [134]. A recently published paper, which focused on examining the prognostic potential of various chemokines, found significantly higher concentrations of CCL-2 in patients with both acute exacerbations of IPF and a stable form of the disease, compared to a control group of subjects [135]. The same study concluded that CCL2 levels, among other chemokines, showed neither correlation with lung function nor patient survival [135].

5.3 CXC chemokine 13 (CXCL13)

CXC chemokine 13 (CXCL13) is a protein secreted by dendritic cells and the main mediator in attracting B lymphocytes to inflammatory lesions. Antigen-stimulated B lymphocytes undergo a process of gradual maturation, so these cells, as well as altered, differentiated B lymphocytes, are present in patients with IPF [136]. Increased CXCL13 mRNA has been isolated in the lungs of patients with IPF compared to control subjects, and serum levels of CXCL13 were increased in patients with IPF compared to control subjects. Elevated CXCL13 protein levels are associated with increased mortality in patients with IPF. The highest levels of CXCL13 were found in IPF patients with acute exacerbations or pulmonary hypertension [137].

5.4 Toll-like receptor 3

The toll-like receptor is a transmembrane glycoprotein receptor expressed predominantly endosomal. Recent studies show an association between Toll-like receptors and aberrant fibrogenesis characteristic of idiopathic pulmonary fibrosis [138]. These receptors recognize molecular patterns that can be potentially dangerous and promote adequate immune response [138]. The Toll-like receptor 3 L412F polymorphism is associated with defective TLR3 activation, which causes mortality in IPF [139]. The association of this mutation with accelerated decline in lung function and consequent early death has been proven. This information can be critical in identifying patients with a rapidly progressive phenotype [140]. Toll-like receptor 3 belongs to the group of receptors that have a significant role in innate immunity. It mediates the innate immune response to tissue injury or infection by inducing NF-κB activation and type 1 interferon production [141]. Toll-like receptors recognize patterns from bacterial, viral, protozoal, and fungal pathogens, which are most important for their survival [141]. The Toll-like receptor 3 is a receptor that recognizes viral double-stranded RNA (dsRNA) and regulates the pro-inflammatory response and IFN-1 production [142]. In studies on fibroblasts in IPF, the unregulated proliferation of primary fibroblasts was observed and decreased production of IFN-β mediated by TLR3 receptors [139]. Activation of TLR3 receptors in primary fibroblasts has an antifibrotic effect and leads to a decrease in TGF-β production, increased collagen production, and increased metalloproteinase activity [143, 144].

The TLR signaling pathway during the reactive response to viruses acts as a blocker of fibroproliferation, so TLR3 signaling deficiency can cause an inadequate lung response to viral pathogens and expose them to chronic cycles of damage and repair considered the basis of IPF pathology [144].

5.5 Toll-interactin protein (TOLLIP)

Toll-interactin protein (TOLLIP) is a protein whose expression in the lungs has been observed in type II alveolar cells, macrophages, and basal cells. This protein has a role in important signaling pathways associated with lung diseases, including IL-1β, IL-13, TLR, and TGF-β [145].

It has been found that the rs111521887 and rs5743894 gene variants located in TOLLIP introns are associated with 40–50% reduced TOLLIP gene expression in the lungs and susceptibility to IPF [146]. Interestingly, the rs5743890_G allele is related to increased mortality in IPF, although it is associated with decreased IPF susceptibility, which suggests that the genetic basis is related to different clinical outcomes [39]. This indicates the heterogeneity and complexity of the pathogenesis of IPF [146]. TOLLIP is an important regulator of innate immune responses mediated by Toll-like receptors and the TGF-β1 signaling pathway through TGF-β1 receptor degradation [92]. It antagonizes the TGF-β signaling pathway by degrading the TGF-β1 receptor [147]. This TLR inhibitory protein is potentially useful for detecting various responses to the treatment of IPF in different genotypes [148].

Decreased TOLLIP expression increases proinflammatory cytokines IL-6 and TNF production in macrophages after TLR stimulation [149]. These data suggest that TOLLIP expression may be protective by reducing the proinflammatory and profibrotic cascade [144].

5.6 Defensins

Defensins are small antimicrobial peptides mainly secreted by neutrophils and epithelial cells, which affect some gram-positive and gram-negative bacteria, as well as viruses [92]. Comparative analysis of gene expression from blood and lung tissue samples of patients with stable IPF and those with acute exacerbation of IPF revealed increased gene expression for alpha-defensins 3 and 4 in IPF with acute disease exacerbation [150].

Alpha-defensins are activated by MMP7, whose gene expression is also increased in the lungs of patients with IPF [22]. It has been found that serum levels of alpha defensin are higher in patients with IPF than in healthy subjects and are associated with the deterioration of the disease [150, 151].

5.7 S100A4

S100 calcium-binding protein A4 (S100A4, fibroblast-specific protein-1) belongs to the S100 family containing calcium-binding motifs. S100A4 promotes lung fibrosis via proliferation and activation of fibroblasts and promotes the transition of fibroblasts to myofibroblasts [152].

Akiyama et al. [153] have shown the clinical significance of serum S100A4 in IPF patients. They revealed an independent association of higher S100A4 levels with a higher disease progression rate and a higher mortality rate, suggesting that S100A4 may be promising in the prognosis and management of IPF. The presence of higher levels of S100A4 in the serum of participants with IPF was linked with a significantly lower progression-free survival and higher 2-year mortality.

5.8 S100A8/A9

S100A8/A9 belongs to the S100 family of calcium-binding proteins derived from neutrophils and monocytes, which modulate the immune response [154]. In the pathogenesis of pulmonary fibrosis, the role of these proteins is based on the proliferation of fibroblasts, the influence on their differentiation, and the increase in collagen production by mentioned cells [155]. Concentrations of S100A8 and A9 are, as recent research results show, significantly higher in patients with acute disease exacerbation than in healthy patients, as well as in patients with confirmed IPF without acute exacerbation [156]. Patients with higher concentrations of these two biomarkers had a significantly poorer three-month survival rate, so S100A8 and S100A9 proved to be significant prognostic markers [156].

5.9 S100A12

S100A12 is a member of the S100 family of calcium-binding proteins that has a significant role in regulating inflammatory processes and immune response. Its proinflammatory activity includes chemotaxis and activation of the intracellular signaling cascade, leading to cytokine and oxidative stress production [157]. In a study with a relatively large number of patients with IPF, serum concentrations of S100A12 in IPF were high and correlated with poor disease prognosis [158].

5.10 Anti-heat shock protein-72 antibodies (AHSP-72)

HSP production is regulated by various stress effects on cells, as well as their damage. They are located on the cell surface and have a role in transmitting information and modulation of the immune response [159]. Various autoantibodies to HSP have been found in patients with autoimmune diseases. What singled out HSP and autoantibodies to these proteins as potential biomarkers in IPF is, inter alia, the fact that cell cultures have been found to have the ability to activate monocytes and increase IL-8 production by these cells [158, 160]. IL-8, as a pro-inflammatory chemokine, further acts as a chemoattractant on neutrophils and activates them [161]. This interleukin is considered one of the major mediators in the pathogenesis of IPF, and its higher serum concentrations and BAL of these patients are associated with more extensive pulmonary fibrosis [162].

The results of a study conducted by Mills et al. indicate that IPF patients did not show a significant increase in serum antiHSP-72 antibodies compared to healthy subjects, nor did the concentration of the identical immunoglobulins differ between IPF and other interstitial lung diseases. However, in the bronchoalveolar lavage, an increase in the concentration of total antibodies (classes G, A, and M), but not of class G itself, is associated with a better disease outcome, i.e., it was observed in patients with slower disease progression [163]. These results contrast with the data from the previous study, which showed that the increase in the concentration of autoantibodies to HSP-70 in IPF patients was associated with a poor disease outcome [164]. This discrepancy in the conclusions can be justified by applying different methods, i.e., the antigens used to isolate antibodies and the non-homogeneous groups in the research of Kahloon et al. in terms of age, gender and ethnicity. It is undeniable that these proteins and autoantibodies directed at them have their place in the pathogenesis of IPF, but further research is needed to elucidate the role and potential use of these biomarkers in pulmonary fibrosis.

5.11 YKL-40

YKL-40 is a glycoprotein, a member of the chitinase and chitin-like protein family, expressed in many tissues, especially those characterized by high metabolic activity [165]. The exact biological role of YKL40 is not fully known, but it is involved in various pathophysiological processes as an inflammatory glycoprotein, including cell proliferation, migration, and tissue remodeling [166].

YKL-40 is mainly expressed in alveolar epithelial cells and macrophages, and its values are elevated in the serum and lungs of patients with IPF [165]. In addition, high concentrations of YKL-40 are detected in other diseases accompanied by high levels of fibrosis, such as liver cirrhosis, Crohn's disease, and systemic sclerosis [165]. Elevated levels of YKL-40 in serum and bronchoalveolar lavage are associated with a higher risk of death in patients with IPF, although there is a weak correlation between these concentrations [104]. Also, YKL-40 values are inversely related to lung function in asthma, sarcoidosis, and IPF [165]. YKL-40 is not a marker specific for IPF, although the cut-off value of 79 ng/ml is mentioned in the literature and associated with a poorer prognosis [105]. Compared to the short-term prognostic markers SP-D and CCL18, YKL-40 has the highest predictive value 3–4 years after diagnosis, so a potential combination of these markers could allow a better assessment of survival [165].

5.12 Vimentin/anti-vimentin antibodies

Vimentin is a cytoskeleton protein in cells of mesenchymal origin which is considered responsible for increased cell invasiveness so that one can assume its importance in fibroblast invasion into the so-called fibrous foci in the lungs of IPF patients [167]. This filament is essential to the process of wound healing, so its overexpression results in increased cell invasiveness and excessive scar tissue formation [167, 168].

Immunochemical staining of tissue samples from IPF patients showed that vimentin was significantly more expressed in the cells at the periphery of the fibrous focus than in the center. In the same study, it was found that in the fasting state, as an inducer of the autophagy process, fibroblasts originating from IPF patients expressed vimentin more than control group fibroblasts, while the process of autophagy was lacking [169].

The defect of the autophagy process has already been associated with the development of idiopathic pulmonary fibrosis, where there is no removal of parts of the extracellular matrix by their implementation in autophagosomes and the destruction of these products after fusion with lysosomes [170, 171].

The antiangiogenetic, as well as the antitumor agent WFA (withaferin A), can bind to vimentin, covalently modify it, and cause its aggregation [172]. Treatment of IPF fibroblasts with this agent increased the number of autophagosomes in these cells, i.e., it stimulated autophagy. In addition, the expression of vimentin and type I collagen were reduced, and the inhibition of vimentin reduced the invasiveness of fibroblasts [169]. All these facts confirm the role of vimentin in pulmonary fibrosis and its importance in the progression of the disease.

Various cells involved in the development of pulmonary fibrosis secrete vimentin under the influence of TGF-β1 [173]. This secreted cytoskeletal protein was found in significantly higher IPF patients than in the healthy, control group [174]. Over-expression of otherwise immunologically inert molecules leads to their higher immunogenicity [175]. This is confirmed by the results of a 2017 study that proved anti-vimentin autoantibodies in IPF patients in a much higher concentration than is the case with other lung diseases and healthy subjects. Patients with poorer clinical and poor disease outcomes had higher circulating concentrations of anti-vimentin antibodies features [174].

5.13 T-lymphocytes

As mentioned above, the central event in the development of IPF is an excessive reaction to repeated damage to alveolar epithelial cells with the formation of scar tissue that replaces the functional one [176]. Pulmonary fibrosis was considered a non-immune disease, but more and more evidence speak in favor of the role of the immune system in initiating the onset of fibrotic changes, as well as in the progression of fibrosis.

Regulatory T-lymphocytes are CD4+ T-cells that participate in immunosuppression and prevent the development of an immune response to the body's antigens (autotolerance) [177]. These cells can produce various cytokines, including IL-10 and TGF-β1, and therefore may have the potential to both suppress and promote the onset of fibrotic changes [148].

Activation of these T-lymphocytes increases the expression of semaphorin seven, which has a chemotactic effect on macrophages, stimulates the production of proinflammatory cytokines, and regulates collagen production by fibrocytes [178]. Increased expression of semaphorin seven on regulatory T cells has been found in IPF [179].

The cell population of Th2 lymphocytes (T-helper cells) and their product IL-13, which have long been known to have a role in allergic diseases and the pathogenesis of asthma, are now also associated with the development of IPF. Namely, this interleukin affects the extracellular matrix production and induces tissue fibrosis, which has been shown in animal models, where increased expression of IL-13 had profibrotic effects [180]. Studies show an increased concentration of this cytokine in the blood of patients with IPF and the correlation of these concentrations with disease progression [181]. These claims are consistent with the results of studies performed on mice lacking the IL-13 gene in which the induction of pulmonary fibrosis by bleomycin was inhibited [182].

5.14 Soluble receptor for advanced glycosylated end products (sRAGE)

The soluble receptor for advanced glycation end-products (sRAGE) acts as a decoy for capturing advanced glycation end-products (AGEs) and inhibits the activation of the oxidative stress and apoptotic pathways. The study of Manichaikul et al. [183] found that adults with IPF have lower sRAGE levels. They were associated with greater disease severity and a higher death rate or lung transplant at one year compared with healthy controls. Additionally, lower plasma sRAGE levels in patients with IPF and other ILDs when compared with healthy controls Lower sRAGE levels were associated with disease severity. In their study, Cabrera Cesar et al. [184] provide evidence, for the first time, for the possible use of AGE as a differential diagnostic biomarker to distinguish between IPF and connective tissue disease-associated interstitial lung disease (CTD-ILD). The role of RAGE in human and experimental models of IPF did not fully understand [185].

Machahua et al. [186] evaluated the AGEs, and sRAGE levels in serum as a potential biomarker in IPF, demonstrate that the increase of AGE/sRAGE ratio is higher in IPF. AGE/sRAGE increase correlates with respiratory functional progression (FVC and DLCO values); changes in serum AGEs and sRAGE correlated with % change of FVC, DLCO, and TLC during the follow-up.

No difference in AGE or RAGE expression was observed in lungs with non-specific interstitial pneumonia compared to that in the controls. Levels of circulating AGEs also increased significantly in the lungs of patients with IPF compared to those with NSIP and normal control [187].

6. Markers of endothelial damage

Aberrant angiogenesis is implicated in the pathogenesis of pulmonary fibrosis, and mediators of this process are VEGF, endothelin 1, interleukin 8.

6.1 Vascular endothelial growth factor (VEGF)

Vascular endothelial growth factor-A (VEGF-A) is the predominantly expressed member of the VEGF family and is often denoted as VEGF. It is a tyrosine kinase glycoprotein and is one of the most potent factors that stimulate angiogenesis. VEGF is elevated in IPF compared with healthy controls [137, 188].

Barratt et al. [189] report that the levels of VEGF-A165b protein were found to be dramatically elevated in the lung tissue of patients with IPF, is produced mostly by the alveolar epithelium but also by macrophages, lymphocytes, and fibroblasts.

Ando et al. reported reduced VEGF-A in the BALF of IPF patients compared to controls [190]. VEGF-A levels in peripheral blood are associated with the severity and progression of IPF [191]. Enhanced expression of VEGF-A is correlated with increased alveolar-capillary density in non-fibrotic regions of IPF lungs [192].

Nintedanib, therapeutics for IPF, acts by targeting VEGF receptor signaling, slows IPF progression, but the utility of VEGF as a marker of treatment success is not determined [193, 194].

6.2 Endothelin 1 (ET-1)

Endothelin-1 (ET-1) is a vasoactive peptide that plays a central role in lung fibrosis. ET-1 drives fibroblast activation, proliferation, differentiation into myofibroblast - processes that lead to excessive collagen deposition [195]. Barlo et al. [196] revealed that ET-1 in serum was significantly increased in IPF patients compared with healthy control subjects until it was significantly decreased in bronchoalveolar lavage fluid (BALF).

6.3 Interleukin-8 (IL-8)

Interleukin-8 (IL-8) is produced by phagocytes when exposed to inflammatory stimuli and promotes angiogenesis [191]. IL-8 levels were significantly higher in IPF exacerbated patients, and an increase in IL-8 by one pg/ml increases the odds of death by 6.7% in IPF patients [197]. Schupp et al. [198] found significantly higher levels of IL-8 in BAL samples from IPF-AE patients compared to stable IPF patients. Xaubet et al. [199] found that the percentage of IL-8–positive bronchoalveolar lavage macrophages was significantly higher in areas of IPF lung with extensive fibrosis defined by HRCT scans compared with BALF from healthy volunteers.

7. Multimarker approach

The literature supports the concept of combining multiple markers and/or clinical parameters in clinical decision support. Biomarker panels consisting of two or more suspected biomarkers may potentially indicate a higher likelihood of IPF than any single biomarker, more effectively differentiate IPF patients from healthy volunteers and patients with other pulmonary diseases, define prognosis at the time of diagnosis, identify responses to therapy.

For example, the improved predictive value of the combination of biomarkers SP-A and SP-D in IPF was observed [200]. Rosas et al. [86] found that the combination of serum MMP1 and MMP7 levels distinguish IPF from other chronic lung diseases more than either protein on its own. Also, the combination of five proteins (MMP-7, MMP-1, MMP-8, Insulin-like Growth Factor Binding Protein 1(IGFBP1) and tumor necrosis factor receptor superfamily, member 1a (TNFRSF1A)) could distinguish with high sensitivity and specificity IPF patients from normal controls. White et al. [63] showed that a combined serum biomarker panel combining SP-D, MMP-7, and osteopontin differentiated IPF patients from other types of ILD (except for rheumatoid arthritis–associated ILD) more readily than each biomarker, and this biomarker index may improve diagnostic confidence in IPF. Hamai et al. [201] found that a combination of MMP-7 and KL-6 potentially support the diagnosis of IPF and might improve survival prediction in patients with IPF. Recently published study Xue et al. [202], found that KL-6, CCL3, and CXCL13 significantly improves the diagnosis of idiopathic interstitial pneumonia. IPF patients with a high level of SP-D but low KL-6 in their serum had a better prognosis [203]. A panel of mi-RNAs including miR-302c, miR-423, miR-210, miR-376C, and miR-185 has been shown to be associated with disease severity, differentiating fast from slow IPF progressors [204].

The next step was to examine the combination of clinical parameters and molecular biomarkers to achieve more accurate results regarding the prognosis of IPF. Kinder et al. [84] reported on a significant improvement in their prediction model of 1-year mortality in surgical lung biopsy-proven IPF, when serum levels of SP-A and SP-D were added to the clinical predictors of mortality alone [205]. Richards et al. [206] evaluated a panel of 92 proteins in a retrospective derivation cohort of IPF patients and tested significant findings in an independent validation cohort of IPF patients, and identified five biomarkers (MMP-7, intercellular adhesion molecule-1, Interleukin-8, vascular cell adhesion protein −1, S100A12) associated with disease progression or mortality. Combining clinical parameters and plasma protein concentrations (gender, FVC%, DLCO%, MMP-7), they constructed peripheral blood risk index-PCMI, distinguishing high and low mortality risk subgroups in the derivation was accurately predictive of mortality in the validation cohort. Song et al. [65] found that the predictive model of survival includes biomarkers (MMP7, SPA, KL6) and clinical variables (FVC%, DLCO%, age, change in FVC at six months) is better than the model based on clinical parameters.

Herazo-Maya et al. [207] have recently identified a 52-gene signature in peripheral blood mononuclear cells of patients with IPF, and y further validated in six different cohorts of patients with IPF. They developed a SAMS (Scoring Algorithm for Molecular Subphenotypes) risk scoring system based on the 52-gene signature. Applying SAMS, low risk and high-risk groups of IPF patients with significant differences in outcome (mortality or transplant-free survival). This 52-gene signature could be valuable in predicting response to therapy.

In testing the idea that a combination of clinical and biological parameters can improve IPF patients' outcomes prediction, Adegunsoye et al. [208] derived a clinical-molecular risk (CMR) score (CA-125, MMP7, YKL-40, OPN, age, and percent predicted FVC) for treatment exposed patients. They found that a clinical-molecular signature of IPF transplant-free survival may provide a reliable predictor of outcome risk in anti-fibrotic treated patients. This risk score may help identify individuals at risk of poor outcomes despite antifibrotic initiation and open the discussion of the application of CMS risk score before initiation of antifibrotic therapy to identify patients warranting closer clinical monitoring or earlier lung transplant referral [209].

8. Conclusions

Within the last decade, a broad range of molecular biomarkers for IPF has been reported. Until now, despite a large number of publications about IPF biomarkers, their use in routine is not recommended in international clinical practice yet. The successful translation of molecular biomarkers into clinical practice requires validation in large, multi-center, prospective studies with long-term, longitudinal follow-up, standardization of assays, serial measurements of biomarkers, and interventional trials that show changes related to clinical IPF state.

However, most data about IPF biomarkers originate from small-sized, single-center studies of the retrospective design, cross-sectional with measurements at a single time-point, and often in Asiatic cohorts of patients where their use is more common. This raises questions about the generalizability of the results obtained in Asiatic cohorts as well as about the determination of an optimal cut-off. Their accuracy should also be confirmed in non/Asiatic, Caucasian cohorts to routinely apply them in the management of IPF.

Furthermore, diagnostic criteria for IPF have recently changed, and most of the studies published before did not systematically use HRCT or histology. However, using these stringent criteria, confident data regarding biomarkers value could be obtained. Also, the gold standard for measuring disease activity is missing.

The validation of useful and accurate diagnostic markers could reduce uncertainty and the use of the invasive procedure. Inter-assay disagreement can represent a confounding factor in the interpretation of test results in different studies, and the definition of an optimal cut-off is very important.

Finally, as already touched on in the chapter, investigators are resorting to panels of multiple biomarkers to differentiate IPF patients more effectively from healthy volunteers or patients with other pulmonary diseases. The use of a biomarker index composed of multiple biomarkers already studied separately, with the aim of improving diagnostic accuracy in distinguishing IPF from other ILDs or healthy controls, is promising.

There is evidence of extremely strong genetic association in IPF. Recent advances in genetic sequencing and bioinformatics have made it much easier to detect genetic variants rapidly. It seems that in the near future, we will be able to analyze genetic markers to gain prognostic information for IPF patients or help screen at-risk patients with a familial history that do not exhibit signs or symptoms of IPF.

The utilization of high-throughput sequencing to detect microbial and/or viral genetic material in bronchoalveolar lavage fluid or lung tissue samples has amplified the ability to identify and quantify specific microbial and viral populations [210].

Use of liquid biopsy, which allows the isolation of circulating cell-free DNA from blood, could be very important in the discrimination of patients affected by IPF from those with other ILDs [211].

Discovery, validation, and implementation of clinically useful molecular biomarkers discovered through omics (genomics, epigenomics, transcriptomics, proteomics, and metabolomics) will facilitate precision medicine in IPF [212–214].

Soon, we expect the results of many clinical trials evaluating as primary or secondary outcomes known and new biomarkers that will convince clinicians of the value of using biomarkers at multiple stages of the diagnosis and personalized management of IPF.

Conflict of interest

The authors declare no conflict of interest.

Author details

Sanja Stankovic[1,2]*, Mihailo Stjepanovic[1,3] and Milika Asanin[1,3]

1 University Clinical Center of Serbia, Belgrade, Serbia

2 Faculty of Medical Sciences, University of Kragujevac, Serbia

3 Medical Faculty, University of Belgrade, Serbia

*Address all correspondence to: sanjast2013@gmail.com

IntechOpen

References

[1] Martinez FJ, Collard HR, Pardo A, Raghu G, Richeldi L, Selman M, et al. Idiopathic pulmonary fibrosis. Nat Rev Dis Primer 2017;3:17074. doi. org/10.1038/nrdp.2017.74.

[2] Olson AL, Gifford AH, Inase N, Fernández Pérez ER, Suda T. The epidemiology of idiopathic pulmonary fibrosis and interstitial lung diseases at risk of a progressive-fibrosing phenotype. Eur Respir Rev. 2018 ;27(150):180077. doi: 10.1183/16000617.0077-2018.

[3] Duchemann B, Annesi-Maesano I, Jacobe de Naurois C, Sanyal S, Brillet PY, Brauner M, et al. Prevalence and incidence of interstitial lung diseases in a multi-ethnic county of Greater Paris. Eur Respir J. 2017;50(2):1602419. doi: 10.1183/13993003.02419-2016.

[4] Wuyts WA, Dahlqvist C, Slabbynck H, Schlesser M, Gusbin N, Compere C, et al. Baseline clinical characteristics, comorbidities and prescribed medication in a real-world population of patients with idiopathic pulmonary fibrosis: the PROOF registry. BMJ Open Respir Res. 2018;5(1):e000331. doi: 10.1136/bmjresp-2018-000331.

[5] Kulkarni T, Duncan SR. Acute exacerbation of idiopathic pulmonary fibrosis: who to treat, how to treat. Curr Pulmonol Rep. 2019 ;8(4):123-130. doi: 10.1007/s13665-019-00238-7.

[6] Sgalla G, Iovene B, Calvello M, Ori M, Varone F, Richeldi L. Idiopathic pulmonary fibrosis: pathogenesis and management. Respir Res. 2018;19(1):32. doi: 10.1186/s12931-018-0730-2.

[7] Moua T, Lee AS, Ryu JH. Comparing effectiveness of prognostic tests in idiopathic pulmonary fibrosis. Expert Rev Respir Med. 2019 ;13(10):993-1004. doi: 10.1080/17476348.2019.1656069.

[8] Ley B, Collard HR, King TE Jr. Clinical course and prediction of survival in idiopathic pulmonary fibrosis. Am J Respir Crit Care Med. 2011;183(4):431-40. doi: 10.1164/rccm.201006-0894CI.

[9] Alfaro TM, Robalo Cordeiro C. Comorbidity in idiopathic pulmonary fibrosis - what can biomarkers tell us? Ther Adv Respir Dis. 2020;14:1753466620910092. doi: 10.1177/1753466620910092.

[10] Mori Y, Kondoh Y. What parameters can be used to identify early idiopathic pulmonary fibrosis? Respir Investig. 2021;59(1):53-65. doi: 10.1016/j.resinv.2020.10.008.

[11] Kishaba T. Evaluation and management of idiopathic pulmonary fibrosis. Respir Investig. 2019;57(4):300-311. doi: 10.1016/j.resinv.2019.02.003.

[12] Raghu G, Remy-Jardin M, Myers JL, Richeldi L, Ryerson CJ, et al; American Thoracic Society, European Respiratory Society, Japanese Respiratory Society, and Latin American Thoracic Society. Diagnosis of Idiopathic Pulmonary Fibrosis. An Official ATS/ERS/JRS/ALAT Clinical Practice Guideline. Am J Respir Crit Care Med. 2018;198(5):e44-e68. doi: 10.1164/rccm.201807-1255ST.

[13] Wells AU, Desai SR, Rubens MB, Goh NS, Cramer D, Nicholson AG, et al. Idiopathic pulmonary fibrosis: a composite physiologic index derived from disease extent observed by computed tomography. Am J Respir Crit Care Med. 2003 ;167(7):962-9. doi: 10.1164/rccm.2111053.

[14] Ley B, Ryerson CJ, Vittinghoff E, Ryu JH, Tomassetti S, Lee JS, et al. A multidimensional index and staging system for idiopathic pulmonary fibrosis. Ann Intern Med. 2012 ;156(10):

684-91. doi: 10.7326/0003-4819-156-10-201205150-00004.

[15] Nathan SD, Albera C, Bradford WZ, Costabel U, Glaspole I, Glassberg MK, et al. Effect of pirfenidone on mortality: pooled analyses and meta-analyses of clinical trials in idiopathic pulmonary fibrosis. Lancet Respir Med. 2017 ;5(1): 33-41. doi: 10.1016/S2213-2600(16) 30326-5.

[16] van den Blink B, Wijsenbeek MS, Hoogsteden HC. Serum biomarkers in idiopathic pulmonary fibrosis. Pulm Pharmacol Ther. 2010;23(6):515-20. doi: 10.1016/j.pupt.2010.08.001.

[17] Behr J, Günther A, Bonella F, Dinkel J, Fink L, Geiser T, et al. S2K Guideline for Diagnosis of Idiopathic Pulmonary Fibrosis. Respiration. 2021;100(3):238-271. doi: 10.1159/ 000512315.

[18] American Thoracic Society; European Respiratory Society. American Thoracic Society/European Respiratory Society International Multidisciplinary Consensus Classification of the Idiopathic Interstitial Pneumonias. This joint statement of the American Thoracic Society (ATS), and the European Respiratory Society (ERS) was adopted by the ATS board of directors, June 2001 and by the ERS Executive Committee, June 2001. Am J Respir Crit Care Med. 2002 ;165(2):277-304. doi: 10.1164/ajrccm.165.2.ats01.

[19] Raghu G, Collard HR, Egan JJ, Martinez FJ, Behr J, Brown KK, et al.; ATS/ERS/JRS/ALAT Committee on Idiopathic Pulmonary Fibrosis. An official ATS/ERS/JRS/ALAT statement: idiopathic pulmonary fibrosis: evidence-based guidelines for diagnosis and management. Am J Respir Crit Care Med. 2011;183(6):788-824. doi: 10.1164/ rccm.2009-040GL.

[20] Prasse A, Müller-Quernheim J. Non-invasive biomarkers in pulmonary

fibrosis. Respirology. 2009;14(6): 788-95. doi: 10.1111/j.1440-1843. 2009.01600.x.

[21] Ray P, Le Manach Y, Riou B, Houle TT. Statistical evaluation of a biomarker. Anesthesiology. 2010;112(4):1023-40. doi: 10.1097/ ALN.0b013e3181d47604.

[22] Ley B, Brown KK, Collard HR. Molecular biomarkers in idiopathic pulmonary fibrosis. Am J Physiol Lung Cell Mol Physiol. 2014;307(9):L681-91. doi: 10.1152/ajplung.00014.2014.

[23] Jee AS, Sahhar J, Youssef P, Bleasel J, Adelstein S, Nguyen M, Corte TJ. Review: Serum biomarkers in idiopathic pulmonary fibrosis and systemic sclerosis associated interstitial lung disease - frontiers and horizons. Pharmacol Ther. 2019;202:40-52. doi: 10.1016/j.pharmthera.2019.05.014.

[24] Strimbu K, Tavel JA. What are biomarkers? Curr Opin HIV AIDS. 2010;5(6):463-6. doi: 10.1097/ COH.0b013e32833ed177.

[25] Ou FS, Michiels S, Shyr Y, Adjei AA, Oberg AL. Biomarker Discovery and Validation: Statistical Considerations. J Thorac Oncol. 2021;16(4):537-545. doi: 10.1016/j.jtho.2021.01.1616.

[26] Panteghini M. Cardiac: is this biomarker ready for the prime time? Scand J Clin Lab Invest Suppl. 2010;242:66-72. doi: 10.3109/00365513. 2010.493394.

[27] Hayton C, Terrington D, Wilson AM, Chaudhuri N, Leonard C, Fowler SJ. Breath biomarkers in idiopathic pulmonary fibrosis: a systematic review. Respir Res. 2019;20(1):7. doi: 10.1186/s12931-019-0971-8.].

[28] Chiba H, Otsuka M, Takahashi H. Significance of molecular biomarkers in idiopathic pulmonary fibrosis: a mini

review. Respir Investig. 2018;56:384-91. doi.org/10.1016/j.resinv.2018.06.001.

[29] Horimasu Y, Hattori N, Ishikawa N, Kawase S, Tanaka S, Yoshioka K, et al. Different MUC1 gene polymorphisms in German and Japanese ethnicities affect serum KL-6 levels. Respir Med. 2012;106(12):1756-64. doi: 10.1016/j. rmed.2012.09.001.

[30] Kokosi MA, Margaritopoulos GA, Wells AU. Personalised medicine in interstitial lung diseases: Number 6 in the Series "Personalised medicine in respiratory diseases" Edited by Renaud Louis and Nicolas Roche. Eur Respir Rev. 2018;27(148):170117. doi: 10.1183/16000617.0117-2017.

[31] d'Alessandro M, Bergantini L, Cameli P, Vietri L, Lanzarone N, Alonzi V, et al. Krebs von den Lungen-6 as a biomarker for disease severity assessment in interstitial lung disease: a comprehensive review. Biomark Med. 2020;14(8):665-674. doi: 10.2217/ bmm-2019-0545.

[32] Sokai A, Tanizawa K, Handa T, Kanatani K, Kubo T, Ikezoe K, et al. Importance of serial changes in biomarkers in idiopathic pulmonary fibrosis. ERJ Open Res. 2017;3(3):00019-2016. doi: 10.1183/23120541.00019-2016.

[33] Wakamatsu K, Nagata N, Kumazoe H, Oda K, Ishimoto H, Yoshimi M, et al.. Prognostic value of serial serum KL-6 measurements in patients with idiopathic pulmonary fibrosis. Respir Investig. 2017;55(1):16-23. doi: 10.1016/j. resinv.2016.09.003.

[34] Bennett D, Salvini M, Fui A, Cillis G, Cameli P, Mazzei MA, et al. Calgranulin B and KL-6 in bronchoalveolar lavage of patients with IPF and NSIP. Inflammation. 2019;42(2):463-470. doi: 10.1007/ s10753-018-00955-2.

[35] Qiu M, Chen Y, Ye Q. Risk factors for acute exacerbation of idiopathic pulmonary fibrosis: A systematic review and meta-analysis. Clin Respir J. 2018;12(3):1084-1092. doi: 10.1111/ crj.12631.

[36] Elhai M, Avouac J, Allanore Y. Circulating lung biomarkers in idiopathic lung fibrosis and interstitial lung diseases associated with connective tissue diseases: Where do we stand? Semin Arthritis Rheum. 2020;50(3):480-491. doi: 10.1016/j. semarthrit.2020.01.006.

[37] Aloisio E, Braga F, Puricelli C, Panteghini M. Prognostic role of Krebs von den Lungen-6 (KL-6) measurement in idiopathic pulmonary fibrosis: a systematic review and meta-analysis. Clin Chem Lab Med. 2021;59(8):1400-1408. doi: 10.1515/ cclm-2021-0199.

[38] Ballester B, Milara J, Cortijo J. Mucins as a new frontier in pulmonary fibrosis. J Clin Med. 2019;8(9):1447. doi: 10.3390/jcm8091447.

[39] Campo I, Zorzetto M, Bonella F. Facts and promises on lung biomarkers in interstitial lung diseases. Expert Rev Respir Med. 2015;9(4):437-57. doi: 10.1586/17476348.2015.1062367.

[40] Kim KC. Role of epithelial mucins during airway infection. Pulm Pharmacol Ther. 2012;25(6):415-9. doi: 10.1016/j.pupt.2011.12.003.

[41] Seibold MA, Wise AL, Speer MC, Steele MP, Brown KK, Loyd JE, et al. A common MUC5B promoter polymorphism and pulmonary fibrosis. N Engl J Med. 2011;364(16):1503-12. doi: 10.1056/NEJMoa1013660.

[42] Boucher RC. Idiopathic pulmonary fibrosis-a sticky business. N Engl J Med. 2011;364(16):1560-1. doi: 10.1056/ NEJMe1014191.

[43] Seibold MA, Wise AL, Speer MC, Steele MP, Brown KK, Loyd JE, et al. A common MUC5B promoter polymorphism and pulmonary fibrosis. N Engl J Med. 2011;364(16):1503-12. doi: 10.1056/NEJMoa1013660.

[44] Kropski JA, Blackwell TS, Loyd JE. The genetic basis of idiopathic pulmonary fibrosis. Eur Respir J. 2015;45(6):1717-27. doi: 10.1183/09031936.00163814.

[45] Zhu QQ, Zhang XL, Zhang SM, Tang SW, Min HY, Yi L, Xu B, Song Y. Association between the MUC5B promoter polymorphism rs35705950 and idiopathic pulmonary fibrosis: A meta-analysis and trial sequential analysis in Caucasian and Asian populations. Medicine (Baltimore). 2015 ;94(43):e1901. doi: 10.1097/MD.0000000000001901.

[46] Nakano Y, Yang IV, Walts AD, Watson AM, Helling BA, Fletcher AA, et al. MUC5B promoter variant rs35705950 affects MUC5B expression in the distal airways in idiopathic pulmonary fibrosis. Am J Respir Crit Care Med. 2016;193(4):464-6. doi: 10.1164/rccm.201509-1872LE.

[47] Helling BA, Gerber AN, Kadiyala V, Sasse SK, Pedersen BS, Sparks L, et al. Regulation of MUC5B expression in idiopathic pulmonary fibrosis. Am J Respir Cell Mol Biol. 2017;57(1):91-99. doi: 10.1165/rcmb.2017-0046OC.

[48] Peljto AL, Zhang Y, Fingerlin TE, Ma SF, Garcia JG, Richards TJ, et al. Association between the MUC5B promoter polymorphism and survival in patients with idiopathic pulmonary fibrosis. JAMA. 2013;309(21):2232-9. doi: 10.1001/jama.2013.5827.

[49] d'Alessandro M, Bergantini L, Torricelli E, Cameli P, Lavorini F, Pieroni M, et al. Systematic review and metanalysis of oncomarkers in IPF patients and serial changes of oncomarkers in a prospective Italian real-life case series. Cancers (Basel). 2021;13(3):539. doi: 10.3390/cancers13030539.

[50] Rusanov V, Kramer MR, Raviv Y, Medalion B, Guber A, Shitrit D. The significance of elevated tumor markers among patients with idiopathic pulmonary fibrosis before and after lung transplantation. Chest. 2012;141(4):1047-1054. doi: 10.1378/chest.11-0284.

[51] Scarà S, Bottoni P, Scatena R. CA 19-9: Biochemical and clinical aspects. Adv Exp Med Biol. 2015;867:247-60. doi: 10.1007/978-94-017-7215-0_15.

[52] Fahim A, Crooks MG, Wilmot R, Campbell AP, Morice AH, Hart SP. Serum carcinoembryonic antigen correlates with severity of idiopathic pulmonary fibrosis. Respirology. 2012;17(8):1247-52. doi: 10.1111/j.1440-1843.2012.02231.x.

[53] Yin BW, Lloyd KO. Molecular cloning of the CA125 ovarian cancer antigen: identification as a new mucin, MUC16. J Biol Chem. 2001;276(29):27371-5. doi: 10.1074/jbc.M103554200.

[54] Maher TM, Oballa E, Simpson JK, Porte J, Habgood A, Fahy WA, et al. An epithelial biomarker signature for idiopathic pulmonary fibrosis: an analysis from the multicentre PROFILE cohort study. Lancet Respir Med. 2017;5(12):946-955. doi: 10.1016/S2213-2600(17)30430-7.

[55] Balestro E, Castelli G, Bernardinello N, Cocconcelli E, Biondini D, Fracasso F, et al. CA 19-9 serum levels in patients with end-stage idiopathic pulmonary fibrosis (IPF) and other interstitial lung diseases (ILDs): Correlation with functional decline. Chron Respir Dis. 2020;17: 1479973120958428. doi: 10.1177/1479973120958428.

[56] Mason RJ, Greene K, Voelker DR. Surfactant protein A and surfactant protein D in health and disease. Am J Physiol. 1998;275(1):L1-13. doi: 10.1152/ajplung.1998.275.1.L1.

[57] Whitsett JA, Wert SE, Weaver TE. Alveolar surfactant homeostasis and the pathogenesis of pulmonary disease. Annu Rev Med. 2010;61: 105-19. doi: 10.1146/annurev.med.60.041807.123500.

[58] Greene KE, King TE Jr, Kuroki Y, Bucher-Bartelson B, Hunninghake GW, Newman LS, et al. Serum surfactant proteins-A and -D as biomarkers in idiopathic pulmonary fibrosis. Eur Respir J. 2002;19(3):439-46. doi: 10.1183/09031936.02.00081102.

[59] Maitra M, Wang Y, Gerard RD, Mendelson CR, Garcia CK. Surfactant protein A2 mutations associated with pulmonary fibrosis lead to protein instability and endoplasmic reticulum stress. J Biol Chem. 2010;285(29):22103-13. doi: 10.1074/jbc.M110.121467.

[60] Bridges JP, Xu Y, Na CL, Wong HR, Weaver TE. Adaptation and increased susceptibility to infection associated with constitutive expression of misfolded SP-C. J Cell Biol. 2006;172(3):395-407. doi: 10.1083/jcb.200508016.

[61] Lawson WE, Cheng DS, Degryse AL, Tanjore H, Polosukhin VV, Xu XC, et al. Endoplasmic reticulum stress enhances fibrotic remodeling in the lungs. Proc Natl Acad Sci U S A. 2011;108(26):10562-7. doi: 10.1073/pnas.1107559108.

[62] Collard HR, Calfee CS, Wolters PJ, Song JW, Hong SB, Brady S, et al. Plasma biomarker profiles in acute exacerbation of idiopathic pulmonary fibrosis. Am J Physiol Lung Cell Mol Physiol. 2010;299(1):L3-7. doi: 10.1152/ajplung.90637.2008.

[63] White ES, Xia M, Murray S, Dyal R, Flaherty CM, Flaherty KR, et al. Plasma surfactant protein-D, matrix metalloproteinase-7, and osteopontin index distinguishes idiopathic pulmonary fibrosis from other idiopathic interstitial pneumonias. Am J Respir Crit Care Med. 2016;194(10):1242-1251. doi: 10.1164/rccm.201505-0862OC.

[64] Wang K, Ju Q, Cao J, Tang W, Zhang J. Impact of serum SP-A and SP-D levels on comparison and prognosis of idiopathic pulmonary fibrosis: A systematic review and meta-analysis. Medicine (Baltimore). 2017 Jun;96(23):e7083. doi: 10.1097/MD.0000000000007083.

[65] Song JW, Do KH, Jang SJ, Colby TV, Han S, Kim DS. Blood biomarkers MMP-7 and SP-A: predictors of outcome in idiopathic pulmonary fibrosis. Chest. 2013;143(5):1422-1429. doi: 10.1378/chest.11-2735.

[66] Brasch F, Johnen G, Winn-Brasch A, Guttentag SH, Schmiedl A, Kapp N, et al. Surfactant protein B in type II pneumocytes and intra-alveolar surfactant forms of human lungs. Am J Respir Cell Mol Biol. 2004;30(4):449-58. doi: 10.1165/rcmb.2003-0262OC.

[67] Guttentag SH, Beers MF, Bieler BM, Ballard PL. Surfactant protein B processing in human fetal lung. Am J Physiol. 1998;275(3):L559-66. doi: 10.1152/ajplung.1998.275.3.L559.

[68] Kahn N, Rossler AK, Hornemann K, Muley T, Grünig E, Schmidt W, et al. C-proSP-B: A possible biomarker for pulmonary diseases? Respiration. 2018;96(2):117-126. doi: 10.1159/000488245.

[69] Doyle IR, Nicholas TE, Bersten AD. Partitioning lung and plasma proteins: circulating surfactant proteins as biomarkers of alveolocapillary permeability. Clin Exp Pharmacol

Physiol. 1999;26(3):185-97. doi:
10.1046/j.1440-1681.1999.03015.x.

[70] Almuntashiri S, Zhu Y, Han Y,
Wang X, Somanath PR, Zhang D. Club
Cell Secreted Protein CC16: potential
applications in prognosis and therapy
for pulmonary diseases. J Clin Med.
2020;9(12):4039. doi: 10.3390/
jcm9124039.

[71] Rokicki W, Rokicki M, Wojtacha J,
Dżeljijli A. The role and importance of
club cells (Clara cells) in the
pathogenesis of some respiratory
diseases. Kardiochir Torakochirurgia
Pol. 2016;13(1):26-30. doi: 10.5114/
kitp.2016.58961.

[72] Buendía-Roldán I, Ruiz V, Sierra P,
Montes E, Ramírez R, Vega A, et al.
Increased Expression of CC16 in
Patients with Idiopathic Pulmonary
Fibrosis. PLoS One. 2016;11(12):
e0168552. doi: 10.1371/journal.
pone.0168552.

[73] Lee HW, Blasco MA, Gottlieb GJ,
Horner JW 2nd, Greider CW,
DePinho RA. Essential role of mouse
telomerase in highly proliferative
organs. Nature. 1998;392(6676):569-74.
doi: 10.1038/33345.

[74] Zvereva MI, Shcherbakova DM,
Dontsova OA. Telomerase: structure,
functions, and activity regulation.
Biochemistry (Mosc). 2010;75(13):1563-
83. doi: 10.1134/s0006297910130055.

[75] Courtwright AM, El-Chemaly S.
Telomeres in interstitial lung disease:
The short and the long of It. Ann Am
Thorac Soc. 2019;16(2):175-181. doi:
10.1513/AnnalsATS.201808-508CME.

[76] Cronkhite JT, Xing C, Raghu G,
Chin KM, Torres F, Rosenblatt RL,
et al. Telomere shortening in familial
and sporadic pulmonary fibrosis.
Am J Respir Crit Care Med.
2008;178(7):729-37. doi: 10.1164/
rccm.200804-550OC.

[77] Stuart BD, Lee JS, Kozlitina J,
Noth I, Devine MS, Glazer CS, et al.
Effect of telomere length on survival in
patients with idiopathic pulmonary
fibrosis: an observational cohort study
with independent validation. Lancet
Respir Med. 2014;2(7):557-65. doi:
10.1016/S2213-2600(14)70124-9.

[78] Alder JK, Chen JJ, Lancaster L,
Danoff S, Su SC, Cogan JD,
Vulto I, Xie M, Qi X, Tuder RM,
Phillips JA 3rd, Lansdorp PM, Loyd JE,
Armanios MY. Short telomeres are a
risk factor for idiopathic pulmonary
fibrosis. Proc Natl Acad Sci U S A.
2008;105(35):13051-6. doi: 10.1073/
pnas.0804280105.

[79] Campbell ID, Humphries MJ.
Integrin structure, activation, and
interactions. Cold Spring Harb Perspect
Biol. 2011;3(3):a004994. doi: 10.1101/
cshperspect.a004994.

[80] Tatler AL, Jenkins G. TGF-β
activation and lung fibrosis. Proc Am
Thorac Soc. 2012;9(3):130-6. doi:
10.1513/pats.201201-003AW.

[81] Horan GS, Wood S, Ona V,
Li DJ, Lukashev ME, Weinreb PH, et al.
Partial inhibition of integrin alpha(v)
beta6 prevents pulmonary fibrosis
without exacerbating inflammation.
Am J Respir Crit Care Med.
2008;177(1):56-65. doi: 10.1164/
rccm.200706-805OC.

[82] Saini G, Porte J, Weinreb PH,
Violette SM, Wallace WA,
McKeever TM, et al. αvβ6 integrin may
be a potential prognostic biomarker in
interstitial lung disease. Eur Respir J.
2015;46(2):486-94. doi: 10.1183/
09031936.00210414.

[83] Mahalanobish S, Saha S, Dutta S,
Sil PC. Matrix metalloproteinase: An
upcoming therapeutic approach for
idiopathic pulmonary fibrosis.
Pharmacol Res. 2020;152:104591.
doi: 10.1016/j.phrs.2019.104591.

[84] Visse R, Nagase H. Matrix metalloproteinases and tissue inhibitors of metalloproteinases: structure, function, and biochemistry. Circ Res. 2003;92(8):827-39. doi: 10.1161/01. RES.0000070112.80711.3D.

[85] Craig VJ, Zhang L, Hagood JS, Owen CA. Matrix metalloproteinases as therapeutic targets for idiopathic pulmonary fibrosis. Am J Respir Cell Mol Biol. 2015;53(5):585-600. doi: 10.1165/rcmb.2015-0020TR.

[86] Rosas IO, Richards TJ, Konishi K, Zhang Y, Gibson K, Lokshin AE, et al. MMP1 and MMP7 as potential peripheral blood biomarkers in idiopathic pulmonary fibrosis. PLoS Med. 2008;5(4):e93. doi: 10.1371/ journal.pmed.0050093.

[87] Pardo A, Gibson K, Cisneros J, Richards TJ, Yang Y, Becerril C, et al. Up-regulation and profibrotic role of osteopontin in human idiopathic pulmonary fibrosis. PLoS Med. 2005;2(9):e251. doi: 10.1371/journal. pmed.0020251.

[88] Richards TJ, Park C, Chen Y, Gibson KF, Peter Di Y, Pardo A, et al. Allele-specific transactivation of matrix metalloproteinase 7 by FOXA2 and correlation with plasma levels in idiopathic pulmonary fibrosis. Am J Physiol Lung Cell Mol Physiol. 2012;302(8):L746-54. doi: 10.1152/ ajplung.00319.2011.

[89] Zuo F, Kaminski N, Eugui E, Allard J, Yakhini Z, Ben-Dor A, et al. Gene expression analysis reveals matrilysin as a key regulator of pulmonary fibrosis in mice and humans. Proc Natl Acad Sci U S A. 2002;99(9):6292-7. doi: 10.1073/ pnas.092134099.

[90] Morais A, Beltrão M, Sokhatska O, Costa D, Melo N, Mota P, et al. Serum metalloproteinases 1 and 7 in the diagnosis of idiopathic pulmonary fibrosis and other interstitial pneumonias. Respir Med. 2015;109(8):1063-8. doi: 10.1016/j. rmed.2015.06.003.

[91] Bauer Y, White ES, de Bernard S, Cornelisse P, Leconte I, Morganti A, et al. MMP-7 is a predictive biomarker of disease progression in patients with idiopathic pulmonary fibrosis. ERJ Open Res. 2017;3(1):00074-2016. doi: 10.1183/23120541.00074-2016.

[92] Tzouvelekis A, Herazo-Maya J, Sakamoto K, Bouros D. Biomarkers in the evaluation and management of idiopathic pulmonary fibrosis. Curr Top Med Chem. 2016;16(14):1587-98. doi: 10.2174/1568026616666150930120959.

[93] Kadota J, Mizunoe S, Mito K, Mukae H, Yoshioka S, Kawakami K, et al. High plasma concentrations of osteopontin in patients with interstitial pneumonia. Respir Med. 2005;99(1):111-7. doi: 10.1016/j. rmed.2004.04.018.

[94] Goyal M, Jaswal S, Garg K, Gupta S, Dey S, Dutta K. Diagnostic role of osteopontin in interstitial lung disease. J Health Sci Med Res 2021;39(3):181-189 doi: 10.31584/jhsmr.2021780.

[95] Gui X, Qiu X, Xie M, Tian Y, Min C, Huang M, et al. Prognostic value of serum osteopontin in acute exacerbation of idiopathic pulmonary fibrosis. Biomed Res Int. 2020;2020:3424208. doi: 10.1155/2020/3424208.

[96] Foster MW, Morrison LD, Todd JL, Snyder LD, Thompson JW, Soderblom EJ, et al. Quantitative proteomics of bronchoalveolar lavage fluid in idiopathic pulmonary fibrosis. J Proteome Res. 2015;14(2):1238-49. doi: 10.1021/pr501149m.

[97] Yoshihara T, Nanri Y, Nunomura S, Yamaguchi Y, Feghali-Bostwick C, Ajito K, et al. Periostin plays a critical role in the cell cycle in lung fibroblasts.

Respir Res. 2020;21(1):38. doi: 10.1186/s12931-020-1299-0.

[98] Ohta S, Okamoto M, Fujimoto K, Sakamoto N, Takahashi K, Yamamoto H, et al; Consortium for Development of Diagnostics for Pulmonary Fibrosis Patients (CoDD-PF). The usefulness of monomeric periostin as a biomarker for idiopathic pulmonary fibrosis. PLoS One. 2017;12(3):e0174547. doi: 10.1371/journal.pone.0174547.

[99] Okamoto M, Izuhara K, Ohta S, Ono J, Hoshino T. Ability of periostin as a new biomarker of idiopathic pulmonary fibrosis. Adv Exp Med Biol. 2019;1132:79-87. doi: 10.1007/978-981-13-6657-4_9.

[100] Naik PK, Bozyk PD, Bentley JK, Popova AP, Birch CM, Wilke CA, et al.; COMET Investigators. Periostin promotes fibrosis and predicts progression in patients with idiopathic pulmonary fibrosis. Am J Physiol Lung Cell Mol Physiol. 2012;303(12):L1046-56. doi: 10.1152/ajplung.00139.2012.

[101] Chen L, Li S, Li W. LOX/LOXL in pulmonary fibrosis: potential therapeutic targets. J Drug Target. 2019;27(7):790-796. doi: 10.1080/1061186X.2018.1550649.

[102] Chien JW, Richards TJ, Gibson KF, Zhang Y, Lindell KO, Shao L, et al. Serum lysyl oxidase-like 2 levels and idiopathic pulmonary fibrosis disease progression. Eur Respir J. 2014;43(5):1430-8. doi: 10.1183/09031936.00141013.

[103] Annunziata M, Granata R, Ghigo E. The IGF system. Acta Diabetol. 2011;48(1):1-9. doi: 10.1007/s00592-010-0227-z.

[104] Le Roith D. Seminars in medicine of the Beth Israel Deaconess Medical Center. Insulin-like growth factors. N Engl J Med. 1997;336(9):633-40. doi: 10.1056/NEJM199702273360907.

[105] Guiot J, Bondue B, Henket M, Corhay JL, Louis R. Raised serum levels of IGFBP-1 and IGFBP-2 in idiopathic pulmonary fibrosis. BMC Pulm Med. 2016;16(1):86. doi: 10.1186/s12890-016-0249-6.

[106] Kelley KM, Oh Y, Gargosky SE, Gucev Z, Matsumoto T, Hwa V, et al. Insulin-like growth factor-binding proteins (IGFBPs) and their regulatory dynamics. Int J Biochem Cell Biol. 1996;28(6):619-37. doi: 10.1016/1357-2725(96)00005-2.

[107] Jones JI, Clemmons DR. Insulin-like growth factors and their binding proteins: biological actions. Endocr Rev. 1995;16(1):3-34. doi: 10.1210/edrv-16-1-3.

[108] Russo VC, Azar WJ, Yau SW, Sabin MA, Werther GA. IGFBP-2: The dark horse in metabolism and cancer. Cytokine Growth Factor Rev. 2015;26(3):329-46. doi: 10.1016/j.cytogfr.2014.12.001.

[109] Jaffar J, Unger S, Corte TJ, Keller M, Wolters PJ, Richeldi L, et al. Fibulin-1 predicts disease progression in patients with idiopathic pulmonary fibrosis. Chest. 2014;146(4):1055-1063. doi: 10.1378/chest.13-2688.

[110] Ge Q, Chen L, Jaffar J, Argraves WS, Twal WO, Hansbro P, et al. Fibulin1C peptide induces cell attachment and extracellular matrix deposition in lung fibroblasts. Sci Rep. 2015;5:9496. doi: 10.1038/srep09496.

[111] Liu G, Cooley MA, Jarnicki AG, Hsu AC, Nair PM, Haw TJ, et al. Fibulin-1 regulates the pathogenesis of tissue remodeling in respiratory diseases. JCI Insight. 2016;1(9):e86380. doi: 10.1172/jci.insight.86380.

[112] Magnini D, Montemurro G, Iovene B, Tagliaboschi L, Gerardi RE, Lo Greco E, et al. Idiopathic pulmonary fibrosis: molecular endotypes of fibrosis

stratifying existing and emerging therapies. Respiration. 2017;93(6):379-395. doi: 10.1159/000475780.

[113] Hynes RO. The extracellular matrix: not just pretty fibrils. Science. 2009;326(5957):1216-9. doi: 10.1126/science.1176009.

[114] Leeming DJ, Sand JM, Nielsen MJ, Genovese F, Martinez FJ, Hogaboam CM, et al. Serological investigation of the collagen degradation profile of patients with chronic obstructive pulmonary disease or idiopathic pulmonary fibrosis. Biomark Insights. 2012;7:119-26. doi: 10.4137/BMI.S9415.

[115] Organ LA, Duggan AR, Oballa E, Taggart SC, Simpson JK, Kang'ombe AR, et al. Biomarkers of collagen synthesis predict progression in the PROFILE idiopathic pulmonary fibrosis cohort. Respir Res. 2019;20(1):148. doi: 10.1186/s12931-019-1118-7.

[116] Jenkins RG, Simpson JK, Saini G, Bentley JH, Russell AM, Braybrooke R, et al. Longitudinal change in collagen degradation biomarkers in idiopathic pulmonary fibrosis: an analysis from the prospective, multicentre PROFILE study. Lancet Respir Med. 2015;3(6):462-72. doi: 10.1016/S2213-2600(15)00048-X.

[117] Kakugawa T, Yokota S, Ishimatsu Y, Hayashi T, Nakashima S, Hara S, et al. Serum heat shock protein 47 levels are elevated in acute exacerbation of idiopathic pulmonary fibrosis. Cell Stress Chaperones. 2013;18(5):581-90. doi: 10.1007/s12192-013-0411-5.

[118] Yokota S, Kubota H, Matsuoka Y, Naitoh M, Hirata D, Minota S, et al. Prevalence of HSP47 antigen and autoantibodies to HSP47 in the sera of patients with mixed connective tissue disease. Biochem Biophys Res Commun. 2003;303(2):413-8. doi: 10.1016/s0006-291x(03)00352-8.

[119] Nakayama S, Mukae H, Sakamoto N, Kakugawa T, Yoshioka S, Soda H, et al. Pirfenidone inhibits the expression of HSP47 in TGF-beta1-stimulated human lung fibroblasts. Life Sci. 2008;82(3-4):210-7. doi: 10.1016/j.lfs.2007.11.003.

[120] King TE Jr, Pardo A, Selman M. Idiopathic pulmonary fibrosis. Lancet. 2011;378(9807):1949-61. doi: 10.1016/S0140-6736(11)60052-4.

[121] Roy SG, Nozaki Y, Phan SH. Regulation of alpha-smooth muscle actin gene expression in myofibroblast differentiation from rat lung fibroblasts. Int J Biochem Cell Biol. 2001;33(7):723-34. doi: 10.1016/s1357-2725(01)00041-3.

[122] Willis BC, Liebler JM, Luby-Phelps K, Nicholson AG, Crandall ED, du Bois RM, et al. Induction of epithelial-mesenchymal transition in alveolar epithelial cells by transforming growth factor-beta1: potential role in idiopathic pulmonary fibrosis. Am J Pathol. 2005;166(5):1321-32. doi: 10.1016/s0002-9440(10)62351-6.

[123] Phillips RJ, Burdick MD, Hong K, Lutz MA, Murray LA, Xue YY, et al. Circulating fibrocytes traffic to the lungs in response to CXCL12 and mediate fibrosis. J Clin Invest. 2004;114(3):438-46. doi: 10.1172/JCI20997.

[124] Heukels P, van Hulst JAC, van Nimwegen M, Boorsma CE, Melgert BN, van den Toorn LM, et al. Fibrocytes are increased in lung and peripheral blood of patients with idiopathic pulmonary fibrosis. Respir Res. 2018;19(1):90. doi: 10.1186/s12931-018-0798-8.

[125] Moeller A, Gilpin SE, Ask K, Cox G, Cook D, Gauldie J, et al Circulating fibrocytes are an indicator of poor prognosis in idiopathic pulmonary fibrosis. Am J Respir Crit Care Med. 2009;179(7):588-94. doi: 10.1164/rccm.200810-1534OC.

[126] Prasse A, Pechkovsky DV, Toews GB, Schäfer M, Eggeling S, Ludwig C, et al. CCL18 as an indicator of pulmonary fibrotic activity in idiopathic interstitial pneumonias and systemic sclerosis. Arthritis Rheum. 2007;56(5):1685-93. doi: 10.1002/art.22559.

[127] Prasse A, Probst C, Bargagli E, Zissel G, Toews GB, Flaherty KR, et al. Serum CC-chemokine ligand 18 concentration predicts outcome in idiopathic pulmonary fibrosis. Am J Respir Crit Care Med. 2009;179(8):717-23. doi: 10.1164/rccm.200808-1201OC.

[128] Hieshima K, Imai T, Baba M, Shoudai K, Ishizuka K, Nakagawa T, et al. A novel human CC chemokine PARC that is most homologous to macrophage-inflammatory protein-1 alpha/LD78 alpha and chemotactic for T lymphocytes, but not for monocytes. J Immunol. 1997;159(3):1140-9. PMID: 9233607.

[129] Wynn TA. Fibrotic disease and the T(H)1/T(H)2 paradigm. Nat Rev Immunol. 2004;4(8):583-94. doi: 10.1038/nri1412.

[130] Saito Y, Azuma A, Matsuda K, Kamio K, Abe S, Gemma A. Pirfenidone exerts a suppressive effect on CCL18 expression in U937-derived macrophages partly by inhibiting STAT6 phosphorylation. Immunopharmacol Immunotoxicol. 2016;38(6):464-471. doi: 10.1080/08923973.2016.1247852.

[131] Neighbors M, Cabanski CR, Ramalingam TR, Sheng XR, Tew GW, Gu C, et al. Prognostic and predictive biomarkers for patients with idiopathic pulmonary fibrosis treated with pirfenidone: post-hoc assessment of the CAPACITY and ASCEND trials. Lancet Respir Med. 2018;6(8):615-626. doi: 10.1016/S2213-2600(18)30185-1.

[132] Baran CP, Opalek JM, McMaken S, Newland CA, O'Brien JM Jr, Hunter MG, et al. Important roles for macrophage colony-stimulating factor, CC chemokine ligand 2, and mononuclear phagocytes in the pathogenesis of pulmonary fibrosis. Am J Respir Crit Care Med. 2007;176(1):78-89. doi:10.1164/rccm.200609-1279OC.

[133] Moore BB, Murray L, Das A, Wilke CA, Herrygers AB, Toews GB. The role of CCL12 in the recruitment of fibrocytes and lung fibrosis. Am J Respir Cell Mol Biol. 2006;35(2):175-81. doi:10.1165/rcmb.2005-0239OC.

[134] Suga M, Iyonaga K, Ichiyasu H, Saita N, Yamasaki H, Ando M. Clinical significance of MCP-1 levels in BALF and serum in patients with interstitial lung diseases. Eur Respir J. 1999;14(2):376-82. doi:10.1034/j.1399-3003.1999.14b23.x

[135] Gui X, Qiu X, Tian Y, Xie M, Li H, Gaoet Y et al. Prognostic value of IFN-γ, sCD163, CCL2 and CXCL10 involved in acute exacerbation of idiopathic pulmonary fibrosis. Int Immunopharmacol. 2019;70:208-15. doi:10.1016/j.intimp.2019.02.039

[136] Xue J, Kass DJ, Bon J, Vuga L, Tan J, Csizmadia E, et al. Plasma B lymphocyte stimulator and B cell differentiation in idiopathic pulmonary fibrosis patients. J Immunol. 2013;191(5):2089-95. doi: 10.4049/jimmunol.1203476.

[137] Vuga LJ, Tedrow JR, Pandit KV, Tan J, Kass DJ, Xue J, et al. C-X-C motif chemokine 13 (CXCL13) is a prognostic biomarker of idiopathic pulmonary fibrosis. Am J Respir Crit Care Med. 2014;189(8):966-74. doi: 10.1164/rccm.201309-1592OC.

[138] O'Dwyer DN, Armstrong ME, Kooblall M, Donnelly SC. Targeting defective Toll-like receptor-3 function and idiopathic pulmonary fibrosis. Expert Opin Ther Targets. 2015;19(4):507-14. doi: 10.1517/14728222.2014.988706.

[139] O'Dwyer DN, Armstrong ME, Trujillo G, Cooke G, Keane MP, Fallon PG, et al. The Toll-like receptor 3 L412F polymorphism and disease progression in idiopathic pulmonary fibrosis. Am J Respir Crit Care Med. 2013;188(12):1442-50. doi: 10.1164/rccm.201304-0760OC.

[140] Hambly N, Shimbori C, Kolb M. Molecular classification of idiopathic pulmonary fibrosis: personalized medicine, genetics and biomarkers. Respirology. 2015;20(7):1010-22. doi: 10.1111/resp.12569.

[141] Kawai T, Akira S. The role of pattern-recognition receptors in innate immunity: update on Toll-like receptors. Nat Immunol. 2010;11(5):373-84. doi: 10.1038/ni.1863.

[142] Alexopoulou L, Holt AC, Medzhitov R, Flavell RA. Recognition of double-stranded RNA and activation of NF-kappaB by Toll-like receptor 3. Nature. 2001;413(6857):732-8. doi: 10.1038/35099560.

[143] Fang F, Ooka K, Sun X, Shah R, Bhattacharyya S, Wei J, et al A synthetic TLR3 ligand mitigates profibrotic fibroblast responses by inducing autocrine IFN signaling. J Immunol. 2013;191(6):2956-66. doi: 10.4049/jimmunol.1300376.

[144] Michalski JE, Schwartz DA. Genetic Risk Factors for Idiopathic Pulmonary Fibrosis: Insights into Immunopathogenesis. J Inflamm Res. 2021;13:1305-1318. doi: 10.2147/JIR.S280958.

[145] Li X, Kim SE, Chen TY, Wang J, Yang X, Tabib T, et al. Toll interacting protein protects bronchial epithelial cells from bleomycin-induced apoptosis. FASEB J. 2020;34(8):9884-9898. doi: 10.1096/fj.201902636RR.

[146] Noth I, Zhang Y, Ma SF, Flores C, Barber M, Huang Y, et al. Genetic variants associated with idiopathic pulmonary fibrosis susceptibility and mortality: a genome-wide association study. Lancet Respir Med. 2013;1(4):309-317. doi: 10.1016/S2213-2600(13)70045-6.

[147] Zhu L, Wang L, Luo X, Zhang Y, Ding Q, Jiang X, et al. Tollip, an intracellular trafficking protein, is a novel modulator of the transforming growth factor-β signaling pathway. J Biol Chem. 2012;287(47):39653-63. doi: 10.1074/jbc.M112.388009.

[148] Inchingolo R, Varone F, Sgalla G, Richeldi L. Existing and emerging biomarkers for disease progression in idiopathic pulmonary fibrosis. Expert Rev Respir Med. 2019;13(1):39-51. doi: 10.1080/17476348.2019.1553620.

[149] Didierlaurent A, Brissoni B, Velin D, Aebi N, Tardivel A, Käslin E, et al. Tollip regulates proinflammatory responses to interleukin-1 and lipopolysaccharide. Mol Cell Biol. 2006;26(3):735-42. doi: 10.1128/MCB.26.3.735-742.2006.

[150] Konishi K, Gibson KF, Lindell KO, Richards TJ, Zhang Y, Dhir R, et al. Gene expression profiles of acute exacerbations of idiopathic pulmonary fibrosis. Am J Respir Crit Care Med. 2009;180(2):167-75. doi: 10.1164/rccm.200810-1596OC.

[151] Mukae H, Iiboshi H, Nakazato M, Hiratsuka T, Tokojima M, Abe K, et al. Raised plasma concentrations of alpha-defensins in patients with idiopathic pulmonary fibrosis. Thorax. 2002;57(7):623-8. doi: 10.1136/thorax.57.7.623.

[152] Zhang W, Ohno S, Steer B, Klee S, Staab-Weijnitz CA, Wagner D, et al. S100a4 Is secreted by alternatively activated alveolar macrophages and promotes activation of lung fibroblasts in pulmonary fibrosis. Front Immunol. 2018 ;9:1216. doi:10.3389/fimmu.2018.01216.

[153] Akiyama N, Hozumi H, Isayama T, Okada J, Sugiura K, Yasui H, et al. Clinical significance of serum S100 calcium-binding protein A4 in idiopathic pulmonary fibrosis. Respirology. 2020;25(7):743-749. doi: 10.1111/resp.13707

[154] Pruenster M, Vogl T, Roth J, Sperandio M. S100A8/A9: From basic science to clinical application. Pharmacol Ther. 2016;167:120-31. doi:10.1016/j.pharmthera.2016.07.015.

[155] Araki K, Kinoshita R, Tomonobu N, Gohara Y, Tomida S, Takahashiet Y al. The heterodimer S100A8/A9 is a potent therapeutic target for idiopathic pulmonary fibrosis. J Mol Med (Berl). 2021;99(1):131-45. doi:10.1007/s00109-020-02001-x

[156] Tanaka K, Enomoto N, Hozumi H, Isayama T, Naoi H, Aono Y et al. Serum S100A8 and S100A9 as prognostic biomarkers in acute exacerbation of idiopathic pulmonary fibrosis [published online ahead of print, 2021 Jun 18]. Respir Investig. 2021;S2212-5345(21)00089-7. doi:10.1016/j.resinv.2021.05.008.

[157] Tzouvelekis A, Herazo-Maya JD, Ryu C, Chu JH, Zhang Y, Gibson KF, et al. S100A12 as a marker of worse cardiac output and mortality in pulmonary hypertension. Respirology. 2018;23(8):771-779. doi: 10.1111/resp.13302.

[158] Richards TJ, Kaminski N, Baribaud F, Flavin S, Brodmerkel C, Horowitz D, et al. Peripheral blood proteins predict mortality in idiopathic pulmonary fibrosis. Am J Respir Crit Care Med. 2012;185(1):67-76. doi: 10.1164/rccm.201101-0058OC.

[159] Calderwood SK, Mambula SS, Gray PJ Jr, Theriault JR. Extracellular heat shock proteins in cell signaling. FEBS Lett. 2007;581(19):3689-94. doi: 10.1016/j.febslet.2007.04.044.

[160] Purcell AW, Todd A, Kinoshita G, Lynch TA, Keech CL, Gething MJ, et al. Association of stress proteins with autoantigens: a possible mechanism for triggering autoimmunity? Clin Exp Immunol. 2003;132(2):193-200. doi: 10.1046/j.1365-2249.2003.02153.x.

[161] Fichtner F, Koslowski R, Augstein A, Hempel U, Röhlecke C, Kasper M. Bleomycin induces IL-8 and ICAM-1 expression in microvascular pulmonary endothelial cells. Exp Toxicol Pathol. 2004;55(6):497-503. doi: 10.1078/0940-2993-00345.

[162] Carré PC, Mortenson RL, King TE Jr, Noble PW, Sable CL, Riches DW. Increased expression of the interleukin-8 gene by alveolar macrophages in idiopathic pulmonary fibrosis. A potential mechanism for the recruitment and activation of neutrophils in lung fibrosis. J Clin Invest. 1991;88(6):1802-10. doi: 10.1172/JCI115501.

[163] Mills R, Mathur A, Nicol LM, Walker JJ, Przybylski AA, Mackinnon AC, et al. Intrapulmonary autoantibodies to HSP72 are associated with improved outcomes in IPF. J Immunol Res. 2019;2019:1845128. doi: 10.1155/2019/1845128.

[164] Kahloon RA, Xue J, Bhargava A, Csizmadia E, Otterbein L, Kass DJ, et al. Patients with idiopathic pulmonary fibrosis with antibodies to heat shock protein 70 have poor prognoses. Am J Respir Crit Care Med. 2013;187(7):768-75. doi: 10.1164/rccm.201203-0506OC.

[165] Korthagen NM, van Moorsel CH, Barlo NP, Ruven HJ, Kruit A, Heron M, et al. Serum and BALF YKL-40 levels are predictors of survival in idiopathic pulmonary fibrosis. Respir Med. 2011;105(1):106-13. doi: 10.1016/j.rmed.2010.09.012.

[166] Tong X, Ma Y, Liu T, Li Z, Liu S, Wu G, et al. Can YKL-40 be used as a

biomarker for interstitial lung disease?: A systematic review and meta-analysis. Medicine (Baltimore). 2021;100(17):e25631. doi: 10.1097/MD.0000000000025631.

[167] Li H, Chang L, Du WW, Gupta S, Khorshidi A, Sefton M, et al. Anti-microRNA-378a enhances wound healing process by upregulating integrin beta-3 and vimentin. Mol Ther. 2014;22(10):1839-50. doi: 10.1038/mt.2014.115.

[168] Eckes B, Colucci-Guyon E, Smola H, Nodder S, Babinet C, Krieg T, et al. Impaired wound healing in embryonic and adult mice lacking vimentin. J Cell Sci. 2000;113 (Pt 13):2455-62. PMID: 10852824.

[169] Surolia R, Li FJ, Wang Z, Li H, Dsouza K, Thomas V, et al. Vimentin intermediate filament assembly regulates fibroblast invasion in fibrogenic lung injury. JCI Insight. 2019;4(7):e123253. doi: 10.1172/jci.insight.123253.

[170] Araya J, Kojima J, Takasaka N, Ito S, Fujii S, Hara H, et al. Insufficient autophagy in idiopathic pulmonary fibrosis. Am J Physiol Lung Cell Mol Physiol. 2013;304(1):L56-69. doi: 10.1152/ajplung.00213.2012.

[171] O'Dwyer DN, Ashley SL, Moore BB. Influences of innate immunity, autophagy, and fibroblast activation in the pathogenesis of lung fibrosis. Am J Physiol Lung Cell Mol Physiol. 2016;311(3):L590-601. doi: 10.1152/ajplung.00221.2016.

[172] Bargagna-Mohan P, Hamza A, Kim YE, Khuan Abby Ho Y, Mor-Vaknin N, Wendschlag N, et al. The tumor inhibitor and antiangiogenic agent withaferin A targets the intermediate filament protein vimentin. Chem Biol. 2007;14(6):623-34. doi: 10.1016/j.chembiol.2007.04.010.

[173] Meng X, Ezzati P, Wilkins JA. Requirement of podocalyxin in TGF-beta induced epithelial mesenchymal transition. PLoS One. 2011;6(4):e18715. doi: 10.1371/journal.pone.0018715.

[174] Li FJ, Surolia R, Li H, Wang Z, Kulkarni T, Liu G, et al. Autoimmunity to vimentin is associated with outcomes of patients with idiopathic pulmonary fibrosis. J Immunol. 2017;199(5):1596-1605. doi: 10.4049/jimmunol.1700473.

[175] Kurts C, Sutherland RM, Davey G, Li M, Lew AM, Blanas E, et al. CD8 T cell ignorance or tolerance to islet antigens depends on antigen dose. Proc Natl Acad Sci U S A. 1999;96(22):12703-7. doi: 10.1073/pnas.96.22.12703.

[176] Moore MW, Herzog EL. Regulatory T Cells in idiopathic pulmonary fibrosis: Too much of a good thing? Am J Pathol. 2016;186(8):1978-1981. doi: 10.1016/j.ajpath.2016.06.002.

[177] Josefowicz SZ, Lu LF, Rudensky AY. Regulatory T cells: mechanisms of differentiation and function. Annu Rev Immunol. 2012;30:531-64. doi: 10.1146/annurev.immunol.25.022106.141623.

[178] Holmes S, Downs AM, Fosberry A, Hayes PD, Michalovich D, Murdoch P, et al. Sema7A is a potent monocyte stimulator. Scand J Immunol. 2002;56(3):270-5. doi: 10.1046/j.1365-3083.2002.01129.x.

[179] Kang HR, Lee CG, Homer RJ, Elias JA. Semaphorin 7A plays a critical role in TGF-beta1-induced pulmonary fibrosis. J Exp Med. 2007;204(5):1083-93. doi: 10.1084/jem.20061273.

[180] Kolodsick JE, Toews GB, Jakubzick C, Hogaboam C, Moore TA, McKenzie A, et al. Protection from fluorescein isothiocyanate-induced fibrosis in IL-13-deficient, but not IL-4-deficient, mice results from impaired collagen synthesis by fibroblasts. J Immunol.

2004;172(7):4068-76. doi: 10.4049/jimmunol.172.7.4068.

[181] Murray LA, Zhang H, Oak SR, Coelho AL, Herath A, Flaherty KR, et al. Targeting interleukin-13 with tralokinumab attenuates lung fibrosis and epithelial damage in a humanized SCID idiopathic pulmonary fibrosis model. Am J Respir Cell Mol Biol. 2014;50(5):985-94. doi: 10.1165/rcmb.2013-0342OC.

[182] Liu T, Jin H, Ullenbruch M, Hu B, Hashimoto N, Moore B, et al. Regulation of found in inflammatory zone 1 expression in bleomycin-induced lung fibrosis: role of IL-4/IL-13 and mediation via STAT-6. J Immunol. 2004;173(5):3425-31. doi: 10.4049/jimmunol.173.5.3425.

[183] Manichaikul A, Sun L, Borczuk AC, Onengut-Gumuscu S, Farber EA, Mathai SK, et al. Plasma soluble receptor for advanced glycation end products in idiopathic pulmonary fibrosis. Ann Am Thorac Soc. 2017;14(5):628-635. doi: 10.1513/AnnalsATS.201606-485OC

[184] Cabrera Cesar E, Lopez-Lopez L, Lara E, Hidalgo-San Juan MV, Parrado Romero C, et al. Serum biomarkers in differential diagnosis of idiopathic pulmonary fibrosis and connective tissue disease-associated interstitial lung disease. J Clin Med. 2021;10(14):3167. doi: 10.3390/jcm10143167.

[185] Perkins TN, Oury TD. The perplexing role of RAGE in pulmonary fibrosis: causality or casualty? Ther Adv Respir Dis. 2021;15:17534666211016071. doi: 10.1177/17534666211016071.

[186] Machahua C, Montes-Worboys A, Planas-Cerezales L, Buendia-Flores R, Molina-Molina M, Vicens-Zygmunt V. Serum AGE/RAGEs as potential biomarker in idiopathic pulmonary fibrosis. Respir Res. 2018;19(1):215. doi: 10.1186/s12931-018-0924-7.

[187] Kyung SY, Byun KH, Yoon JY, Kim YJ, Lee SP, Park JW, et al. Advanced glycation end-products and receptor for advanced glycation end-products expression in patients with idiopathic pulmonary fibrosis and NSIP. Int J Clin Exp Pathol. 2013;7(1):221-8. PMID: 24427342; PMCID: PMC3885476.

[188] Smadja DM, Nunes H, Juvin K, Bertil S, Valeyre D, Gaussem P, et al. Increase in both angiogenic and angiostatic mediators in patients with idiopathic pulmonary fibrosis. Pathol Biol (Paris). 2014 ;62(6):391-4. doi: 10.1016/j.patbio.2014.07.006.

[189] Barratt SL, Blythe T, Jarrett C, Ourradi K, Shelley-Fraser G, Day MJ, et al. Differential expression of VEGF-Axxx isoforms is critical for development of pulmonary fibrosis. Am J Respir Crit Care Med 2017;196:479-493.

[190] Ando M, Miyazaki E, Ito T, Hiroshige S, Nureki SI, Ueno T, et al. Significance of serum vascular endothelial growth factor level in patients with idiopathic pulmonary fibrosis. Lung. 2010;188(3):247-52. doi: 10.1007/s00408-009-9223-x.

[191] Simler NR, Brenchley PE, Horrocks AW, Greaves SM, Hasleton PS, Egan JJ. Angiogenic cytokines in patients with idiopathic interstitial pneumonia. Thorax. 2004;59(7):581-5. doi: 10.1136/thx.2003.009860.

[192] Ebina M, Shimizukawa M, Shibata N, Kimura Y, Suzuki T, Endo M, et al. Heterogeneous increase in CD34-positive alveolar capillaries in idiopathic pulmonary fibrosis. Am J Respir Crit Care Med. 2004;169(11):1203-8. doi: 10.1164/rccm.200308-1111OC.

[193] Wollin L, Wex E, Pautsch A, Schnapp G, Hostettler KE, Stowasser S, Kolb M. Mode of action of nintedanib in the treatment of idiopathic pulmonary fibrosis. Eur Respir J 2015;45:1434-1445.

[194] Flynn M, Baker S, Kass DJ. Idiopathic pulmonary fibrosis biomarkers: Clinical utility and a way of understanding disease pathogenesis. Current Biomarker Findings 2015; 5:21-33.

[195] Ross B, D'Orléans-Juste P, Giaid A. Potential role of endothelin-1 in pulmonary fibrosis: from the bench to the clinic. Am J Respir Cell Mol Biol. 2010;42(1):16-20. doi: 10.1165/rcmb.2009-0175TR.

[196] Barlo NP, van Moorsel CH, Kazemier KM, van den Bosch JM, Grutters JC. Potential role of endothelin-1 in pulmonary fibrosis: from the bench to the clinic. Am J Respir Cell Mol Biol. 2010;42(5):633. doi: 10.1165/rcmb.2009-0410OC.

[197] Papiris SA, Tomos IP, Karakatsani A, Spathis A, Korbila I, Analitis A, et al. High levels of IL-6 and IL-8 characterize early-on idiopathic pulmonary fibrosis acute exacerbations. Cytokine. 2018;102:168-172. doi: 10.1016/j.cyto.2017.08.019.

[198] Schupp JC, Binder H, Jäger B, Cillis G, Zissel G, Müller-Quernheim J, et al. Macrophage activation in acute exacerbation of idiopathic pulmonary fibrosis. PLoS One. 2015;10(1):e0116775. doi: 10.1371/journal.pone.0116775.

[199] Xaubet A, Agustí C, Luburich P, Barberá JA, Carrión M, Ayuso MC, et al. Interleukin-8 expression in bronchoalveolar lavage cells in the evaluation of alveolitis in idiopathic pulmonary fibrosis. Respir Med. 1998;92(2):338-44. doi: 10.1016/s0954-6111(98)90118-4.

[200] Takahashi H, Fujishima T, Koba H, Murakami S, Kurokawa K, Shibuya Y, et al. Serum surfactant proteins A and D as prognostic factors in idiopathic pulmonary fibrosis and their relationship to disease extent. Am J Respir Crit Care Med. 2000 ;162(3 Pt 1):1109-14. doi: 10.1164/ajrccm.162.3.9910080.

[201] Hamai K, Iwamoto H, Ishikawa N, Horimasu Y, Masuda T, Miyamoto S, et al. Comparative Study of Circulating MMP-7, CCL18, KL-6, SP-A, and SP-D as Disease Markers of Idiopathic Pulmonary Fibrosis. Dis Markers. 2016;2016:4759040. doi: 10.1155/2016/4759040.

[202] Xue M, Guo Z, Cai C, Sun B, Wang H. Evaluation of the diagnostic efficacies of serological markers KL-6, SP-A, SP-D, CCL2, and CXCL13 in idiopathic interstitial pneumonia. Respiration. 2019;98(6):534-545. doi: 10.1159/000503689.

[203] Hisata S, Kimura Y, Shibata N, Ono S, Kobayashi T, Chiba S, et al. Normal range of KL-6/MUC1 independent of elevated SP-D indicates a better prognosis in the patients with honeycombing on high-resolution computed tomography. Pulm Med. 2011;2011:806014. doi: 10.1155/2011/806014.

[204] Oak SR, Murray L, Herath A, Sleeman M, Anderson I, Joshi AD, et al. A micro RNA processing defect in rapidly progressing idiopathic pulmonary fibrosis. PLoS One. 2011;6(6):e21253. doi: 10.1371/journal.pone.0021253.

[205] Kinder BW, Brown KK, McCormack FX, Ix JH, Kervitsky A, Schwarz MI, et al. Serum surfactant protein-A is a strong predictor of early mortality in idiopathic pulmonary fibrosis. Chest. 2009;135(6):1557-1563. doi: 10.1378/chest.08-2209.

[206] Richards TJ, Kaminski N, Baribaud F, Flavin S, Brodmerkel C, Horowitz D, et al. Peripheral blood proteins predict mortality in idiopathic pulmonary fibrosis. Am J Respir Crit Care Med. 2012 ;185(1):67-76. doi: 10.1164/rccm.201101-0058OC.

[207] Herazo-Maya JD, Sun J, Molyneaux PL, Li Q, Villalba JA, Tzouvelekis A, et al. Validation of a 52-gene risk profile for outcome

prediction in patients with idiopathic pulmonary fibrosis: an international, multicentre, cohort study. Lancet Respir Med. 2017;5(11):857-868. doi: 10.1016/S2213-2600(17)30349-1.

[208] Adegunsoye A, Alqalyoobi S, Linderholm A, Bowman WS, Lee CT, Pugashetti JV, et al. Circulating plasma biomarkers of survival in antifibrotic-treated patients with idiopathic pulmonary fibrosis. Chest. 2020;158(4):1526-1534. doi: 10.1016/j.chest.2020.04.066.

[209] Swaminathan AC, Todd JL. That Was Then, This Is Now: A Fresh Look at Idiopathic pulmonary fibrosis biomarkers in the antifibrotic era. Chest. 2020;158(4):1321-1322. doi: 10.1016/j.chest.2020.05.564.

[210] Ntolios P, Tzilas V, Bouros E, Avdoula E, Karakasiliotis I, Bouros D, Steiropoulos P. The role of microbiome and virome in idiopathic pulmonary fibrosis. Biomedicines. 2021;9(4):442. doi: 10.3390/biomedicines9040442.

[211] Pallante P, Malapelle U, Nacchio M, Sgariglia R, Galati D, Capitelli L, et al. Liquid biopsy is a promising tool for genetic testing in idiopathic pulmonary fibrosis. Diagnostics (Basel). 2021;11(7):1202. doi: 10.3390/diagnostics11071202.

[212] Yang IV, Schwartz DA. Epigenetics of idiopathic pulmonary fibrosis. Transl Res. 2015;165(1):48-60. doi: 10.1016/j.trsl.2014.03.011.

[213] Khan T, Dasgupta S, Ghosh N, Chaudhury K. Proteomics in idiopathic pulmonary fibrosis: the quest for biomarkers. Mol Omics. 2021;17(1): 43-58. doi: 10.1039/d0mo00108b.

[214] Newton CA, Herzog EL. Molecular markers and the promise of precision medicine for interstitial lung disease. Clin Chest Med. 2021;42(2):357-364. doi: 10.1016/j.ccm.2021.03.011.

Chapter 3

Diagnosis of IPF

Pahnwat T. Taweesedt, Kejal Gandhi, Reena Shah and Salim Surani

Abstract

Idiopathic pulmonary fibrosis (IPF) is a chronic, progressive interstitial lung fibrosis with an unknown cause commonly seen in the elderly. Obtaining histories such as past medical history, exposure history, occupational history, and family history can be crucial parts to help to find other pulmonary fibrosis causes. Not only that, but thorough physical examination can rule out pulmonary fibrosis related to other diseases. Several diagnostic modalities have helped to improve the IPF assessment, including computer tomographic scan, histopathology, bronchoscopy lavage, serological testing, and serum biomarkers. Diagnostic of exclusion is required. The consensus from multidisciplinary IPF experts' discussion from various societies recommends the clinical practice for IPF diagnosis to help define this condition. In this book chapter, we will discuss the evidence for each of the diagnostic techniques for IPF.

Keywords: pulmonary fibrosis, IPF, telomere-related mutation, Hermansky-Pudlak syndrome, HRCT, UIP, IPF diagnosis, familial IPF, cryobiopsy

1. Introduction

Idiopathic pulmonary fibrosis (IPF) is a chronic, progressive, irreversible, fibrotic lung disease with unidentifiable etiology. IPF is commonly seen in the elderly aged group [1]. IPF associates with high morbidity and mortality. It is crucial to diagnose IPF, as specific antifibrotic therapy may improve survival from 2 to 5 years to 6.9–7.9 years [2].

In 2000, the American Thoracic Society (ATS), the European Respiratory Society (ERS), and American College of Chest Physician (ACCP) first collaborated and published a consensus statement for IPF diagnosis and treatment based on an experts' opinions. This initial definition of IPF included criteria such as usual interstitial pneumonia (UIP) finding on thoracic or open lung biopsy, restrictive lung function in patients with chronic fibrosing interstitial pneumonia after excluding other causes [3].

Eleven years later, ATS, ERS, the Japanese Respiratory Society (JRS), and the Latin American Thoracic Association (ALAT) updated the guidelines with clinical, imaging, and histopathological findings in IPF diagnostic criteria based on the international evidence-based data [4]. Among patients for whom IPF was suspected, three high-resolution computed tomography (HRCT) pattens were reported; "UIP," "possible UIP," and "inconsistent with UIP" [4]. Surgical lung biopsy (SLB) was recommended in patients with suspected IPF who have the last two HRCT patterns [4]. SLB pattern is primarily divided into "UIP," "probable UIP", "possible UIP", "unclassifiable fibrosis," and "not UIP" [4]. Recommendations from French, German and Swiss have been proposed in 2013 and 2017, respectively [5].

In 2018, the consensus statement from Fleischner Society and clinical practice guideline ATS/ERS/JRS/ALAT for UIP/IPF diagnosis were published with numbers of similar main components (**Table 1**) [6, 7]. With more support data from observational studies and randomized controlled trials than 2011 guidelines, diagnosis and treatment recommendations were improved from 2011. Recently, the German respiratory society updated the German guidelines for the diagnosis of IPF in 2021 [8].

Not only HRCT and SLB, but clinical manifestations, history, and other diagnostic modalities have also been proposed to help with IPF diagnosis.

		Fleischner Society consensus statement	**ATS/ERS/JRS/ALAT 2018 CPG**
HRCT findings		**Typical UIP**	UIP
	Location	Subpleural & basal predominance	
	Pattern	Honeycombing ± traction bronchiectasis	
	Biopsy	Not recommended	
		Probable UIP	
	Location	Subplerual & basal prodominance	
	Pattern	Traction bronchiectasis	
	Biopsy	Not recommended	Recommended (conditional)
		Indeterminate for UIP	
	Location	Diffuse or variable	Subpleural & Basal predominant
	Pattern	Non-UIP features	Distortion, groud glass opacity
	Biopsy	Recommended	
		Non-IPF	**Alternative diagnosis**
	Pattern	Feature of other diseases	
	Biopsy	Recommended	
Histological findings		**Definite UIP**	UIP
	Location	Subplerual & paraseptal prodominance	
	Pattern	Architecture remodeling, dense/patchy fibrosis, fibroblast foci	
		Probable UIP	
	Pattern	Honeycombing ± fibroblastic foci	
		Indeterminate for UIP	
	Pattern	Centrilobular injury/scarring foci Mild lymphoid hyperplasia/diffuse inflammation Diffuse homogenous fibrosis	Fibrosis ± architectural distortion Some UIP
			Alternative diagnosis
	Pattern	UIP + finding highly suggestive of another diagnosis or non-UIP	Feature of other diseases

ATS: American Thoracic Society; CPG: clinical practice gruidline, ERS: European Respiratory Society; IPF: idiopathic pulmonary fibrosis, JRS: Japanese Respiratory Society; ALAT: Latin American Thoracic Society; HRCT: high-resolution computed tomography; UIP: usual interstitial pneumonia.

Table 1.
Comparison of the 2018 Fleischner society consensus statement and clinical practice guideline from ATS/ERS/JRS/ALAT 2018 for UIP/IPF diagnosis [6, 7].

Multidisciplinary discussion is of utmost importance. Due to the rapidly growing of new data in the IPF field, guidelines from worldwide pulmonary societies consensus are necessary. We will discuss the current evidence that has been used to improve the diagnosis of IPF.

2. Clinical presentation, risk factors, and history

2.1 Clinical presentation and past medical history

IPF is typically present at age above 50 years and is predominant in men [1, 9]. Lungs are the only organ involvement in IPF. Gradual onset of shortness of breath on exertion is the most common symptom that accounts for up to 86% of the patients with IPF, which can progress to shortness of breath at rest. Chronic non-productive cough can be found in up to 75% of the cases [10]. Other symptoms include fatigue and decreased appetite. As IPF requires the diagnosis of exclusion, autoimmune diseases, connective tissue disease-related symptoms (e.g., arthralgia, dry eyes, Raynaud phenomenon), medications, radiation history, environment exposure (e.g., home, workplace, frequent visit places, hobbies), occupation, family history should be inquired in detailed to rule out any identifiable conditions. The physical exam is usually remarkable for bibasilar crackles and rales [6]. Digital clubbing was described in 20–30% of IPF cases [8].

Smoking is an undeniable risk factor of IPF in several studies [11]. Up to 70% of patients with IPF have a smoking history. Ever tobacco smoking or even second-hand smoking cases had a higher risk of developing IPF, although the latter had lower odds [9]. The pathogenesis of smoking as the risk factor of IPF is suggested to be due to oxidative stress [12].

Chronic obstructive pulmonary disease, co-morbidity that smoking is a potent risk factor, was found in one-third of the IPF cases. Gastroesophageal reflux disease (GERD) was noted in 60–90% of the patients with IPF and was thought to cause micro-aspiration that may precipitate IPF and acute exacerbation. The majority of GERD in IPF patients are asymptomatic. Nonetheless, the relationship between GERD and IPF remains controversial as there was no significant relationship after controlling for smoking in meta-regression [13]. Diabetes was positively correlated with IPF, but causal relationships still cannot determinate [14]. The presence of obstructive sleep apnea in patients with IPF was noted to be more than 50%, but true prevalence still cannot be concluded due to the small number of participants in those studies [15]. Chronic human herpes virus-7, human herpes virus-8, Ebstein-Barr virus, and cytomegalovirus infection could increase the risk of IPF [2]. However, acute infection of these viruses did not associate with IPF [2].

2.2 Environmental and occupational risk factors

The environmental exposure was reported in up to 27% [10]. Various occupa-tional exposure has been revealed to be associated with IPF (**Table 2**). Silica, wood dust, metal dust/fumes, and vapors/gases/dust/fume had population attributable fractions of 3,4, 8, and 26%, respectively [16]. Deposition of dust and fumes from metal in the lung may give rise to the disturbance in the immune system. IPF risk has been reported to be increased with the longer duration of work exposure. In a meta-analysis of case–control studies by Park et al., metal dust, wood dust, pesticide had a high odds ratio (OR) in the IPF group [11]. However, textile dust, stone, and sand dust did not significantly increase the risk of IPF in this meta-analysis study [11]. The agriculture sector and farming workers showed an increased risk of IPF

Potential risk factors for IPF
Tobacco Smoking
Chronic viral infection (human herpes virus-7, human herpes virus-8, Ebstein-Barr virus, cytomegalovirus)
Exposure (e.g., metal dust, wood dust, pesticide)
Agriculture and farming worker
Family history of pulmonary fibrosis

Table 2.
Potential risk factors for IPF.

Family history related to IPF
Familial pulmonary fibrosis
Hermansky-Pudlak syndrome
Telomere-related mutation

Table 3.
Family history related to IPF.

with an OR of 1.88 (95% CI 1.17–3.04). In contrast, demolition and building construction, and woodworker carpentry did not significantly increase the risk of IPF [11].

2.3 Family history

Although IPF cases occur sporadically, familial cases have been reported, such as familial pulmonary fibrosis (FPF), Hermansky-Pudlak syndrome (HPS), and telomere-related mutation (**Table 3**). Genetic testing is recommended in patients with early-onset (less than 50 years old) pulmonary fibrosis and positive family history.

FPF is defined by two or more people in the family with a confirmed history of pulmonary fibrosis [17]. It accounts for less than five to up to 25 percent of IPF cases [18]. Pulmonary fibrosis in the family had a significant association with IPF cases with an OR of 12.6 (95% confidence interval 6.5–24.2) [9]. In addition to aiding diagnosis, family history helps predict survival. Transplant-free survival in patient-reported FPF is less in patients with IPF than patients with interstitial lung disease (ILD) other than IPF [18].

HPS, an autosomal recessive disorder, was first described in 1959 by Frantisek Hermansky and Paulus Pudlak [19]. This syndrome is characterized by oculocutaneous albinism, inflammatory bowel disease, platelet dysfunction, and pulmonary fibrosis. Pulmonary fibrosis is commonly found in HPS-1, HPS-2, and HPS-4 genetic types and affected middle-aged (HPS-1 and HPS-4) or children (HPS-2) [19].

Telomere-related mutation in IPF includes TERT, TERC, TINF2, NAF1, PARN, DKC1, and RTEL1 [20]. Premature shortening of the telomere, a region at the ends of the chromosome with repetitive DNA sections, may lead to the accelerated aging process in IPF. Screening for short telomeres should be done in patients with extrapulmonary organ involvements associated with short telomere syndrome, especially patients considered for a lung transplant. Patients with shortened telomeres have decreased lung transplant-free survival and faster disease progression [20].

3. Imaging

High-resolution CT scan (HRCT) plays a central role in the diagnosis of IPF. As described earlier, diagnosis of IPF requires exclusion of other known causes of ILD in addition to the presence of UIP pattern on HRCT. If HRCT shows a definitive UIP pattern, further surgical lung biopsy is not required for diagnosis. HRCT patterns in suspected IPF patients can be divided into four patterns: UIP, intermediate UIP, probable UIP, and alternative diagnosis (**Table 4**). All the patterns are characterized by their distribution and lung parenchymal appearance [6].

UIP is the hallmark pattern of IPF. It has characteristic bilateral, peripheral, lower lobe predominance with parenchymal findings of honeycombing and traction bronchiectasis along with fine reticular opacities in the absence of extensive ground-glass opacities. Honeycombing is defined as a group of cystic airspaces 3 to 10 mm in diameter, with well-defined, thick walls. It is absent in intermediate and probable UIP patterns. Traction bronchiectasis or bronchiolectasis ranges from non-tapering of the bronchial wall to marked airway dilatation and varicosity in the presence of parenchymal distortion [6]. A typical UIP pattern is only observed in 50% of IPF patients. Thus, the IPF spectrum varies from typical UIP patterns to atypical findings such as ground-glass opacities, nodules, consolidation, or atypical distribution [21]. Mild ground glass opacities and the reticular pattern can be seen in UIP. However, presence of GGO out of proportion to the reticular pattern is inconsistent with UIP.

Acute exacerbation of IPF is characterized by acute onset dyspnea and hypoxemia and development of bilateral ground-glass opacities and/or consolidation on a

UIP	Probable UIP	Indeterminate UIP	Alternative diagnosis

• Basal and subpleural predominance with heterogenous distribution
• Honeycombing with or without traction bronchiectasis and bronchiolectasis, with superimposed mild GGO, reticular pattern
	• Basal and subpleural predominance with heterogenous distribution
	• Reticular pattern with traction bronchiectasis
	• ± Mild GGO
	• No honeycombing
		• The basal and subpleural predominance
		• Subtle reticular pattern, with mild GGO or early distortion
		• No honeycombing
		• CT features and/ or distribution does not suggest an alternative diagnosis
			• Parenchymal features:
			  ○ Cysts
			  ○ Predominant GGO
			  ○ Nodules
			  ○ Diffuse/ Centrilobular nodules
			  ○ Consolidation
			  ○ Marked mosaic attenuation
			• Predominant Distribution:
			  ○ Peribronchovascular
			  ○ Perilymphatic
			  ○ Upper/mid-lung
			• Other:
			  ○ Pleural plaques (asbestosis)
			  ○ Pleural thickening/ effusions (CTD)
			  ○ Distal clavicular erosions (RA)
			  ○ Extensive lymph node involvement

UIP = usual interstitial pneumonia; GGO = ground glass opacities; CT = computed tomography; CTD = connective tissue disease; RA = rheumatoid arthritis.

Table 4.
HRCT pattern categories.

UIP background. The clinical course of IPF can be correlated with progressive lung parenchymal changes seen on serial HRCT scans. However, there is no consensus on the role of serial HRCT scans in established patients to determine prognosis [22].

4. Lab assay

Serological testing is recommended in all patients with newly identified ILD to exclude identifiable connective tissue disease (CTD) [6]. CTD-associated ILD investigations include erythrocytes sedimentation rate, C-reactive protein, anti-nuclear antibodies, rheumatoid factors, anti-cyclic citrullinated peptide, myositis panel, muscle enzymes, and anti-neutrophil cytoplasmic antibodies. Other serologic testing may be obtained based on clinical signs and symptoms such as anti-U1 ribonucleoprotein, anti-PM/Scl75 (polymyositis/scleroderma 75), anti-PM/Scl100, anti-Ku, anti-nuclear matrix protein 2, anti-transcriptional intermediary factor 1-gamma, anti-signal recognition particle, anti-small ubiquitin-related modifier-activating enzyme, anti-3-hydroxy-3-methylglutaryl-CoA reductase, and anti-melanoma differentiation-associated protein 5 (**Table 5**) [8].

5. Bronchoscopic approach

Cellular analysis from bronchoalveolar lavage (BAL) fluid is suggested in suspected IPF cases with probable UIP, indeterminate UIP, or an alternative diagnosis pattern on HRCT. This work-up is not suggested for patients with HRCT patterns of UIP [6]. BAL is not used for the IPF diagnosis by itself but might support the detection of other conditions (**Tables 6 and 7**).

Systemic sclerosis	anti–Scl70/topoisomerase-1, anti-centromere, anti-RNA polymerase III, anti-Th/To, U3 RNP (fibrillarin), and anti-Ku
Sjögren syndrome	anti-Ro and anti-La
Myositis	Creatine phosphokinase, myoglobin, aldolase, antisynthetase antibodies (anti-Jo-1 and others), anti-MDA5, anti-PM/Scl75, anti-PM/Scl100, anti-TIF1- γ, anti-SEP, anti-HMGCR, anti NXP2, anti-U1RNP
Rheumatoid arthritis	Rheumatoid factor, anti-cyclic citrullinated peptide
Vasculitis	Antineutrophil cytoplasmic antibodies, anti myeloperoxidase antibodies, antiproteinase 3 antibodies

Table 5.
Laboratory workup for common connective tissue disease-related interstitial lung diseases.

BAL	Macrophages	Lymphocytes	Neutrophils	Eosinophils	CD4/CD8
Healthy individual	>85%	10–15%	<3%	≤1%	49–83%
IPF	49–83%	7–27%	6–22%	2–8%	1–3%

Table 6.
Comparison of cellular analysis from bronchoalveolar lavage between a healthy individual and IPF [6].

Lymphocytic predominance	Sarcoidosis, HP, NSIP, Drug-induced, Radiation, COP, Lymphoproliferative disorders, CTD
Neutrophilic predominance	CTD, IPF, aspiration, infection, bronchitis, asbestosis, ARDS/DAD
Eosinophilic predominance	Eosinophilic pneumonia, Drug-induced, BM transplant, asthma, ABPA, Hodgkin, infection

Table 7.
Cellular analysis of bronchoalveolar lavage in different conditions.

6. Histopathology

Multiple lung biopsies from few lobes are suggested in suspected IPF cases with probable UIP, indeterminate UIP, or alternative diagnosis patterns on HRCT. SLB is preferred over transbronchial lung biopsy and cryobiopsy. SLB be done by video-assisted thoracoscopic surgical (VATS) technique over open thoracotomy. When patients have a UIP pattern on HRCT, lung biopsy is not recommended in clinically suspected IPF patients after excluded other potential ILD etiologies. In these cases, diagnosis of IPF can be made without histopathology proof.

Similar to the HRCT pattern, histopathology patterns in suspected IPF individuals can be categorized into four groups; UIP, probable UIP, indeterminate UIP, and alternative diagnosis (**Table 8**) [6]. Classic "UIP" is the principal histopathologic feature of IPF. It frequently demonstrates dense fibrosis in paraseptal and subpleural areas of the lung with distortion of architecture, often resulting in microscopic honeycombing pattern accompanied by unaffected lung parenchyma in the low-magnification photomicrograph. For higher-magnification photomicrographs, fibroblast foci and patchy fibrosis are characteristics of UIP. The honeycombing pattern on biopsy is defined as fibrosed cystic airspace.

Accurate diagnosis of IPF requires the synopsis consideration of clinical manifestation, HRCT, and biopsy results (**Table 9**). When the HRCT pattern of clinically suspected IPF patients is not classic UIP or discordant with biopsy result, the multidiscipline decision from different subspecialties discussion such as pulmonologist, radiologist, and pathologist is suggested [6].

UIP	Probable UIP	Indeterminate UIP	Alternative diagnosis
• Predominant subpleural ± paraseptal involvement • Distortion of lung architecture with dense fibrosis ± honeycombing • Fibroblast foci • Patchy fibrosis • No features of an alternative diagnosis	• Honeycombing ——or—— • Some features of UIP but to the extent that if not possible for UIP diagnosis + No features of an alternative diagnosis	• Fibrosis ± distortion of lung architecture + Non-UIP pattern or Interstitial inflammation, chronic fibrous pleuritis, OP, granuloma, hyaline membranes, airway-centered • Some features of UIP + alternative diagnosis features	• Other IIPs features in all biopsies • Indicative of other disease such as LAM, sarcoidosis, HP

HP = hypersensitivity pneumonitis; IIPs = Idiopathic interstitial pneumonias; LAM = Lymphangioleiomyomatosis; OP = organizing pneumonia; UIP = usual interstitial pneumonia.

Table 8.
Histopathologic feature of idiopathic pulmonary fibrosis [6].

Biopsy result					
	Clinically suspected IPF after exclusion of other ILD causes	UIP	Probable UIP	Indeterminate for UIP	Alternative diagnosis
HRCT finding	**UIP**	IPF			
		A biopsy is not recommended			
	Probable UIP	IPF	IPF	Likely IPF	Not IPF
	Indeterminate for UIP	IPF	Likely IPF	Not IPF	Not IPF
	Alternative diagnosis	Likely IPF	Not IPF	Not IPF	Not IPF

HRCT = high-resolution computed tomography; IPF=Idiopathic pulmonary fibrosis; UIP = usual interstitial pneumonia.

Table 9.
Diagnosis of IPF using surgical lung biopsy result and high-resolution computed tomography finding [6].

7. Genetic biomarker

Genetic factors affecting the susceptibility to IPF mainly depend on whether a patient has sporadic IPF or familial IPF. With the increase in the use of genome sequencing, multiple gene variants have been associated with IPF. Common variants with modest effects have been associated with sporadic IPF, whereas rare gene variants with more significant impact have been associated with a familial form of IPF.

7.1 Genetic variants associated with sporadic IPF

Mucin 5B (MUC5B) variant is a common variant associated with sporadic IPF. It is a glycoprotein involved in mucociliary clearance. A MUC5B promoter single nucleotide polymorphism (rs35705950) increases the susceptibility to developing IPF four-fold [23]. Despite this, MUC5B promoter SNP is associated with decreased mortality in IPF patients. However, it is not associated with systemic scleroderma-related ILD can increase the risk of ILD in rheumatoid arthritis patients, especially in those having CT findings of UIP.

Toll interacting protein (TOLLIP) is a regulator of toll-like receptor (TLR), and variation in this gene leads to a decrease in TLR mRNA expression and increased risk of pulmonary infection [24]. TT TOLLIP genotype ((rs3750920) is associated with improved survival with N-acetyl cysteine treatment [25]. However, the other minor allele of TOLLIP (rs5743890) decreases the susceptibility to IPF development but is associated with increased mortality from IPF [26].

Desmoplakin (DSP) encodes for desmoplakin, an adhesion molecule between 2 cells and tethers the cytoskeleton to the cell membrane. Two variants in DSP have been identified in which one variant (rs2744371) is protective, whereas the other variant (rs2076295) increases the susceptibility to IPF [27].

A-kinase Anchoring protein 13 (AKAP13) is a regulator of rhoA, which is involved in the profibrotic signaling pathway. Single nucleotide polymorphism in AKAP13 has also been associated with an increased risk of IPF. AKAP 13 mRNA expression was higher in the lung biopsy section of IPF patients compared to controls [28].

7.2 Genetic factors associated with familial IFP

Various surfactant-producing gene mutations have been identified, such as SFPT-C and SFPT-A2 associated with IPF in families. Transcription and translation of the SFPT-C gene leads to pro-SPC formation, which is further processed in the endoplasmic reticulum before being secreted in the alveolar space. SFPT-C mutation leads to the formation of pro-SPC. However, it cannot be further processed and folded, leading to protein accumulation within the endoplasmic reticulum and thus, activating unfolded protein response (UPR) within the cell. Unfolded protein response helps to protect the cell and also enhances protein folding chaperones. However, prolonged standing activation of UPR system leads to alveolar epithelial cell death through apoptosis [29]. Studies have shown markers for endothelium reticulum stress and UPR pathway activation even in the absence of SFPT-C mutation. These studies demonstrate that this pathway may contribute to the pathogenesis of IPF [30]. Similarly, SFTP-A2 gene mutations have been identified in a family with 15 members who had familial IPF, bronchoalveolar carcinoma, or underlying lung disease. SFTP-A2 also accumulates mutant surfactant protein A within the endoplasmic reticulum, leading to stress and ultimate activation of the apoptotic pathway [31].

Telomerase complex mutations have been identified in families with UIP. Telomeres are the tandem repeats of TTAGGG found at both ends of chromosomes, protecting the end of chromosomes during cell division. Telomerase helps maintain these telomeres length. Telomerase mutation leads to the shortening of telomere in the alveolar epithelial cells, which was found to be involved in the disease process. Telomere shortening has also been observed in peripheral leukocytes in these patients. New studies have shown shortened telomere length in patients with sporadic IPF and non-telomerase complex mutation IPF, indicating it might play a role in the pathogenesis of IPF [32].

Other molecular biomarkers such as elevated levels of matrix metalloproteinase 7 (MMP 7), mucin 1 (KL-6), CC chemokine ligand 18 (CCL 18), cancer antigen have also been associated with disease progression but have limited clinical value at present and requires further studies [33].

Thus, the use of genetic and biologic biomarkers can further help understand the pathogenesis of IPF and develop future targeted therapies. However, currently, more studies are required to use these markers for diagnostic purposes.

8. Conclusion

When encountering patients with clinical context and tempo of disease compatible with IPF, excluding identifiable causes by acquiring history and serology is recommended. Other investigations such as biomarkers may aid the defining of IPF. After that, IPF diagnosis can be made with the UIP pattern shown by HRCT. In patients with HRCT patterns of non-UIP, a surgical lung biopsy will assist the diagnosis. When a definite diagnosis cannot be concluded by UIP pattern from HRCT or biopsy result, the mutual agreement from the multidisciplinary discussion is recommended to help diagnose IPF.

Author details

Pahnwat T. Taweesedt[1], Kejal Gandhi[2], Reena Shah[3] and Salim Surani[4,5]*

1 Corpus Christi Medical Center, Corpus Christi, TX, USA

2 Department of Medicine, Georgetown University/Medstar Washington Hospital Center, Washington, DC, USA

3 Aga Khan University Hospital, Nairobi, Kenya

4 Texas A&M University, TX, USA

5 Research Collaborator, Mayo Clinic, Rochester, MN, USA

*Address all correspondence to: srsurani@hotmail.com

IntechOpen

References

[1] Esposito DB, Lanes S, Donneyong M, Holick CN, Lasky JA, Lederer D, et al. Idiopathic pulmonary fibrosis in United States automated claims. Incidence, prevalence, and algorithm validation. American Journal of Respiratory and Critical Care Medicine. Nov 2015;**192**(10):1200-1207

[2] Sheng G, Chen P, Wei Y, Yue H, Chu J, Zhao J, et al. Viral infection increases the risk of idiopathic pulmonary fibrosis: A meta-analysis. Chest. May 2020;**157**(5):1175-1187

[3] American Thoracic Society. Idiopathic pulmonary fibrosis: Diagnosis and treatment. International consensus statement. American Thoracic Society (ATS), and the European Respiratory Society (ERS). American Journal of Respiratory and Critical Care Medicine. Feb 2000;**161**(2 Pt 1):646-664

[4] Raghu G, Collard HR, Egan JJ, Martinez FJ, Behr J, Brown KK, et al. An official ATS/ERS/JRS/ALAT statement: Idiopathic pulmonary fibrosis: Evidence-based guidelines for diagnosis and management. American Journal of Respiratory and Critical Care Medicine. Mar 2011;**183**(6):788-824

[5] Funke-Chambour M, Azzola A, Adler D, Barazzone-Argiroffo C, Benden C, Boehler A, et al. Idiopathic pulmonary fibrosis in Switzerland: Diagnosis and treatment. Respiration. 2017;**93**(5):363-378

[6] Raghu G, Remy-Jardin M, Myers JL, Richeldi L, Ryerson CJ, Lederer DJ, et al. Diagnosis of idiopathic pulmonary fibrosis. An official ATS/ERS/JRS/ALAT clinical practice guideline. American Journal of Respiratory and Critical Care Medicine. Sep 2018;**198**(5):e44-e68

[7] Lynch DA, Sverzellati N, Travis WD, Brown KK, Colby TV, Galvin JR, et al. Diagnostic criteria for idiopathic pulmonary fibrosis: A Fleischner society white paper. The Lancet Respiratory Medicine. Feb 2018;**6**(2):138-153

[8] Behr J, Günther A, Bonella F, Dinkel J, Fink L, Geiser T, et al. S2K guideline for diagnosis of idiopathic pulmonary fibrosis. Respiration. 2021;**100**(3):238-271

[9] Abramson MJ, Murambadoro T, Alif SM, Benke GP, Dharmage SC, Glaspole I, et al. Occupational and environmental risk factors for idiopathic pulmonary fibrosis in Australia: Case-control study. Thorax. Oct 2020;**75**(10):864-869

[10] Behr J, Kreuter M, Hoeper MM, Wirtz H, Klotsche J, Koschel D, et al. Management of patients with idiopathic pulmonary fibrosis in clinical practice: The INSIGHTS-IPF registry. The European Respiratory Journal. Jul 2015;**46**(1):186-196

[11] Park Y, Ahn C, Kim T-H. Occupational and environmental risk factors of idiopathic pulmonary fibrosis: A systematic review and meta-analyses. Scientific Reports. Mar 2021;**11**(1):4318

[12] Oh CK, Murray LA, Molfino NA. Smoking and idiopathic pulmonary fibrosis. Pulmonary Medicine. 2012;**2012**:808260

[13] Bédard Méthot D, Leblanc É, Lacasse Y. Meta-analysis of gastroesophageal reflux disease and idiopathic pulmonary fibrosis. Chest. Jan 2019;**155**(1):33-43

[14] Bai L, Zhang L, Pan T, Wang W, Wang D, Turner C, et al. Idiopathic pulmonary fibrosis and diabetes mellitus: A meta-analysis and systematic review. Respiratory Research. Jun 2021;**22**(1):175

[15] Schiza SE, Bouloukaki I, Bolaki M, Antoniou KM. Obstructive sleep apnea

in pulmonary fibrosis. Current Opinion in Pulmonary Medicine. Sep 2020;**26** (5):443-448

[16] Blanc PD, Annesi-Maesano I, Balmes JR, Cummings KJ, Fishwick D, Miedinger D, et al. The occupational burden of nonmalignant respiratory diseases. An official American Thoracic Society and European Respiratory Society statement. American Journal of Respiratory and Critical Care Medicine. Jun 2019;**199**(11):1312-1334

[17] Borie R, Kannengiesser C, Sicre de Fontbrune F, Gouya L, Nathan N, Crestani B. Management of suspected monogenic lung fibrosis in a specialised Centre. European Respiratory Review: An Official Journal of the European Respiratory Society. Jun 2017;**26**(144): 160122

[18] Cutting CC, Bowman WS, Dao N, Pugashetti JV, Garcia CK, Oldham JM, et al. Family history of pulmonary fibrosis predicts worse survival in patients with interstitial lung disease. Chest. May 2021;**159**(5): 1913-1921

[19] Yokoyama T, Gochuico BR. Hermansky-Pudlak syndrome pulmonary fibrosis: A rare inherited interstitial lung disease. European Respiratory Review: An Official Journal of the European Respiratory Society. Mar 2021;**30**(159):200193

[20] Courtwright AM, El-Chemaly S. Telomeres in interstitial lung disease: The short and the long of it. Annals of the American Thoracic Society. Feb 2019;**16**(2):175-181

[21] Souza CA, Müller NL, Flint J, Wright JL, Churg A. Idiopathic pulmonary fibrosis: Spectrum of high-resolution CT findings. American Journal of Roentgenology [Internet]. 2005;**185**(6):1531–1539. Available from: https://doi.org/10.2214/ AJR.04.1599

[22] Fujimoto K, Taniguchi H, Johkoh T, Kondoh Y, Ichikado K, Sumikawa H, et al. Acute exacerbation of idiopathic pulmonary fibrosis: High-resolution CT scores predict mortality. European Radiology [Internet]. 2012;**22**(1):83–92. Available from: https://doi.org/10.1007/ s00330-011-2211-6

[23] Lee M-G, Lee YH. A meta-analysis examining the association between the MUC5B rs35705950 T/G polymorphism and susceptibility to idiopathic pulmonary fibrosis. Inflammation Research [Internet]. 2015;**64**(6):463–470. Available from: https://doi.org/ 10.1007/s00011-015-0829-6

[24] Shah JA, Vary JC, Chau TTH, Bang ND, Yen NTB, Farrar JJ, et al. Human TOLLIP regulates TLR2 and TLR4 signaling and its polymorphisms are associated with susceptibility to tuberculosis. Journal of Immunology [Internet]. Aug 15, 2012;**189**(4):1737–1746. Available from: http://www. jimmunol.org/content/189/4/1737. abstract

[25] Oldham JM, Ma S-F, Martinez FJ, Anstrom KJ, Raghu G, Schwartz DA, et al. TOLLIP, MUC5B, and the response to N-Acetylcysteine among individuals with idiopathic pulmonary fibrosis. American Journal of Respiratory and Critical Care Medicine [Internet]. Sep 2, 2015;**192**(12):1475–1482. Available from: https://doi.org/10.1164/ rccm.201505-1010OC

[26] Noth I, Zhang Y, Ma S-F, Flores C, Barber M, Huang Y, et al. Genetic variants associated with idiopathic pulmonary fibrosis susceptibility and mortality: A genome-wide association study. The Lancet Respiratory Medicine. 2013;**1**(4):309-317

[27] Mathai SK, Pedersen BS, Smith K, Russell P, Schwarz MI, Brown KK, et al. Desmoplakin variants are associated with idiopathic pulmonary fibrosis. American Journal of Respiratory and

Critical Care Medicine [Internet]. 2015; **193**(10):1151–1160. Available from: https://doi.org/10.1164/rccm.201509 -1863OC

[28] Allen RJ, Porte J, Braybrooke R, Flores C, Fingerlin TE, Oldham JM, et al. Genetic variants associated with susceptibility to idiopathic pulmonary fibrosis in people of European ancestry: A genome-wide association study. The Lancet Respiratory Medicine. 2017; 5(11):869-880

[29] Lawson WE, Crossno PF, Polosukhin V V, Roldan J, Cheng D-S, Lane KB, et al. Endoplasmic reticulum stress in alveolar epithelial cells is prominent in IPF: Association with altered surfactant protein processing and herpesvirus infection. American Journal of Physiology-Lung Cellular and Molecular Physiology [Internet]. 2008; **294**(6):L1119–L1126. 10.1152/ajplung. 00382.2007

[30] Korfei M, Ruppert C, Mahavadi P, Henneke I, Markart P, Koch M, et al. Epithelial endoplasmic reticulum stress and apoptosis in sporadic idiopathic pulmonary fibrosis. American Journal of Respiratory and Critical Care Medicine. 2008;**178**(8):838-846

[31] Wang Y, Kuan PJ, Xing C, Cronkhite JT, Torres F, Rosenblatt RL, et al. Genetic defects in surfactant protein A2 are associated with pulmonary fibrosis and lung Cancer. American Journal of Human Genetics [Internet]. 2009;**84**(1):52–59. Available from: 10.1016/j.ajhg.2008.11.010

[32] Cronkhite JT, Xing C, Raghu G, Chin KM, Torres F, Rosenblatt RL, et al. Telomere shortening in familial and sporadic pulmonary fibrosis. American Journal of Respiratory and Critical Care Medicine. 2008;**178**(7):729-737

[33] Neighbors M, Cabanski CR, Ramalingam TR, Sheng XR, Tew GW, Gu C, et al. Prognostic and predictive biomarkers for patients with idiopathic pulmonary fibrosis treated with pirfenidone: Post-hoc assessment of the CAPACITY and ASCEND trials. The Lancet Respiratory Medicine. Aug 2018; **6**(8):615-626

Section 3

Treatment

Chapter 4

Pharmacological Management of Idiopathic Pulmonary Fibrosis

Ladan Panahi, George Udeani, Andrew Scott Tenpas,
Theresa Ofili, Elizabeth Marie Aguilar, Sarah Burchard,
Alexandra Ruth Ritenour, April Jacob Chennat,
Nehal Ahmed, Chairat Atphaisit, Crystal Chi,
Jesus Cruz III, Monica D. Deleon, Samantha Lee, Zack Mayo,
Mackenzie Mcbeth, Mariel Morales, Jennifer N. Nwosu,
Kelly Palacios, Jaycob M. Pena and Nitza Vara

Abstract

Idiopathic pulmonary fibrosis (IPF) is a common interstitial lung disease (ILD) caused by environmental exposures, infections, or traumatic injuries and subsequent epithelial damage. Since IPF is a progressively fatal disease without remission, treatment is both urgent and necessary. The two medications indicated solely for treatment include the tyrosine kinase inhibitor nintedanib (Ofev®) and the anti-fibrotic agent pirfenidone (Esbriet®). This chapter discusses in detail the current treatment options for clinical management of IPF, specifically the mentioned two pharmacotherapeutic agents that decrease physiological progression and likely improve progression-free survival. The chapter also discusses the evolution of drug therapy in IPF management and the drawbacks and limitations learned throughout historical trials and observational studies.

Keywords: drug therapy, pharmacological management, idiopathic pulmonary fibrosis, review

1. Introduction

Idiopathic pulmonary fibrosis (IPF) is a common interstitial lung disease (ILD) caused by environmental exposures, infections, or traumatic injuries and subsequent epithelial damage [1, 2]. It is characterized by fibroblast activation, followed by excessive secretion of extracellular matrix in the bronchial walls and alveolar interstitium [3]. This uncontrolled deposition leads to stiffening of lung tissue, which impairs diffusion of gases and reduces blood oxygenation [3, 4]. More prevalent among males and adults over 65 years old, it has a high incidence in North America and Europe [1]. Smoking, family history, and genetic mutations associated with telomere length maintenance have been linked to increased risk of developing IPF, as well as the history of gastroesophageal reflux disease and obstructive sleep apnea [1].

Patients typically present with chronic, progressive dyspnea, and dry cough [5]. Their history may include long-term smoke or workplace exposure such as inhalation of wood or metal particulates [6]. On physical examination, bibasilar inspiratory crackles ("velcro rales") and finger clubbing may be seen [4, 7]. Pulmonary function tests (PFTs) usually demonstrate reduced lung capacity and reduced diffusion capacity for carbon monoxide, indicating restrictive disease and abnormal gas exchange [4, 8]. Exclusion of other interstitial lung diseases—including autoimmune diseases—is required before a diagnosis can be made. Additionally, the presence of a honeycomb fibrosis pattern on high-resolution computed tomography is necessary [4, 8]. Patients commonly have at least one comorbidity, such as chronic obstructive pulmonary disease (COPD), pulmonary hypertension, lung cancer, and diabetes mellitus [4, 8].

IPF is characterized by irreversible and potentially fatal lung deterioration [8, 9]. Patients may experience different rates of disease progression, ranging from gradual deterioration to stable periods lasting months or years. Symptoms associated with progression include worsening dyspnea, hypoxemia, and pulmonary hypertension, as well as fatal exacerbations, where respiratory function declines acutely and unpredictably [8, 9]. Although the disease course varies among patients, prognosis remain poor, with an average life expectancy of 3–5 years after diagnosis [4, 9].

2. Standards of care

Since IPF is a progressively fatal disease without remission, treatment is both urgent and necessary [10, 11]. The two medications indicated solely for treatment include the tyrosine kinase inhibitor nintedanib (Ofev®) and the anti-fibrotic agent pirfenidone (Esbriet®) [4, 12]. Both were approved in 2014 after clinical trials suggested that they halted the decline in lung function, including a decline in forced vital capacity (FVC) by 50% over a 1-year period [4, 11]. Moreover, they have been shown to be safe and effective in reducing severe respiratory episodes often seen in IPF [4].

Treatment regimens for COPD, heart disease, and smoking cessation are also recommended to reduce respiratory strain if experienced concurrently [4, 13]. Patients suffering from hypoxemia and IPF often receive supplemental oxygen [4, 14]. Pulmonary rehabilitation, physical therapy, and oxygen are all recommended to improve exercise tolerance and duration, reduce dyspnea, prevent the development of pulmonary hypertension, and improve overall lung capacity [4].

Lung transplantation remains a viable option for those who meet the criteria for the procedure [11]. It must be considered earlier in disease progression, with early evaluation to maximize eligibility [4, 11]. Past treatments like warfarin, N-acetylcysteine, prednisone, and azathioprine are no longer recommended due to an overall lack of treatment efficacy [4, 15]. Furthermore, these pharmacotherapeutic options should be avoided in IPF until high-quality randomized control trials prove efficacy since they have failed to show relevant reductive changes in FVC, adverse events, or death [16].

3. Non-pharmacological management and supportive care

Though current drug therapies demonstrate a reduction in acute exacerbations due to their cytotoxic and immunosuppressive side effect profiles, non-drug measures are often considered. Unfortunately, patients opting for mechanical ventilation—often as a bridge to lung transplantation—suffer from low survival rates [17]. Poor prognostic indicators include a decline in 6-minute walk (6 MW) distance greater than 150 meters within one year, a decrease in FVC greater than 10% within 6 months, and a decline in diffusing capacity for carbon monoxide (DLCO) greater than 15% within 6 months [4].

Improvements in both quality of life and 6 MW distance can be seen in those undergoing pulmonary rehabilitation [4]. Length of survival is highly variable; patients diagnosed with mild, moderate, and severe diseases survive an average of 55.6, 38.7, and 27.4 months, respectively [4]. Ultimately, transplantation remains the only option for those with advanced IPF; those who do not undergo this procedure often have poorer outcomes [4, 12]. Approximately 66% of transplant recipients live for more than 3 years postsurgery, while 53% survive greater than 5 years [4]. Transplantation does carry certain complications such as cancer, infections, primary graft dysfunction, cytomegalovirus, and allograft rejection are all commonly seen [12]. Moreover, supplemental oxygen has been shown to improve symptom control during exercise, while lung transplantation may increase survival rates and improve patients' overall quality of life [14].

Since drug therapy is merely supportive therapy, patients are encouraged to take alternative measures to decrease their risk, including smoking cessation, supplemental oxygen, and pulmonary rehabilitation [4]. Ongoing GERD has been thought to worsen IPF, but the use of antacids based on clinical trials remains inconclusive [4]. Although the relation of GERD to IPF is still unknown, the prevalence of GERD and erosive esophagitis are observed more commonly in patients with IPF than in the general population [18, 19].

Lastly, patients should receive pneumonia and influenza vaccinations as part of complementary therapy, though there is no proven benefit for the previously mentioned interventions [14]. Although there is no documented outcome benefit with vaccination in the IPF setting, preventing pulmonary infections is essential as extrapulmonary comorbidities through interactions with environmental factors by various mechanisms are thought to contribute to IPF [20]. Vaccinations are especially recommended for post-transplantation patients since they may be more susceptible immunologically. In outpatient settings, pulmonary hypertension should be controlled with supplemental oxygen [21]. Unless a patient participates in a clinical trial, alternative therapies should be avoided.

4. Previous therapies

Although commonly used for their anti-inflammatory effects, corticosteroids do not improve clinical outcomes in IPF [14, 22]. When used as monotherapy, they show no survival benefit and actually increased risk of morbidity with long-term use [7, 14]. A regimen consisting of prednisone, azathioprine, and N-acetylcysteine (NAC) was once accepted therapy [7, 14]. However, trial data revealed that, compared to placebo, the combination increased risk of death and hospitalization [7, 14].

Ambrisentan (Letairis®), a potent type-A selective endothelin receptor antagonist, was once thought to decrease time to disease progression [7]. However, the ARTEMIS-IPF trial examined its use in IPF patients, finding it to be ineffective and associated with increased risk of hospitalizations and disease progression [7]. The trial was eventually terminated when an interim analysis found minimal efficacy [7]. Recent guidelines no longer recommend the anticoagulant warfarin since it was associated with a higher risk of mortality compared to placebo [7, 14].

5. Current therapy: nintedanib

After numerous studies yielded conflicting results, new treatment options were developed, including two novel anti-fibrotic agents capable of slowing disease progression [4]. Pirfenidone and nintedanib both demonstrated a significant reduction in annual FVC decline and improved survival [7].

Nintedanib (Ofev®), an oral tyrosine kinase inhibitor, inhibits the fibroblast proliferation leading to progression of lung fibrosis [3, 4]. It may also inhibit other growth factor receptors, including tyrosine kinase vascular endothelial growth factor receptor and platelet-derived growth factor receptor [3, 4, 7]. This multi-faceted inhibition makes it a first-line agent for IPF [3, 7]. The standard dose is 150 mg twice daily taken with food to increase bioavailability [4, 7]. However, dosing can be withheld or lowered to 100 mg twice daily if side effects become intolerable [7]. Once controlled, standard dosing can be resumed [7]. If adverse reactions persist, however, discontinuation should be considered [7]. The most common side effects associated with its use include diarrhea, nausea, and vomiting [7]. Other important side effects include weight loss and drug-induced hepatotoxicity, designated by a 3–5 fold increase in AST/ALT, with or without severe liver damage. Discontinuation or dose reduction is based on the presence of severe liver damage; details relating to specific therapeutic steps can be found in **Table 1**. Adverse reactions should be monitored alongside signs of increased bleeding, especially in those taking anticoagulants.

Bioavailability	5% **Increases by 20% when given with food**
Half-life	9.5 hours
Protein Binding	97.8%
Volume of Distribution	Greater than 1000 L
Metabolism	Hydrolytic cleavage by esterases (Major) CYP3A4 (Minor)
Elimination	More than 90% of the dose eliminated via biliary/fecal excretion
Drug Interactions	P-glycoprotein (P-gp), CYP3A4 inducers
Dose Adjustments	**Baseline hepatic impairment**: • Child-Pugh Class A: Reduce dose to 100 mg twice daily. • Child-Pugh Class B or C: Nintedanib not recommended. **Treatment-induced hepatotoxicity**: • If AST or ALT increases to 3–5 times ULN, without signs of severe liver damage: Hold therapy or reduce dose to 100 mg twice daily. If values return to baseline, treatment may be restarted at a lower dose (100 mg twice daily), then increased to the full dose (150 mg twice daily). • If AST / ALT greater than three times ULN—with signs/symptoms of severe liver damage—or AST/ALT greater than five times ULN: Discontinue therapy
Monitoring Parameters	• LFTs for the first 3 months of treatment • GI effects for first 3 months of treatment • Bleeding events • Cardiovascular events • Pregnancy test before initiation for those of childbearing age

Table 1.
Nintedanib pharmacokinetic parameters and special considerations [4].

Arterial thromboembolic events have been noted in patients taking nintedanib, and caution should be exercised in those at high risk for cardiovascular events [4]. Basic pharmacokinetics and special population dosing can be found in **Table 1** [4].

6. Current therapy: pirfenidone

Pirfenidone (Esbriet®) is an oral synthetic pyridine derivative with anti-fibrotic and anti-inflammatory properties [7, 12, 23, 24]. Its anti-fibrotic effects arise from down-regulation of transforming growth factor (TGF) β and tumor necrosis factor (TNF) α [7, 23, 25]. It may inhibit fibroblast proliferation, expression of heat-shock protein 47, and collagen synthesis as well [7, 23–25]. Clinically, pirfenidone reduces worsening of FVC and may reduce risk of hospitalization [7, 23, 26]. Several studies like CAPACITY, ASCEND and RECAP have confirmed its long-term safety, efficacy, and favorable tolerability [7, 12].

Common side effects and clinical pharmacology can be found in **Table 2**. Most prevalent are gastrointestinal (GI) and skin-related adverse drug effects, which generally wane after the first 6 months and do not impact a patient's ability to continue and maintain a high-dose intensity [12]. Several side effects like fatigue, photosensitivity, and GI distress may require dose reductions [7, 12]. Fatigue, in particular, is observed

Bioavailability	Unknown
Half-Life	3.0 hours
Protein binding	Mean of 50–58% at concentrations of 1–10 μg/mL.
Volume of Distribution	Mean of 59–71 L following oral administration
Dosage and Administration	Recommend titration to 801 mg three times daily (2403 mg/day) with food
Metabolism and Excretion	Primarily metabolized in the liver and bio-transformed by CYP1A2 Roughly 80% dose excreted in urine as metabolite 5-carboxy-pirfenidone
Common side effects	Nausea, rash, dyspnea, diarrhea, fatigue, bronchitis, upper respiratory tract infections, dizziness, photosensitivity
Interactions	• CYP1A2 inhibitors (ciprofloxacin, fluvoxamine) may decrease metabolism and require dosing adjustments or discontinuation. • Grapefruit juice should be used with caution, though study results are inconsistent.
Warnings/Precautions	• Photosensitivity reactions may require dose adjustments. • Limit exposure to sunlight and sunlamps, use sunscreen (SPF ≥ 50) and protective clothing while taking. • GI side effects may be managed with temporary dose reduction, with gradual titration back to full dose. Taking after a full meal may help. • Mild-to-severe fatigue can be managed by dose modifications but may necessitate discontinuation. • Elevated liver enzymes (AST, ALT, bilirubin) occurred in trials and may require dose adjustments or discontinuation.
Monitoring Parameters	• Monitor liver function (AST, ALT, bilirubin) before initiating and each month after for six months, then every three months, or if the patient experiences symptoms of liver injury. • If ALT or AST exceeds 3–5 times ULN—with no symptoms—dose adjustments may be made. If 3–5 times ULN—accompanied with symptoms or hyperbilirubinemia—or > 5× ULN, discontinue permanently.

Bioavailability	Unknown
Special Populations	• Hepatic impairment: Monitor liver function monitored closely and potential for adverse reactions. Use contraindicated in those with severe hepatic dysfunction or end-stage liver disease
	• Renal impairment: Avoid severe kidney impairment (CrCl <30 mL/min) or dialysis.
	• Pregnant and nursing women: Not studied. It should be avoided during pregnancy and when nursing.
	• Geriatrics: No dose adjustments needed.
	• Pediatrics: Not studied.

Table 2.
Pharmacokinetic parameters and special considerations [7, 12, 27–29].

within the first few weeks of treatment and may substantially affect the quality of life. It may be difficult to distinguish from the disease itself, though it can be managed by dose modifications or even discontinuation [7, 12]. Several studies have examined the importance of taking pirfenidone with food [27, 28, 30, 31]. Administration after meals slows absorption and may mitigate GI side effects [7, 12, 27, 28].

Updated practice guidelines recommend both nintedanib and pirfenidone [15]. Though both have been shown safe and effective, a lack of head-to-head trials makes it difficult to recommend one over the other [15]. The two agents have a different mechanism of action, making the prospect of combination therapy intriguing [12, 32]. However, when investigated, it was found that the combination led to greater photosensitivity and GI side effects [12, 32].

7. Acute exacerbations

Acute exacerbations (AE) are defined as an acute downturn in blood oxygenation, increased lung attenuation per computed tomography scan, and acute worsening of dyspnea [33]. Common causes include exposure to particulate matter (PM) ≥ 2.5 μm or crocin peptide released by *S. nepalensis*, bronchoscopy or lung biopsy, and inhalation of water repellant [33–36]. Sources of PM include tobacco smoke, candles, forest fires, and dust [33, 37]. The exact incidence of exacerbations is unknown but is estimated to vary between 5 and 20% [36, 38].

Since AE mortality rates range between 60 and 80% within a 90-day period, most care is strictly palliative in nature [39]. The two primary therapies include corticosteroids like prednisone and cytotoxic medications like cyclophosphamide. However, no proven benefit for these therapies has been demonstrated [40]. In addition, mechanical ventilation should not be employed due to poor outcomes [41]. Novel therapy involving administration of polymyxin B-immobilized fiber column (PMX-DHP), originally developed to manage sepsis by removing plasma endotoxins, has shown increased effectiveness [38, 42]. One limitation of its use is it can lower white blood cell counts via absorption of neutrophils [38, 39]. It remains most effective if administered within 3–7 days of AE onset [38, 39].

8. Clinical evidence for efficacy

The SENSCIS trial was a 52-week randomized, placebo-controlled, double-blind study examining the treatment of systemic sclerosis-associated interstitial lung disease (SSc-ILD) with nintedanib [43, 44]. It was shown to decrease FVC decline rate (mL/year) within the treatment group compared to placebo [3, 43]. An annual difference of −52.4 mL/year for nintedanib versus −93.3 mL/year for placebo was shown at 52 weeks [3, 43]. The INPULSIS trial, a 52-week, randomized, double-blind, phase 3 trial, showed a similar reduction in FVC decline rate with nintedanib versus placebo [3, 45]. TOMORROW, a 52-week, randomized, double-blind, placebo-controlled, phase 2 trial—alongside INPULSIS—showed a decrease in acute exacerbations with nintedanib compared to placebo [4, 45]. The INBUILD trial, a 52-week, randomized, double-blind, placebo-controlled, parallel-group trial, examined patients with progressive fibrosing interstitial lung diseases other than IPF [3, 46]. Treatment groups received nintedanib 150 mg twice daily or placebo [3, 46]. Reduction in FVC decline rate was uniform across the five subgroups [46, 47].

Three major trials have recently examined pirfenidone, including CAPACITY 004, CAPACITY 006, and ASCEND [4, 12]. The two CAPACITY trials were run side-by-side for 72 weeks [48, 49]. CAPACITY 004 showed a significant reduction in FVC decline with pirfenidone, though only a significant difference up to week 48 was seen in CAPACITY 006 [48, 49]. The ASCEND trial, a 52-week, phase 3 trial, found that patients with a predicted FVC > 50% at baseline received benefit from pirfenidone over 1 year, reducing the rate of decline by approximately 50% [4, 49]. ASCEND also analyzed 6 MW distance [49, 50]. There was a significant difference between baseline and week 52 with the two treatments, including a 27.5% reduction in the pirfenidone group [49, 50]. Pooled population data from all three trials showed a 48% reduced risk of death at 1 year compared to placebo [48, 49].

9. Comparison: nintedanib vs. pirfenidone

As mentioned above, both agents have been shown safe and effective in placebo-controlled, randomized trials [51–53]. Both may slow the FVC decline rate by almost 50% over 1 year [51]. The two treatments have also demonstrated remarkable efficacy in minimizing severe respiratory hospitalizations and acute exacerbations [51, 54]. Though both agents may reduce mortality, each cost over $100,000 annually [51, 55].

9.1 Mechanisms of action

Nintedanib has a unique mechanism of action compared to pirfenidone. It inhibits tyrosine kinase, an enzyme that targets growth factor (GF) pathway receptors like fibroblast GF, platelet-derived GF, and vascular endothelial GF [3, 4]. Elevated bleeding risk is seen in patients taking concomitant anticoagulation therapy [7, 15]. Patients should regularly monitor liver function and GI disturbances, including diarrhea [43, 46]. Conversely, pirfenidone inhibits collagen synthesis, downregulates TGF-β, tumor necrosis factor-α, and reduces fibroblast proliferation [7, 24, 26]. Side effects include abnormal liver function, anorexia, nausea, photosensitive rashes, and vomiting [56].

9.2 Dosing

Pirfenidone comes in a 267 mg capsule, initially dosed as one capsule three times daily the first week [56, 57]. During the second week, the dose can be increased to 534 mg three times daily, and—after two weeks—it can be fully titrated to 801 mg three times (2,403 mg or nine pills per day). It is recommended that each dose be taken after a full meal to minimize GI side effects like nausea, dizziness, and vomiting [56, 57]. Patients may be treated with nintedanib first-line if intolerability to pirfenidone occurs [56–58]. The maximum recommended dose is 150 mg twice daily [58, 59].

9.3 Research similarities and differences

In a 1-year evaluation of both medications, there was a slight decrease in FVC, especially in those with comorbidities, which may account for increases in hospitalization and all-cause mortality [60, 61]. In combined studies, pirfenidone displayed a slower rate of FVC decline than nintedanib, helping to explain increased hospitalizations and mortality with its use [60, 61].

9.4 Side effect profiles

Though pirfenidone is frequently associated with GI complications, diarrhea, and involuntary weight loss is more common with nintedanib [57, 58, 61]. Pirfenidone's side effects include dyspepsia, nausea, loss of appetite, phototoxic reactions, and difficulty concentrating. Sunscreen use is recommended when taking it. Conversely, nintedanib displays less nausea but greater transaminase elevations [57, 58, 61]. Pirfenidone is older and better studied more nintedanib, which may explain why its gastrointestinal and cognitive side effects are better understood [57, 58, 61]. Phototoxicity is generally absent with nintedanib [57, 61].

10. Therapeutic drawbacks

Though pirfenidone and nintedanib may slow disease progression, neither will cure IPF or markedly improve current symptoms [4, 62]. Symptom management, especially cough and dyspnea, is crucial to maintaining the quality of life [4, 63]. This is somewhat challenging given the lack of clinical evidence showing improvement in such symptoms and guideline focus on lung function [4, 63].

Both agents have noteworthy side effects. Nintedanib is most frequently associated with diarrhea, nausea, vomiting, and elevated liver enzymes [62]. By comparison, pirfenidone may cause nausea, diarrhea, dyspepsia, anorexia, and gastroesophageal reflux, as well as rash, upper respiratory infections, and fatigue [62, 64].

Another significant burden of IPF is cost [4, 65]. A recent systematic review estimated its annual cost in the United States at $20,000 per patient per year, about three times greater than the national health care resource use per capita [4, 65]. Hospitalizations and acute exacerbations are key drivers of this cost, with an average cost exceeding $16,000 for each IPF-related hospitalization [4, 66]. Due to their specialty drug and brand-only status, pirfenidone and nintedanib remain extremely expensive, with costs exceeding $10,000 per month per agent [4]. However, nintedanib is associated with fewer acute exacerbations and, consequently, decreased medical costs [4, 62, 67]. A recent comparison analysis from the United Kingdom found that the two drugs were comparable in estimated cost and health-related quality of life benefit [4, 68].

It is important to remember that the INBUILD trial was not powered to provide sufficient evidence for the use of nintedanib in rarer, specific fibrosing ILD [47]. However, it can be challenging to recruit patients with these rarer disease states. The fact that nintedanib reduced the rate of disease progression (i.e., FVC decline) in a wide range of progressive fibrosing ILD suggests utility in such populations [47].

11. Novel research/pipeline drugs

In recent decades, our understanding of IPF pathogenicity and management has improved significantly [15, 69]. However, many limitations, such as an inability to translate experimental findings in animal models to human subjects, remain a challenge [69, 70]. Current therapies like nintedanib and pirfenidone are limited to pathways involved in reducing disease progression and physiological decline in those with mild-to-moderate impairment [15, 69]. Second-line treatments capable of improving functional capacity for such patients or benefiting the severely impaired are still needed [15, 70].

Other viable agents have been recently investigated [9]. Increased concentrations of endothelin receptors have been observed in IPF lung tissue [15]. As a result, several clinically significant endothelin receptor antagonists have been previously tested, including ambrisentan, a selective type-A antagonist, and bosentan and macitentan, type-A and type-B antagonists [71, 72]. Nonetheless, recent guidelines strongly discourage the use of ambrisentan given its risk of harm and lack of benefit, along with a conditional recommendation against the use of bosentan and macitentan [15, 73].

The phosphodiesterase-5 inhibitor sildenafil has been investigated due to its role in pulmonary vasodilation and improved gas exchange [15]. Past studies and analyses reported a slight but significant improvement in the degree of dyspnea and quality of life compared to placebo [15]. However, it has failed to demonstrate improvements in mortality, acute exacerbations, and adverse events [15]. Recent guidelines discourage its use, though it continues to be investigated [15, 73].

N-acetylcysteine (NAC), a precursor of the antioxidant glutathione, has also been examined for use in IPF [74]. A pooled analysis compared NAC monotherapy to placebo in IPF patients [15]. Ultimately, there was no significant difference in the rate of death or acute exacerbation, as well as no significant benefit in mortality, quality of life, or adverse outcomes [15]. Current guidelines strongly discourage its use in practice [15, 74].

A recent randomized clinical trial investigated imatinib mesylate (Gleevec®), a tyrosine kinase inhibitor. It showed a statistically significant increased risk of adverse events and no improvement in preventing disease progression or mortality [15, 74]. This distinct lack of benefit has led to its use being discouraged in IPF [15, 74].

Several active interventional and observational trials are currently underway. Recent novel studies suggest that genetic factors may play a crucial role in overall risk, disease progression, and therapeutic response [70, 75]. Future trials and drug development will likely focus more on genetic variation in IPF patients [70, 75].

12. Conclusions

IPF is a common ILD that is progressive and potentially fatal [4, 9]. It is characterized by decreased lung function stemming from abnormal fibrotic processes, ultimately leading to scarring tissue formation, diminished gas exchange, and reduced blood oxygenation [4, 7]. Though there is no known cause, it is more common in males and elderly patients and is associated with risk factors like smoking, environmental exposure, and multiple comorbidities [4, 9]. Due to insufficient understanding of its pathophysiological mechanisms, there are currently no therapies capable of preventing or reversing IPF [7, 9, 76]. Current management includes antifibrotic drugs like nintedanib (Ofev®) and pirfenidone (Esbriet®), which have been shown to slow lung deterioration [4, 7, 13]. Recent investigations examining nintedanib use in other ILDs with progressive phenotypes have shown favorable results, suggesting that such ILDs share similar mechanisms and may thus benefit from similar treatment [3, 77]. Imatinib mesylate (Gleevec®) is not recommended due to the increased risk of adverse events and no improvement in disease progression or mortality [17, 73]. Similarly, the use of ambrisentan (Letairis®)

is discouraged due to lack of effectiveness and increased risk of hospitalization [7]. Other IPF management strategies include smoking cessation, immunization, respiratory rehabilitation, oxygen supplementation, and management of comorbidities [4, 20]. More recent approaches have targeted biological processes linked to IPF, such as aging, oxidative stress, and epithelial-to-mesenchymal cell transition (EMT) [9, 76]. Ultimately, a better understanding of its underlying mechanisms is necessary to develop more effective treatments and reduce mortality [7, 9, 76].

Author details

Ladan Panahi[1,2]*, George Udeani[1,2], Andrew Scott Tenpas[1,2], Theresa Ofili[1,2], Elizabeth Marie Aguilar[1,2], Sarah Burchard[1,2], Alexandra Ruth Ritenour[1,2], April Jacob Chennat[1,2], Nehal Ahmed[1,2], Chairat Atphaisit[1,2], Crystal Chi[1,2], Jesus Cruz III [1,2], Monica D. Deleon[1,2], Samantha Lee[1,2], Zack Mayo[1,2], Mackenzie Mcbeth[1,2], Mariel Morales[1,2], Jennifer N. Nwosu[1,2], Kelly Palacios[1,2], Jaycob M. Pena[1,2] and Nitza Vara[1,2]

1 Department of Pharmacy Practice, Texas A&M Rangel College of Pharmacy, Kingsville, Texas, USA

2 Department of Pharmacy Practice, Texas A&M Rangel College of Pharmacy, College Station, Texas, USA

*Address all correspondence to: panahi@tamu.edu

IntechOpen

References

[1] Lederer DJ, Martinez FJ. Idiopathic pulmonary fibrosis. The New England Journal of Medicine. 2018;**379**(8):797-798. DOI: 10.1056/NEJMc1807508

[2] Thannickal VJ, Toews GB, White ES, Lynch JP 3rd, Martinez FJ. Mechanisms of pulmonary fibrosis. Annual Review of Medicine. 2004;**55**:395-417. DOI: 10.1146/annurev.med.55.091902.103810

[3] Wollin L, Distler JHW, Redente EF, Riches DWH, Stowasser S, Schlenker-Herceg R, et al. Potential of nintedanib in treatment of progressive fibrosing interstitial lung diseases. European Respiratory Journal. 2019;**54**(3):1900161. DOI: 10.1183/13993003.00161-2019

[4] Pleasants R, Tighe RM. Management of idiopathic pulmonary fibrosis. The Annals of Pharmacotherapy. 2019;**53**(12):1238-1248. DOI: 10.1177/1060028019862497

[5] Van Manen MJ, Birring SS, Vancheri C, Cottin V, Renzoni EA, Russell A-M, et al. Cough in idiopathic pulmonary fibrosis. European Respiratory Review. 2016;**25**(141):278-286

[6] Park Y, Ahn C, Kim T-HJS. Occupational and environmental risk factors of idiopathic pulmonary fibrosis: A systematic review and meta-analyses. Scientific Reports. 2021;**11**(1):1-10

[7] Glass DS, Grossfeld D, Renna HA, Agarwala P, Spiegler P, Kasselman LJ, et al. Idiopathic pulmonary fibrosis: Molecular mechanisms and potential treatment approaches. Respiratory Investigation. 2020;**58**(5):320-335. DOI: 10.1016/j.resinv.2020.04.002

[8] Martinez FJ, Collard HR, Pardo A, Raghu G, Richeldi L, Selman M, et al. Idiopathic pulmonary fibrosis. Nature Reviews Disease Primers. 2017;**3**:17074. DOI: 10.1038/nrdp.2017.74

[9] Phan THG, Paliogiannis P, Nasrallah GK, Giordo R, Eid AH, Fois AG, et al. Emerging cellular and molecular determinants of idiopathic pulmonary fibrosis. Cellular and Molecular Life Sciences. 2021;**78**(5):2031-2057. DOI: 10.1007/s00018-020-03693-7

[10] Ley B, Collard HR, King TE Jr. Clinical course and prediction of survival in idiopathic pulmonary fibrosis. American Journal of Respiratory and Critical Care Medicine. 2011;**183**(4):431-440. DOI: 10.1164/rccm.201006-0894CI

[11] Richeldi L, Collard HR, Jones MG. Idiopathic pulmonary fibrosis. Lancet. 2017;**389**(10082):1941-1952. DOI: 10.1016/S0140-6736(17)30866-8

[12] Lancaster LH, de Andrade JA, Zibrak JD, Padilla ML, Albera C, Nathan SD, et al. Pirfenidone safety and adverse event management in idiopathic pulmonary fibrosis. European Respiratory Review. 2017;**26**(146):170057. DOI: 10.1183/16000617.0057-2017

[13] Sgalla G, Iovene B, Calvello M, Ori M, Varone F, Richeldi L. Idiopathic pulmonary fibrosis: Pathogenesis and management. Respiratory Research. 2018;**19**(1):32. DOI: 10.1186/s12931-018-0730-2

[14] Raghu G, Collard HR, Egan JJ, Martinez FJ, Behr J, Brown KK, et al. An official ATS/ERS/JRS/ALAT statement: Idiopathic pulmonary fibrosis: Evidence-based guidelines for diagnosis and management. American Journal of Respiratory and Critical Care Medicine. 2011;**183**(6):788-824. DOI: 10.1164/rccm.2009-040GL

[15] Raghu G, Rochwerg B, Zhang Y, Cuello Garcia CA, Azuma A, Behr J, et al. An Official ATS/ERS/JRS/ALAT clinical practice guideline: Treatment of

idiopathic pulmonary fibrosis. An update of the 2011 clinical practice guideline. American Journal of Respiratory and Critical Care Medicine. 2015;**192**(2):e3-e19. DOI: 10.1164/rccm.201506-1063ST

[16] Sun T, Liu J. Efficacy of N-acetylcysteine in idiopathic pulmonary fibrosis: A systematic review and meta-analysis. Medicine. 2016;**95**(19):e3629

[17] Mooney JJ, Raimundo K, Chang E, Broder MS. Mechanical ventilation in idiopathic pulmonary fibrosis: A nationwide analysis of ventilator use, outcomes, and resource burden. BMC Pulmonary Medicine. 2017;**17**(1):1-9

[18] Raghu G, Freudenberger TD, Yang S, Curtis JR, Spada C, Hayes J, et al. High prevalence of abnormal acid gastro-oesophageal reflux in idiopathic pulmonary fibrosis. The European Respiratory Journal. 2006;**27**(1):136-142. DOI: 10.1183/09031936.06.00037005

[19] el-Serag HB, Sonnenberg A. Comorbid occurrence of laryngeal or pulmonary disease with esophagitis in United States military veterans. Gastroenterology. 1997;**113**(3):755-760. DOI: 10.1016/s0016-5085(97)70168-9

[20] Luppi F, Kalluri M, Faverio P, Kreuter M, Ferrara G. Idiopathic pulmonary fibrosis beyond the lung: Understanding disease mechanisms to improve diagnosis and management. Respiratory Research. 2021;**22**(1):109. DOI: 10.1186/s12931-021-01711-1

[21] Acharya G, Arya S, Badal S, Kumar D, Samdariya S. Pharmacotherapy in idiopathic pulmonary fibrosis. International Journal of Basic & Clinical Pharmacology. 2014;**3**(5):761

[22] Papiris SA, Kagouridis K, Kolilekas L, Papaioannou AI, Roussou A, Triantafillidou C, et al.

Survival in Idiopathic pulmonary fibrosis acute exacerbations: The non-steroid approach. BMC Pulmonary Medicine. 2015;**15**:162. DOI: 10.1186/s12890-015-0146-4

[23] Noble PW, Albera C, Bradford WZ, Costabel U, Glassberg MK, Kardatzke D, et al. Pirfenidone in patients with idiopathic pulmonary fibrosis (CAPACITY): Two randomised trials. Lancet. 2011;**377**(9779):1760-1769. DOI: 10.1016/S0140-6736(11)60405-4

[24] Shi S, Wu J, Chen H, Chen H, Wu J, Zeng F. Single- and multiple-dose pharmacokinetics of pirfenidone, an antifibrotic agent, in healthy Chinese volunteers. Journal of Clinical Pharmacology. 2007;**47**(10):1268-1276. DOI: 10.1177/0091270007304104

[25] Cho ME, Kopp JB. Pirfenidone: An anti-fibrotic therapy for progressive kidney disease. Expert Opinion on Investigational Drugs. 2010;**19**(2):275-283. DOI: 10.1517/13543780903501539

[26] Ley B, Swigris J, Day BM, Stauffer JL, Raimundo K, Chou W, et al. Pirfenidone reduces respiratory-related hospitalizations in idiopathic pulmonary fibrosis. American Journal of Respiratory and Critical Care Medicine. 2017;**196**(6):756-761. DOI: 10.1164/rccm.201701-0091OC

[27] Hu J, Shang D, Xu X, He X, Ni X, Zhang M, et al. Effect of grapefruit juice and food on the pharmacokinetics of pirfenidone in healthy Chinese volunteers: A diet-drug interaction study. Xenobiotica. 2016;**46**(6):516-521. DOI: 10.3109/00498254.2015.1089365

[28] Rubino CM, Bhavnani SM, Ambrose PG, Forrest A, Loutit JS. Effect of food and antacids on the pharmacokinetics of pirfenidone in older healthy adults. Pulmonary Pharmacology & Therapeutics. 2009;**22**(4):279-285. DOI: 10.1016/j.pupt.2009.03.003

[29] Genentech I. Esbriet (Pirfenidone) Capsules and Film-Coated Tablets, for Oral Use [Package Insert]. South San Francisco; 2017

[30] Barranco-Garduno LM, Buendia-Roldan I, Rodriguez JJ, González-Ramírez R, Cervantes-Nevárez AN, Neri-Salvador JC, et al. Pharmacokinetic evaluation of two pirfenidone formulations in patients with idiopathic pulmonary fibrosis and chronic hypersensitivity pneumonitis. Heliyon. 2020;6(10):e05279. DOI: 10.1016/j.heliyon.2020.e05279

[31] Pan L, Belloni P, Ding HT, Wang J, Rubino CM, Putnam WS. A pharmacokinetic bioequivalence study comparing pirfenidone tablet and capsule dosage forms in healthy adult volunteers. Advances in Therapy. 2017;34(9):2071-2082. DOI: 10.1007/s12325-017-0594-8

[32] Ogura T, Taniguchi H, Azuma A, Inoue Y, Kondoh Y, Hasegawa Y, et al. Safety and pharmacokinetics of nintedanib and pirfenidone in idiopathic pulmonary fibrosis. The European Respiratory Journal. 2015;45(5):1382-1392. DOI: 10.1183/09031936.00198013

[33] Tahara M, Fujino Y, Yamasaki K, Oda K, Kido T, Sakamoto N, et al. Exposure to PM2.5 is a risk factor for acute exacerbation of surgically diagnosed idiopathic pulmonary fibrosis: A case-control study. Respiratory Research. 2021;22(1):80. DOI: 10.1186/s12931-021-01671-6

[34] Bennett D, Bargagli E, Refini RM, Pieroni M, Fossi A, Romeo R, et al. Acute exacerbation of idiopathic pulmonary fibrosis after inhalation of a water repellent. International Journal of Occupational Medicine and Environmental Health. 2015;28(4):775-779. DOI: 10.13075/ijomeh.1896.00462

[35] D'Alessandro-Gabazza CN, Kobayashi T, Yasuma T, Toda M, Kim H, Fujimoto H, et al. A Staphylococcus

pro-apoptotic peptide induces acute exacerbation of pulmonary fibrosis. Nature Communications. 2020;11(1):1539. DOI: 10.1038/s41467-020-15344-3

[36] Hyzy R, Huang S, Myers J, Flaherty K, Martinez F. Acute exacerbation of idiopathic pulmonary fibrosis. Chest. 2007;132(5):1652-1658. DOI: 10.1378/chest.07-0299

[37] Tahara M, Fujino Y, Yamasaki K, Oda K, Kido T, Sakamoto N, et al. Exposure to PM 2.5 is a risk factor for acute exacerbation of surgically diagnosed idiopathic pulmonary fibrosis: A case–control study. Respiratory Research. 2021;22(1):1-11

[38] Kishaba T. Acute exacerbation of idiopathic pulmonary fibrosis. Medicina (Kaunas). 2019;55(3):70. DOI: 10.3390/medicina55030070

[39] Kim SY, Park JH, Kim HJ, Jang HJ, Kim HK, Kim SH, et al. Direct hemoperfusion with polymyxin B-immobilized fiber column in a patient with acute exacerbation of idiopathic pulmonary fibrosis. Acute and Critical Care. 2020;35(4):302-306. DOI: 10.4266/acc.2020.00038

[40] Innabi A, Gomez-Manjarres D, Alzghoul BN, Chizinga M, Mehrad B, Patel DC. Cyclophosphamide for the treatment of acute exacerbation of interstitial lung disease: A review of the literature. Sarcoidosis, Vasculitis, and Diffuse Lung Diseases. 2021;38(1):e2021002

[41] Luo Z, Yang L, Liu S, Hu Y, Cao Z, Zhu J, et al. Mechanical ventilation for acute respiratory failure due to idiopathic pulmonary fibrosis versus connective tissue disease-associated interstitial lung disease: Effectiveness and risk factors for death. The Clinical Respiratory Journal. 2020;14(10):918-932

[42] Enomoto N, Mikamo M, Oyama Y, Kono M, Hashimoto D, Fujisawa T, et al.

Treatment of acute exacerbation of idiopathic pulmonary fibrosis with direct hemoperfusion using a polymyxin B-immobilized fiber column improves survival. BMC Pulmonary Medicine. 2015;**15**:15. DOI: 10.1186/ s12890-015-0004-4

[43] Distler O, Highland KB, Gahlemann M, Azuma A, Fischer A, Mayes MD, et al. Nintedanib for systemic sclerosis-associated interstitial lung disease. The New England Journal of Medicine. 2019;**380**(26):2518-2528. DOI: 10.1056/NEJMoa1903076

[44] Maher TM, Mayes MD, Kreuter M, Volkmann ER, Aringer M, Castellvi I, et al. Effect of nintedanib on lung function in patients with systemic sclerosis-associated interstitial lung disease: Further analyses of a randomized, double-blind placebo-controlled trial. Arthritis & Rheumatology. 2021;**73**(4): 671-676. DOI: 10.1002/art.41576

[45] Richeldi L, du Bois RM, Raghu G, Azuma A, Brown KK, Costabel U, et al. Efficacy and safety of nintedanib in idiopathic pulmonary fibrosis. The New England Journal of Medicine. 2014; **370**(22):2071-2082. DOI: 10.1056/ NEJMoa1402584

[46] Wells AU, Flaherty KR, Brown KK, Inoue K, Devaraj A, Richeldi L, et al. Nintedanib in patients with progressive fibrosing interstitial lung diseases-subgroup analyses by interstitial lung disease diagnosis in the INBUILD trial: A randomised, double-blind, placebo-controlled, parallel-group trial. The Lancet Respiratory Medicine. 2020;**8**(5):453-460. DOI: 10.1016/ S2213-2600(20)30036-9

[47] Flaherty KR, Fell CD, Huggins JT, Nunes H, Sussman R, Valenzuela C, et al. Safety of nintedanib added to pirfenidone treatment for idiopathic pulmonary fibrosis. European Respiratory Journal. 2018;**52**(2). DOI: 10.1183/13993003.00230-2018

[48] Gulati S, Luckhardt TR. Updated evaluation of the safety, efficacy and tolerability of pirfenidone in the treatment of idiopathic pulmonary fibrosis. Drug Healthcare and Patient Safety. 2020;**12**:85-94. DOI: 10.2147/ DHPS.S224007

[49] King TE Jr, Bradford WZ, Castro-Bernardini S, Fagan EA, Glaspole I, Glassberg MK, et al. A phase 3 trial of pirfenidone in patients with idiopathic pulmonary fibrosis. The New England Journal of Medicine. 2014; **370**(22):2083-2092. DOI: 10.1056/ NEJMoa1402582

[50] Nathan SD, Costabel U, Albera C, Behr J, Wuyts WA, Kirchgaessler K-U, et al. Pirfenidone in patients with idiopathic pulmonary fibrosis and more advanced lung function impairment. Respiratory Medicine. 2019;**153**:44-51. DOI: 10.1016/j.rmed.2019.04.016

[51] Raghu G, Remy-Jardin M, Myers JL, Richeldi L, Ryerson CJ, Lederer DJ, et al. Diagnosis of idiopathic pulmonary fibrosis. An official ATS/ERS/JRS/ALAT clinical practice guideline. American Journal of Respiratory and Critical Care Medicine. 2018;**198**(5):e44-e68

[52] Varone F, Sgalla G, Iovene B, Bruni T, Richeldi L. Nintedanib for the treatment of idiopathic pulmonary fibrosis. Expert Opinion on Pharmacotherapy. 2018;**19**(2):167-175

[53] Saito S, Alkhatib A, Kolls JK, Kondoh Y, Lasky JA. Pharmacotherapy and adjunctive treatment for idiopathic pulmonary fibrosis (IPF). Journal of Thoracic Disease. 2019;**11**(Suppl 14): S1740

[54] Dempsey TM, Sangaralingham LR, Yao X, Sanghavi D, Shah ND, Limper AH. Clinical effectiveness of antifibrotic medications for idiopathic pulmonary fibrosis. American Journal of Respiratory and Critical Care Medicine. 2019;**200**(2):168-174

[55] Owens GM. Strategies to manage costs in idiopathic pulmonary fibrosis. The American Journal of Managed Care. 2017;**23**(Suppl 11):S191-S196

[56] Costabel U, Bendstrup E, Cottin V, Dewint P, Egan JJJ, Ferguson J, et al. Pirfenidone in idiopathic pulmonary fibrosis: Expert panel discussion on the management of drug-related adverse events. Advances in Therapy. 2014; **31**(4):375-391. DOI: 10.1007/s12325-014-0112-1

[57] Meyer KC, Decker CA. Role of pirfenidone in the management of pulmonary fibrosis. Therapeutics and Clinical Risk Management. 2017;**13**: 427-437. DOI: 10.2147/TCRM.S81141

[58] Brunnemer E, Walscher J, Tenenbaum S, Hausmanns J, Schulze K, Seiter M, et al. Real-world experience with nintedanib in patients with idiopathic pulmonary fibrosis. Respiration. 2018;**95**(5):301-309. DOI: 10.1159/000485933

[59] Fukihara J, Kondoh Y. Nintedanib (OFEV) in the treatment of idiopathic pulmonary fibrosis. Expert Review of Respiratory Medicine. 2016;**10**(12):1247-1254. DOI: 10.1080/17476348.2016.1249854

[60] Belhassen M, Dalon F, Nolin M, Van Ganse E. Comparative outcomes in patients receiving pirfenidone or nintedanib for idiopathic pulmonary fibrosis. Respiratory Research. 2021;**22**(1):135. DOI: 10.1186/s12931-021-01714-y

[61] Cerri S, Monari M, Guerrieri A, Donatelli P, Bassi I, Garuti M, et al. Real-life comparison of pirfenidone and nintedanib in patients with idiopathic pulmonary fibrosis: A 24-month assessment. Respiratory Medicine. 2019;**159**:105803. DOI: 10.1016/j.rmed.2019.105803

[62] Tzouvelekis A, Bonella F, Spagnolo P. Update on therapeutic management of idiopathic pulmonary fibrosis. Therapeutics and Clinical Risk Management. 2015;**11**:359-370. DOI: 10.2147/TCRM.S69716

[63] Ferrara G, Luppi F, Birring SS, Cerri S, Caminati A, Sköld M, et al. Best supportive care for idiopathic pulmonary fibrosis: Current gaps and future directions. European Respiratory Review. 2018;**27**(147). DOI: 10.1183/16000617.0076-2017

[64] Rahaghi FF, Safdar Z, Brown AW, de Andrade JA, Flaherty KR, Kaner RJ, et al. Expert consensus on the management of adverse events and prescribing practices associated with the treatment of patients taking pirfenidone for idiopathic pulmonary fibrosis: A Delphi consensus study. BMC Pulmonary Medicine. 2020;**20**(1):191. DOI: 10.1186/s12890-020-01209-4

[65] Diamantopoulos A, Wright E, Vlahopoulou K, Cornic L, Schoof N, Maher TM. The burden of illness of idiopathic pulmonary fibrosis: A comprehensive evidence review. PharmacoEconomics. 2018;**36**(7):779-807. DOI: 10.1007/s40273-018-0631-8

[66] Mooney JJ, Raimundo K, Chang E, Broder MS. Hospital cost and length of stay in idiopathic pulmonary fibrosis. Journal of Medical Economics. 2017;**20**(5):518-524. DOI: 10.1080/13696998.2017.1282864

[67] Bonella F, Stowasser S, Wollin L. Idiopathic pulmonary fibrosis: Current treatment options and critical appraisal of nintedanib. Drug Design, Development and Therapy. 2015;**9**:6407-6419. DOI: 10.2147/DDDT.S76648

[68] Rinciog C, Watkins M, Chang S, Maher TM, LeReun C, Esser D, et al. A cost-effectiveness analysis of nintedanib in idiopathic pulmonary fibrosis in the UK. PharmacoEconomics. 2017;**35**(4): 479-491. DOI: 10.1007/s40273-016-0480-2

[69] Raghu G. Idiopathic pulmonary fibrosis: Lessons from clinical trials over the past 25 years. European Respiratory Journal. 2017;**50**(4):1701209. DOI: 10.1183/13993003.01209-2017

[70] Mora AL, Rojas M, Pardo A, Selman M. Emerging therapies for idiopathic pulmonary fibrosis, a progressive age-related disease. Nature Reviews Drug Discovery. 2017;**16**(11): 810. DOI: 10.1038/nrd.2017.225

[71] King TE Jr, Brown KK, Raghu G, du Bois RM, Lynch DA, Martinez F, et al. BUILD-3: A randomized, controlled trial of bosentan in idiopathic pulmonary fibrosis. American Journal of Respiratory and Critical Care Medicine. 2011;**184**(1):92-99. DOI: 10.1164/rccm.201011-1874OC

[72] Raghu G, Million-Rousseau R, Morganti A, Perchenet L, Behr J, Music Study Group. Macitentan for the treatment of idiopathic pulmonary fibrosis: The randomised controlled MUSIC trial. The European Respiratory Journal. 2013;**42**(6):1622-1632. DOI: 10.1183/09031936.00104612

[73] Behr J, Gunther A, Bonella F, Geissler K, Koschel D, Kreuter M, et al. German guideline for idiopathic pulmonary fibrosis - Update on Pharmacological Therapies 2017. S2k-Leitlinie Idiopathische Lungenfibrose - Update zur medikamentosen Therapie 2017. Pneumologie. 2018;**72**(2):155-168. DOI: 10.1055/s-0043-123035

[74] Antoniou KM, Margaritopoulos GA, Siafakas NM. Pharmacological treatment of idiopathic pulmonary fibrosis: From the past to the future. European Respiratory Review. 2013;**22**(129):281-291. DOI: 10.1183/09059180.00002113

[75] Kaur A, Mathai SK, Schwartz DA. Genetics in idiopathic pulmonary fibrosis pathogenesis, prognosis, and treatment. Frontiers in Medicine (Lausanne). 2017;**4**:154. DOI: 10.3389/fmed.2017.00154

[76] Veith C, Boots AW, Idris M, van Schooten FJ, van der Vliet A. Redox imbalance in idiopathic pulmonary fibrosis: A role for oxidant cross-talk between NADPH oxidase enzymes and mitochondria. Antioxidants & Redox Signaling. 2019;**31**(14):1092-1115. DOI: 10.1089/ars.2019.7742

[77] Valenzuela C, Torrisi SE, Kahn N, Quaresma M, Stowasser S, Kreuter M. Ongoing challenges in pulmonary fibrosis and insights from the nintedanib clinical programme. Respiratory Research. 2020;**21**(1):7. DOI: 10.1186/s12931-019-1269-6

Section 4

Exacerbation

Chapter 5

Acute Exacerbation of Idiopathic Pulmonary Fibrosis

Nitesh Kumar Jain, Shikha Jain, Hisham Ahmed Mushtaq,
Anwar Khedr, Thoyaja Koritala, Aysun Tekin,
Ramesh Adhikari, Anupam Sule, Samir Gautam,
Vishwanath Pattan, Vikas Bansal, Ali Rabaan,
Kovid Trivedi, Amos Lal, Brian Bartlett, Abbas Jama,
Aishwarya Reddy Korsapati, Mohamed Hassan,
Simon Zec, Adham Mohsen, Amit Munshi Sharma,
Ibtisam Rauf, Mikael Mir, Lia Nandi, Mool Chand,
Hariprasad Reddy Korsapati, Rahul Kashyap,
Salim Surani and Syed Anjum Khan

Abstract

Episodes of Acute exacerbation (AE) of Idiopathic Pulmonary fibrosis (IPF) are important events in the disease trajectory of IPF, associated with punctuated decline in lung function with significant mortality and morbidity associated with it. These episodes are idiosyncratic, and often unpredictable and may have triggers. Our diagnostic criteria for these events, etiology, pathogenesis, risk factors and management continue to evolve over the years, with limited availability of qualitative research data to help guide management. Outcome in general is poor with no well-defined therapy but prevention may be possible with use of Nintedanib. Our chapter aims to explore the contemporary knowledge of the key aspects of this disease entity.

Keywords: acute exacerbation of IPF, idiopathic pulmonary fibrosis, acute exacerbation, drug therapy, treatment, clinical trials, nintedanib, pirfenidone, respiratory failure

1. Introduction

Acute exacerbations of Idiopathic Pulmonary fibrosis (AE-IPF) represent important milestone in the disease course of IPF, which is the most common disease among the group of Idiopathic interstitial pneumonia (IIP). The IPF is more common among males and in the elderly age group [1]. Although the exact etiology of AE-IPF is unknown, there are many important risk factors as well as triggers that have been identified. There is associated accelerated decline in lung function which leads to poor prognosis [1]. It is estimated that about 35 to 46% of deaths in IPF are caused by AE-IPF [2]. In hospital mortality is more than 50% and follow up after hospitalization shows a mortality up to 73% at the end of 90 days [2, 3]. Although treatment with high dose Gluco corticoids have been used extensively, there is lack of controlled well designed trials to support its use and in fact survival has been shown to be decreased with steroids and or other immune suppressants [4, 5]. Some newer anti-fibrotic agents like Pirfenidone and Nintedanib may improve survival, the latter may be helpful in preventing AE-IPF [1, 6, 7].

2. Criteria for diagnosis of AE-IPF

Acute exacerbation of IPF is recognized with the help of a set of criteria laid out by the International IPF Working group network which is as follows [2, 4, 8–12].

"An acute, clinically significant respiratory deterioration characterized by evidence of new widespread alveolar abnormality".

The following four diagnostic criteria have to be met as shown in **Table 1**.

The guidelines also provided certain clarifications that help in making a diagnosis [11].

Events that are clinically considered to meet the definition of acute exacerbation of IPF but fail to meet all four diagnostic criteria owing to missing computed tomography data are to be termed "suspected acute exacerbations." For example, if CT scan shows unilateral ground glass attenuation or data available is incomplete [2].

If the diagnosis of IPF is not previously established, this criterion can be met by the presence of radiologic and/or histopathologic changes consistent with usual interstitial pneumonia pattern on the current evaluation [11].

It is to be noted that the term "idiopathic" was removed from the older definition, as it was seen to be restrictive [11]. Making a distinction between idiopathic and non-idiopathic respiratory events is not easy as there are not well defined clinical or biological criteria [11]. So, although the acute deterioration could be due to an infectious etiology and it is not necessary to rule this out for the purpose of definition, at a practical level infection needs to be diagnosed and treated empirically or definitely as it does have a definite therapeutic recourse [11, 13]. It also follows from this that Broncho alveolar lavage (BAL) is not needed for diagnosis and hence it will help capture more of such events, but at the expense of specificity [11, 13]. BAL may not be needed when HRCT pattern is consistent with UIP, but

A known or concurrent diagnosis of IPF
Clinical respiratory deterioration noted "typically" in the preceding 30 days.
Presence of typical UIP pattern on CT chest including bilateral basilar reticular changes with honeycombing and traction bronchiectasis. Superimposed ground glass attenuation and /or consolidation is necessary in exacerbation. When possible specific UIP pattern may be combined with histopathological information to make a more robust diagnosis.
Absence of heart failure, Pulmonary embolism, fluid overload or any other differential pathology.
Note that endotracheal aspirate is not necessary as per new diagnostic criteria.
The 30-day time limit of clinical deterioration is not strictly enforced.
Exclude other causes of Interstitial Lung disease such as drug toxicity, connective tissue disease, hypersensitivity pneumonitis, etc.

Table 1.
Criteria for diagnosing IPF exacerbation as per working group idiopathic pulmonary fibrosis network (IPF net).

when the Usual interstitial pneumonia (UIP) pattern is indeterminate or suspect then BAL can be useful [12]. Similarly, surgical lung biopsy (SLB) is recommended only when UIP is indeterminate or suspect [12]. However there is considerable morbidity and mortality associated with BAL or surgical biopsy in the context of AE and hence such procedures are to be generally avoided [11].

Similar to Acute lung injury in non-IPF lungs precipitated by triggers such as aspiration, post-operative, medication etc., exacerbation in IPF can be sub-categorized as either "triggered" when a known precipitating etiology is documented or "Idiopathic" when no such etiology is apparent [11].

The new definition also replaced the 30-day time restriction for the acute deterioration to "typically or generally of less than one-month duration" [11]. The phrase "typically less than 1 month" was included to provide precision but allow for the inclusion of exceptions that clinicians believe represent acute exacerbations [11]. A more flexible time interval may lead to "heterogeneity" among clinicians and clinical trial endpoint definitions for acute exacerbation [11].

3. Epidemiology

The incidence of acute exacerbations is variably reported in literature. This is because exacerbations could be more common in certain populations like more elderly people who are also likely to have severe disease, inconsistent definitions and its use, statistical design, follow up time and other factors [2, 9]. Exacerbations are less common in mild to moderate disease compared to severe disease [3, 14]. Reporting can vary depending on the type of study as well. Prospective trials may lack sufficient data to report all exacerbations [2, 4, 8], typically include younger patients with less comorbidities, with mild to moderate disease and therefore may under report incidence [15]. Retrospective studies may over report depending on the criteria used, by including events with pulmonary embolism, heart failure etc. [2, 13, 16].

Suspected exacerbations, which may not satisfy the definition of definitive AE-IPF are also important as they are associated with poor outcomes [4].

A meta-analysis analyzed six trials and reported acute exacerbation rate of 41 acute exacerbations per 1000 patient/years [14]. Rate of acute exacerbations were much lower in trials that included only mild to moderate disease [14].

In a retrospective study from Korea, which included 461 patients with IPF of which 269 cases were biopsy-proven and the median follows up period was 22.9 months, acute exacerbation occurred in 96 (20.8%) patients, and 17 (17.7%) of those acute exacerbation patients experienced multiple episodes of acute exacerbations (range 2–3 episodes). The incidence of acute exacerbation was noted to be 14.2, 18.8 and 20.7 percent at the end of 1, 2 and 3 years respectively [17].

It is to be noted that exacerbation of IPF may even occur in individuals with limited fibrosis and well-preserved lung function [2]. In the STEP-IPF trail, definite AE-IPF was reported as 40 per 1000 patient-years. However, the combined definite and suspected AE-IPF increased the exacerbation rate to 200 per 1000 patient-year [2, 4, 8, 13].

There have been reports of increased rate of AE-IPF in people of Asian descent in the far east such as Japan and Korea, however this has not been proven by randomized control trials [7, 8, 18].

4. Risk factors and pathophysiology

There are many risk factors for acute exacerbation. However, the most important risk factor is advanced disease [2, 14]. Other factors described in literature include low Forced vital capacity [8, 17], recent decline in FVC [19, 20], Low diffusion capacity for carbon monoxide [4], low 6 min walk test [4], pulmonary hypertension [21], poor baseline oxygenation [4, 22], increased dyspnea score [4], younger age group [2], presence of concurrent coronary artery disease [4], higher body mass index [22], previous history of acute exacerbation of IPF [19, 23].

Some important triggers for acute exacerbation have been described.

4.1 Infection

Infections are very common causes of respiratory deterioration. Exacerbations are more common in winter and spring season [24] and in those who are immunosuppressed [2, 25]. Postmortem analysis, multiplex polymerase chain reaction (PCR), pan viral micro array, high output cDNA sequencing and other techniques have demonstrated that infectious etiology is incriminated in many but not all acute exacerbations [23]. Based on the cumulative evidence which demonstrates infection to be causing some but not all acute exacerbations, it is thought to be an important but not exclusive trigger for precipitating acute exacerbations.

4.2 Silent aspiration of gastric contents

Aspiration of gastric contents has been postulated to be a causative factor for IPF and exacerbations in IPF.

In a case control study involving 24 acute exacerbations and 30 controls, Pepsin level in Broncho alveolar lavage (BAL) was found to be fairly commonly present, suggestive of gastric aspiration being fairly common in IPF.8 of the 24 acute exacerbation of IPF patients had very high levels of Pepsin suggesting that aspiration of gastric contents could be a contributor for acute exacerbation [26].

In a study involving 32 patients with asymmetric idiopathic pulmonary fibrosis (AIPF) compared with 64 matched controls with symmetrical IPF, Gastro esophageal reflux disease (GERD) and AE-IPF was significantly higher in patients with AIPF with the left side being less commonly involved [27].

On the contrary, in a post hoc analysis of the two Phase III randomized placebocontrolled INPULSIS trials of Nintedanib in patients with IPF, the rate of decline of FVC in the placebo group was much higher in patients who were taking an antacid (Proton pump inhibitor or H2-receptor antagonists) at baseline when compared to those who were not [difference of − 47.5 mL/year (95% CI: −105.1, 10.1); p = 0.1057] [28].

The data as it is apparent, that although gastro esophageal reflex has been widely debated to be causative, is not very definitive. Therefore, it can be likely that the aspiration of gastro esophageal contents can trigger acute exacerbations like infections but is not the sole causative factor.

4.3 Surgery and other interventions

Many surgical procedures like bronchoscopy and BAL, lung biopsy, lung resection, non-thoracic surgery and others can precipitate acute exacerbation [24, 29–32]. The mechanism of action is unclear but could be related to stress like volutrauma, barotrauma, free oxygen radicals, or intra operative fluid balance.

4.4 Air pollution

Air pollution can be a cause for interstitial lung disease. In a retrospective south Korean longitudinal cohort, out of 505 IPF patients 436 patients were included in the final analysis. 75 patients experienced at least one exacerbation. There were 89 acute exacerbation events occurring over 1699 patient-years, for an incidence rate of 5.2 exacerbations per 100 patient-years [23].

Air pollution data for each of the five pollutants Ozone (O3), Nitrogen di oxide (NO2), particles with a 50% cut-off aerodynamic diameter of <10 μm (PM10), sulfur dioxide (SO2) and carbon monoxide (CO) were measured prospectively at Tele-Monitoring-Systems (TMS) situated throughout Korea. Each TMS recorded hourly measurements of each pollutant during the study period. Mean and maximum exposures of all these 5 pollutants were recorded over the 42-day period prior to the exacerbation period. Acute exacerbation of IPF was significantly associated with important measurement metrics of O3 and NO2 during the exposure period. Mean Ozone and Nitrogen dioxide levels were weakly correlated; however, both were statistically significant independent predictors of AE-IPF [23].

4.5 Medications

Medications can provoke respiratory deterioration in interstitial pneumonia which closely resembles acute exacerbation. Such drugs include everolimus, interferon-gamma and others [33, 34]. Drugs and surgery used to treat Lung cancer patients with interstitial pneumonia did not appear to cause more exacerbations compared to best supportive care and hence should not be withheld when treating Lung cancer with interstitial pneumonia patients [35].

As noted, there have been many triggers associated with acute exacerbation of IPF. However currently the most accepted theory is that exacerbation is thought to be "an acceleration of the underlying inflammatory fibro proliferative disease process". This theory is supported by markers of cell injury as well as genetic expressions.

In one study by Collard et al., 47 patients with acute exacerbation of IPF, 20 patients with stable IPF and 20 patients with acute lung injury were studied. Plasma from these patients were collected and measured for biomarkers of cell activity/injury-receptor for advanced glycation end (RAGE) products, surfactant protein D, KL-6, von Willebrand factor; systemic inflammation-Interleukin-6; and biomarkers of coagulation/fibrinolysis-protein C, thrombomodulin, plasminogen activator inhibitor-1. Plasma from patients with AE-IPF showed higher levels of markers of type II alveolar epithelial cell injury/proliferation, endothelial cell injury, and coagulation/fibrinolysis very much like stable IPF but the response was much more exaggerated. This biomarker profile was different from patients with acute lung injury which was consistent with type I alveolar epithelial injury [36].

In another study, RNA was extracted from 23 stable IPF lungs, 8 IPF lungs with acute exacerbation of IPF and 15 control lungs. The gene expressions were studied. Results indicated that 579 genes were differentially expressed between stable IPF and acute exacerbation of IPF. Functional analysis of these genes was not suggestive of infectious or inflammatory etiology. Gene expression patterns in acute exacerbations of IPF and IPF samples were quite similar and different from the control lung arm [37].

Other immunological theories have also been proposed. Annexin 1 is an antigen found in human body which is increased in patients who have AE of IPF [38]. This antigen can induce both humoral and cell mediated immune responses and certain parts of this antigen have been implicated in the pathogenesis of AE of IPF [38]. Certain molecular studies have also been performed. Heat shock protein 47 (HSP47), has been studied and found to be a good bio marker for collagen production and secretion [39]. In studies comparing stable and AE-IPF patients, serum HSP47 were significantly elevated in AE-IPF patients in comparison to stable IPF patients [39]. Ironically patients who have anti-HSP70 autoantibodies in smaller studies have much poor prognosis due to AE of IPF when compared to controls or even those patients who have IPF but negative anti-HSP70 autoantibodies [40, 41].

Epithelial damage and impaired healing by abundance fibrosis has been an important theory that tries to explain the pathologic damage in IPF patients. When compared to IPF patients, patients with AE of IPF have higher bio markers of neutrophilic damage such as Alpha-defensins which are produced by activated neutrophils [37, 42] and also increased levels of Fibrocytes have been noted which have been found to be associated with worser outcomes in patients with AE of IPF [42, 43].

5. Clinical features

Patients present with worsening respiratory symptoms generally which are less than 30 days in duration. It consists of cough, worsening dyspnea especially on exertion, fever, malaise, and other flu like symptoms. Criteria for diagnosis include PaO2/FiO2 ratio < 225 or a decrease in PaO2 of $\geq$10 mmHg over time [8, 16].

Physical examination is consistent with IPF including bibasilar crackles on auscultation, but with increased respiratory rate [37].

Laboratory testing and imaging are directed to rule out other differentials like congestive heart failure, Myocardial infarction, pulmonary embolism, pulmonary hypertension, pulmonary infections etc. [2, 8]. Accordingly, complete blood count, B-type natriuretic peptide, C-reactive protein, chemistry profile including Blood urea nitrogen and serum creatinine can be performed along with highly sensitive troponins. Laboratory values are consistent with an infectious or inflammatory process but there is no evidence of infection on Blood culture, Urine antigen tests or Broncho alveolar lavage (BAL) if these tests are undertaken [8]. BAL if performed typically shows neutrophilic predominance [8]. BNP is typically elevated in heart failure and pulmonary hypertension [44]. Echo may be beneficial in heart failure and pulmonary hypertension [44]. CRP is typically elevated in infections and inflammation [44]. Pro calcitonin can guide when infection is suspected and even helping with limiting duration of antibiotic use [45]. D-dimer and CT pulmonary angiogram can help with ruling in or ruling out Pulmonary embolism [44].

High resolution computed tomography (HRCT) reveals bilateral ground glass or consolidative opacities superimposed on a background of typical HRCT features of IPF which includes bibasilar reticular opacities, honeycomb changes, and traction bronchiectasis [2].

Acute exacerbation of IPF is essentially a clinical diagnosis aided by predominantly noninvasive test. Although surgical biopsy can be performed for diagnosis which may show diffuse alveolar damage, the mortality and morbidity in the acute situation appear to be prohibitively high and not recommended [46].

6. Treatment and prognosis

Treatment is primarily supportive in nature.

Supplemental oxygen consisting of low flow and high flow oxygen can be used to keep Oxygen saturation (Spo2) more than 92%. Noninvasive ventilation mechanical ventilation (NIMV) and Mechanical ventilation (MV) is used as needed.

In a retrospective review of 19 hospitalized patients with IPF and AE, 1/3rd of patients had an infectious etiology, the percentage of patients who were discharged alive was 37% and only 14.8% of patients were alive at 1 year [47]. Patients with IPF experience AE very commonly. In IPF, about 40% of patients may die due to AE [48, 49]. In another observational study of 112 patients, 56 patients (42.9%) died due to AE [48]. The five-year survival rate of all patients with IPF was 38.3% and the Median survival time was 3.1 years post diagnosis. However, in patients who had an AE, the five-year survival rate was 10.7% and median survival time was 0.6 years [48].

In a pooled data consisting of nine studies, including 135 patients who were intubated for AE of IPF the cumulative mortality was 118 (87%) and short-term mortality (within 3 months of discharge) was 127 (94%) [50]. Therefore AE of IPF is not only common, but also a very poor predictor of survival. Based on these observations, the 2011 IPF guidelines discouraged MV in the vast majority and recommended its use in a selective minority of patients after careful weighing of risks and benefits [11]. However, this data pertains to a time period before 2007. In a study that reported US national data of 1703 patients who received Mechanical ventilation (MV)and 778 patients who received Noninvasive mechanical ventilation (NIMV), mortality was about 50% in those who received MV compared to 30% for those who received NIMV. The mortality of IPF patients treated with MV improved from 58.4% in 2006 to 49.3% in 2012 which was significant [51]. Overall this is suggestive that survival of patients treated with MV has seen a marginal improvement which could be due to various factors such as relative changes in diagnostic criteria and their use, difference in variables used and study design, differences in the severity of disease (patients with decreased FVC have poorer prognosis), judicious selection of patients who were placed on MV and widespread adoption and use of lung protective ventilation strategies [52]. Hence it is imperative that well informed discussions relating to advance care directives are made at the time of diagnosis and re visited when hospitalized [50]. In patients who are candidates for Lung transplant, the use of mechanical ventilation and extra corporeal membrane oxygenation, can be effective and lifesaving [11, 52–55].

Ventilator induced lung injury (VILI) secondary to use of MV results in lung damage and poor prognosis [52]. In IPF, the lungs are fibrotic and non-compliant. Lower PEEP may be more beneficial and protective along with low tidal volume ventilation, hence minimizing both volutrauma and barotrauma [52, 56]. NIMV and high flow oxygen are being increasingly used and may be beneficial [56, 57]. Both NIMV and High flow Oxygen could be beneficial in patients who are not appropriate or choose to forego intubation, the survival may be the same with both modalities [57, 58], with high flow nasal oxygen being better tolerated, allowing patients to even eat and drink [57–59]. Hence they could be very effective means for palliative care [57, 58].

In patients who undergo thoracic surgery, VILI may be a potential etiological mechanism and can be minimized by the aforementioned lung protective ventilation including reducing lung volume, low PEEP, low partial pressure of inspired oxygen (Fio2), and less invasive surgical techniques [52, 56, 60, 61].

Symptoms such as dyspnea are treated with a palliative intent [8, 11]. Oxygen and opioids can also be given for symptom control [8, 11].

In IPF, a combination of inflammation, epithelial cell injury, fibro proliferative repair, and tissue remodeling which interact with the coagulation system help characterize IPF as a procoagulant state [62]. The use of therapeutic anticoagulation such as Warfarin or Alfa-Thrombomodulin has proven to be either harmful or non-beneficial in well conducted studies [63–65]. There is no evidence supporting therapeutic anticoagulation in patients experiencing acute exacerbation [63]. Nevertheless, patients with IPF have almost twice the risk of venous thromboembolism compared to general population and hence pharmacological venous thromboprophylaxis should be routinely used in hospitalized patients [66, 67].

There is not enough evidence of protective role from the use of antacids, but patients who are already using them can continue with their use [68, 69]. Evidence is often contradictory if antacids protect or may potentiate or worsen AE of IPF [70, 71].

Corticosteroids have been used extensively but the practice is driven by expert opinion and anecdotal reports and not driven by good data. Expert guidelines give a weak recommendation to the use of steroids [2, 6]. Acute IPF is characterized by high degree of inflammation with areas of diffuse alveolar damage secondary to Acute Lung injury and organizing pneumonia [9]. Therefore, the use of high dose steroids is intuitively thought to be beneficial [9, 72–74], in spite of absence of good data from randomized control trials [9]. Dosage and duration are also not well defined in literature, although it is typical to use initially high dose corticosteroids followed by a rapid tapering course, as longer duration of steroids may be harmful in IPF [9, 62]. In EXAFIP, a randomized control trial comparing Cyclophosphamide with corticosteroids against placebo with corticosteroids in AE of IPF, the steroid regimen used in all patients was Methylprednisolone 10 mg/kg per day for 3 days followed by a progressive taper to 10 mg per day for patients above 65 kg and 7·5 mg per day for patients below 65 kg at the end of 6 months [75]. Similarly in a RCT involving 77 patients in Japan, Alpha-Thrombomodulin (ART-123) was compared against placebo. All patients received glucocorticoids in two courses of pulse Methylprednisolone (500–1000 mg/day) for 3 days followed by Prednisolone 0.5–1.0 mg/kg/day for 4 days followed by gradual taper [64]. Smaller retrospective studies have shown that using high dose of glucocorticoids used in first 30 days prevent recurrence of exacerbation when compared to lower doses in the same duration or after 30 days but this has not been substantiated by other studies [76, 77]. The use of high dose steroids has been noted to increase survival in non-IPF exacerbation of Interstitial lung disease [76]. It is noteworthy that some studies and even guidelines recommend using no immunosuppressives in select patients, as mortality was no better in the immunosuppressed group when compared to the non-immunosuppressed, with higher incidence of infection in the immune suppressed group, especially in severe disease [11, 14].

Concomitant Immunosuppressive therapy with steroids have also been used and the evidence base for this practice is also not very sound [2, 48]. While treatments such as Alfa-Thrombomodulin and Cyclophosphamide along with concomitant glucocorticoids have been subjected to randomized control trials and have not been shown to improve outcomes [64, 75], others do not have much evidence as they were too small, were uncontrolled, used historical data as control or had no control arm [2]. The latter studies have used medications like Tacrolimus, Cyclosporin-A, Rituximab combined with plasma exchange, Intravenous Immunoglobulin, and polymyxin B-immobilized fiber column (PMX) [6]. Other medications that have been used include Acetylcysteine as standalone therapy, sildenafil, bosentan, interferon-gamma 1b, warfarin, ambrisentan, and imatinib [8].

In a small retrospective study consisting of 11 patients in each group, Corticosteroids alone were compared with Cyclosporin-A and Corticosteroids. The mortality was similar in each group but the Cyclosporin-A group appeared to have longer survival [78]. However in a larger retrospective review with 384 patients in

Cyclosporin-A and high dose Corticosteroids and 7605 patients treated with high dose Corticosteroids alone in Japan, no change in survival was noted [79].

Other considerations include empiric treatment of a course of antibiotics since infectious etiology can be treated but cannot be ruled out conclusively in the vast majority of cases [2]. Procalcitonin has been used in clinical trials and can reduce the duration of antibiotics (8.7 ± 6.6 compared to 14.2 ± 5.2 days in the routine treatment group), without any effect on treatment success, mortality rate, days of hospitalization and ventilation therapy [45]. Tacrolimus, an immunosuppressive drug used widely in solid organ transplant patients including Lung transplant was found to have beneficial survival effects and protection against future exacerbations in small retrospective studies, with lack of data from better designed controlled studies [80]. Direct hemoperfusion with Polymyxin B immobilized fiber column (PMX-DHP) has been used in AE of IPF to absorb endotoxins and reactive oxygen species, among other toxic substances, as well as selectively remove activated neutrophils and preventing activation of monocytes with a goal to limit endothelial damage [81, 82]. PMX-DHP may act by adsorbing harmful cytokines such as vascular endothelial growth factor and may have anti-fibrotic effect [83, 84]. The adsorption of proinflammatory, profibrotic and proangiogenic cytokines is postulated to be an important mechanistic action of PMX-DHP [83]. The use of PMX-DHP along with Corticosteroids has demonstrated improvement in oxygenation, with possible improvement in survival in a multicentric Japanese retrospective study with 73 patient who had AE of IPF [82]. There is a prevailing hypothesis that auto antibodies may have a role in IPF progression. Removal of these auto antibodies by plasma exchange and Rituximab followed by IVIG subsequently may be beneficial in AE-IPF [62, 85]. A small pilot study involving 11 patients has shown the safety and possible efficacy, paving way for a Phase 3 randomized control trial [85].

Interestingly in a retrospective study, patients who were not on any immunosuppression had better survival than those who were on immunosuppression [5].

7. Prognostic score

There has been considerable interest in developing prognostication scores for AE of IPF. A number of markers have been used in different studies and Forced vital capacity %, Diffusion capacity for Carbon monoxide, Pao2/Fio2 (P/F) ratio, HRCT patterns, Acute Physiology and Chronic Health Evaluation II score (APACHE II), Glasgow prognostic score and serum biomarkers like C-reactive protein (CRP), Krebs von den Lungen-6 (KL-6) have all been considered [86]. In a retrospective study of 108 patients, a lower FVC % at baseline (1 year before AE) and P/F ratio on AE presentation were predictive of mortality [86]. In another study of 103 AE-IPF cases, a combination of P/F ratio less than 250 (P), CRP ≥ 5.5 (C), and diffuse HRCT pattern (radiological) (R), together called as PCR index was used to stratify and predict mortality at the end of 3 months [87]. In a systematic review and meta-analysis, 37 studies and 31 prognostic factors were analyzed [88]. Five independent variables after multivariate analysis were found to be helpful with prognostication namely APACHE II score, P/F ratio, LDH level, white blood cell (WBC) count, and oxygen therapy before AE [88]. Interestingly the latter did not find use of FVC or imaging scores to be helpful in terms of prognostication [88]. Prognostication scores and models are certainly good research tools but not commonly used in clinical practise as no intervention other than good supportive care has been found to be useful.

8. Prevention

Prevention of exacerbation in IPF is the most effective strategy as we do not seem to have very effective therapies once the exacerbation gets underway. Avoidance of air pollutants [23], preventing infections like Streptococcal pneumonia and Influenza by vaccination [26, 61], general hygiene measures like handwashing again to prevent infections [52], and judicious use of antacids may be helpful strategies [68, 69].

Many medications have been tested, using prevention of acute exacerbation as an end point. Acetylcysteine monotherapy, bosentan, interferon-gamma, sildenafil, showed no effect [8]. Others like imatinib, ambrisentan, triple therapy (prednisone, azathioprine, acetylcysteine combination) and warfarin showed increased risk of exacerbation [8].

Azuma et al. studied 107 IPF patients in a phase 2 Randomized placebo-controlled trial comparing Pirfenidone and placebo. Although there were no acute exacerbations noted in the Pirfenidone arm compared to placebo [89], the same results could not be reproduced in a phase 3 RCT with 275 patients, showing no difference between the intervention and control arm [18]. In the large phase 3 RCT's, CAPACITY and ASCEND which compared Pirfenidone with placebo yet again, unfortunately AE of IPF as an end point was not studied [90, 91]. Nevertheless, a pooled analysis of the CAPACITY and ASCEND trial did reveal a reduction in non-elective respiratory related hospitalization favoring Pirfenidone [92]. Interestingly Pirfenidone in small studies has proven to be safe and effective in preventing exacerbations in peri operative period in patients who were given 2–4 weeks of medication prior to surgery and continued post operatively when compared against historical controls [93, 94]. Larger RCTs need to be performed for this promising intervention [94].

Another antifibrotic agent Nintedanib was studied after Pirfenidone, which showed a favorable effect against placebo for preventing AE of IPF in the phase 2 TOMORROW trial and phase 3 INPULSIS-2 trial, but no such effect was seen in the phase 3 INPULSIS-1 trial [95, 96]. However the pooled analysis of patients from TOMORROW and INPULSIS trials [6], consisting of 1231 patients (Nintedanib n = 723, placebo n = 508), the hazard ratio for time to first acute exacerbation was 0.53 (95% CI: 0.34, 0.83; p = 0.0047) favoring Nintedanib. The proportion of patients with ≥1 acute exacerbation was 4.6% in the Nintedanib group and 8.7% in the placebo group [6]. Nintedanib can be added after recovering from an exacerbation or continued if it was previously being used.

In a systematic review and meta-analysis, 12,956 patients were included comparing the use of anti fibrotics (Pirfenidone or Nintedanib) vs. nonuse of antifibrotics, which showed that the use of antifibrotics decreased all-cause mortality, RR 0.55 (95% CI, 0.45–0.66). The same review included seven studies involving 2002 treated and 1323 non-treated patients, and showed a decrease in AE, which was statistically significant for Nintedanib (RR 0.62 [95% CI, 0.43–0.89] but only non-significant decrease for Pirfenidone, RR of 0.57 (95% CI, 0.29–1.12) [1].

Overall, the evidence favors Nintedanib over Pirfenidone in terms of preventing AE of IPF. However, there are no head to head comparisons between these two approved medications and real world data could produce results to the contrary [97]. Hence it would be prudent to plan design and conduct appropriate RCT that would give an unambiguous answer to this very important question.

9. Conclusion

Episodes of Acute exacerbation are important events in the disease course of IPF. Up to 40% of deaths in IPF are caused by acute exacerbations. After the initial diagnosis, the median survival of patients with acute exacerbation was much shorter (15.5 months) than that of patients without respiratory deterioration (60.6 months). The 5 year rate of survival of patients with acute exacerbation was 18.4%, whereas 50.0% of patients without respiratory deterioration survived.

While medications like Nintedanib can slow down progression of disease and prevent exacerbations, once diagnosed it has no known effective treatment. Hence more research is needed to alter the disease course of IPF as well as prevent the occurrence of these exacerbations which invariably is an indicator of poor prognosis.

Author details

Nitesh Kumar Jain[1], Shikha Jain[2], Hisham Ahmed Mushtaq[1], Anwar Khedr[1], Thoyaja Koritala[1], Aysun Tekin[3], Ramesh Adhikari[4], Anupam Sule[5], Samir Gautam[6], Vishwanath Pattan[7], Vikas Bansal[3], Ali Rabaan[8], Kovid Trivedi[9], Amos Lal[3], Brian Bartlett[1], Abbas Jama[1], Aishwarya Reddy Korsapati[10], Mohamed Hassan[1], Simon Zec[3], Adham Mohsen[11], Amit Munshi Sharma[12], Ibtisam Rauf[13], Mikael Mir[14], Lia Nandi[15], Mool Chand[1], Hariprasad Reddy Korsapati[1], Rahul Kashyap[3], Salim Surani[16*] and Syed Anjum Khan[1]

1 Mayo Clinic Health System, Mankato, USA

2 MVJ Medical College and Research Hospital, Hoskote, India

3 Mayo Clinic, Rochester, USA

4 Franciscan Health, Lafayette, USA

5 St Joseph Mercy Oakland Hospital, Pontiac, USA

6 Johns Hopkins Hospital, Baltimore, USA

7 Wyoming Medical Center, Casper, USA

8 Johns Hopkins Aramco Healthcare, Dhahran, Saudi Arabia

9 Salem Pulmonary Associates, Salem, USA

10 University of Buckingham Medical School, London, UK

11 Unity Point Health, Sioux City, USA

12 Geisinger Community Medical Center, Scranton, USA

13 St George's University, True Blue, Grenada

14 University of Minnesota, Duluth, Minnesota

15 Kasturba Medical College of Manipal, Karnataka, India

16 Texas A&M University, Corpus Christi, USA

*Address all correspondence to: srsurani@gmail.com or srsurani@hotmail.com

IntechOpen

References

[1] Petnak T, Lertjitbanjong P, Thongprayoon C, Moua T. Impact of Antifibrotic therapy on mortality and acute exacerbation in idiopathic pulmonary fibrosis: A systematic review and Meta-analysis. Chest. 2021;**160**(5): 1751-1763. DOI: 10.1016/j.chest.2021. 06.049

[2] Collard HR, Ryerson CJ, Corte TJ, Jenkins G, Kondoh Y, Lederer DJ, et al. Acute exacerbation of idiopathic pulmonary fibrosis. An international working group report. American Journal of Respiratory and Critical Care Medicine. 2016;**194**:265-275. DOI: 10.1164/rccm.201604-0801CI

[3] Al-hameed FM, Sharma S. Outcome of patients admitted to intensive care unit for acute exacerbation of idiopathic pulmonary fibrosis. Canadian Respiratory Journal. 2004;**11**:379723. DOI: 10.1155/2004/379723

[4] Collard HR, Yow E, Richeldi L, Anstrom KJ, Glazer C. Suspected acute exacerbation of idiopathic pulmonary fibrosis as an outcome measure in clinical trials. Respiratory Research. 2013;**14**:73. DOI: 10.1186/1465-9921-14-73

[5] Papiris SA, Kagouridis K, Kolilekas L, Papaioannou AI, Roussou A, Triantafillidou C, et al. Survival in idiopathic pulmonary fibrosis acute exacerbations: The non-steroid approach. BMC Pulmonary Medicine. 2015;**15**:162. DOI: 10.1186/ s12890-015-0146-4

[6] Richeldi L, Cottin V, du Bois RM, Selman M, Kimura T, Bailes Z, et al. Nintedanib in patients with idiopathic pulmonary fibrosis: Combined evidence from the TOMORROW and INPULSIS (®) trials. Respiratory Medicine. 2016;**113**:74-79. DOI: 10.1016/j. rmed.2016.02.001

[7] Richeldi L, du Bois RM, Raghu G, Azuma A, Brown KK, Costabel U, et al. Efficacy and safety of nintedanib in idiopathic pulmonary fibrosis. The New England Journal of Medicine. 2014;**370**:2071-2082. DOI: 10.1056/ NEJMoa1402584

[8] Leuschner G, Behr J. Acute exacerbation in interstitial lung disease. Frontiers in Medicine. 2017;**4**:1751-1763. DOI: 10.3389/fmed.2017.00176

[9] Ryerson CJ, Cottin V, Brown KK, Collard HR. Acute exacerbation of idiopathic pulmonary fibrosis: Shifting the paradigm. European Respiratory Journal. 2015;**46**:512-520. DOI: 10.1183/13993003.00419-2015

[10] Collard HR, Moore BB, Flaherty KR, Brown KK, Kaner RJ, King TE, et al. Acute exacerbations of idiopathic pulmonary fibrosis. American Journal of Respiratory and Critical Care Medicine. 2007;**176**:636-643. DOI: 10.1164/rccm.200703-463PP

[11] Raghu G, Collard HR, Egan JJ, Martinez FJ, Behr J, Brown KK, et al. Fibrosis AEJACoIP: An official ATS/ ERS/JRS/ALAT statement: Idiopathic pulmonary fibrosis: Evidence-based guidelines for diagnosis and management. American Journal of Respiratory and Critical Care Medicine. 2011;**183**:788-824. DOI: 10.1164/ rccm.2009-040GL

[12] Thomson CC, Duggal A, Bice T, Lederer DJ, Wilson KC, Raghu G. 2018 clinical practice guideline summary for clinicians: Diagnosis of idiopathic pulmonary fibrosis. Annals of the American Thoracic Society. 2019;**16**: 285-290. DOI: 10.1513/AnnalsATS. 201809-604CME

[13] Hambly N, Cox G, Kolb M. Acute exacerbations of idiopathic pulmonary fibrosis: Tough to define; tougher to manage. European Respiratory Journal. 2017;**49**:1700811. DOI: 10.1183/ 13993003.00811-2017

[14] Atkins CP, Loke YK, Wilson AM. Outcomes in idiopathic pulmonary fibrosis: A meta-analysis from placebo controlled trials. Respiratory Medicine. 2014;**108**:376-387. DOI: 10.1016/j.rmed.2013.11.007

[15] Kim DS. Acute exacerbations in patients with idiopathic pulmonary fibrosis. Respiratory Research. 2013;**14**:86. DOI: 10.1186/1465-9921-14-86

[16] Kim DS, Park JH, Park BK, Lee JS, Nicholson AG, Colby T. Acute exacerbation of idiopathic pulmonary fibrosis: Frequency and clinical features. The European Respiratory Journal. 2006;**27**:143-150. DOI: 10.1183/09031936.06.00114004

[17] Song JW, Hong S-B, Lim C-M, Koh Y, Kim DS. Acute exacerbation of idiopathic pulmonary fibrosis: Incidence, risk factors and outcome. European Respiratory Journal. 2011;**37**:356-363. DOI: 10.1183/09031936.00159709

[18] Taniguchi H, Ebina M, Kondoh Y, Ogura T, Azuma A, Suga M, et al. Pirfenidone in idiopathic pulmonary fibrosis. European Respiratory Journal. 2010;**35**:821-829. DOI: 10.1183/09031936.00005209

[19] Reichmann WM, Yu YF, Macaulay D, Wu EQ, Nathan SD. Change in forced vital capacity and associated subsequent outcomes in patients with newly diagnosed idiopathic pulmonary fibrosis. BMC Pulmonary Medicine. 2015;**15**:167. DOI: 10.1186/s12890-015-0161-5

[20] Kondoh Y, Taniguchi H, Ebina M, Azuma A, Ogura T, Taguchi Y, et al. Risk factors for acute exacerbation of idiopathic pulmonary fibrosis— Extended analysis of pirfenidone trial in Japan. Respiratory Investigation. 2015;**53**:271-278. DOI: 10.1016/j.resinv.2015.04.005

[21] Judge EP, Fabre A, Adamali HI, Egan JJ. Acute exacerbations and pulmonary hypertension in advanced idiopathic pulmonary fibrosis. The European Respiratory Journal. 2012;**40**:93-100. DOI: 10.1183/09031936.00115511

[22] Kondoh Y, Taniguchi H, Katsuta T, Kataoka K, Kimura T, Nishiyama O, et al. Risk factors of acute exacerbation of idiopathic pulmonary fibrosis. Sarcoidosis, Vasculitis, and Diffuse Lung Diseases. 2010;**27**:103-110

[23] Johannson KA, Vittinghoff E, Lee K, Balmes JR, Ji W, Kaplan GG, et al. Acute exacerbation of idiopathic pulmonary fibrosis associated with air pollution exposure. The European Respiratory Journal. 2014;**43**:1124-1131. DOI: 10.1183/09031936.00122213

[24] Sakamoto S, Homma S, Mun M, Fujii T, Kurosaki A, Yoshimura K. Acute exacerbation of idiopathic interstitial pneumonia following lung surgery in 3 of 68 consecutive patients: A retrospective study. Internal Medicine. 2011;**50**:77-85. DOI: 10.2169/internalmedicine.50.3390

[25] Petrosyan F, Culver DA, Reddy AJ. Role of bronchoalveolar lavage in the diagnosis of acute exacerbations of idiopathic pulmonary fibrosis: A retrospective study. BMC Pulmonary Medicine. 2015;**15**:70. DOI: 10.1186/s12890-015-0066-3

[26] Lee JS, Song JW, Wolters PJ, Elicker BM, King TE Jr, Kim DS, et al. Bronchoalveolar lavage pepsin in acute exacerbation of idiopathic pulmonary fibrosis. The European Respiratory Journal. 2012;**39**:352-358. DOI: 10.1183/09031936.00050911

[27] Tcherakian C, Cottin V, Brillet PY, Freynet O, Naggara N, Carton Z, et al. Progression of idiopathic pulmonary fibrosis: Lessons from asymmetrical disease. Thorax. 2011;**66**:226-231. DOI: 10.1136/thx.2010.137190

[28] Costabel U, Behr J, Crestani B, Stansen W, Schlenker-Herceg R,

Stowasser S, et al. Anti-acid therapy in idiopathic pulmonary fibrosis: Insights from the INPULSIS (R) trials. Respiratory Research. 2018;**19**:167. DOI: 10.1186/s12931-018-0866-0

[29] Hiwatari N, Shimura S, Takishima T, Shirato K. Bronchoalveolar lavage as a possible cause of acute exacerbation in idiopathic pulmonary fibrosis patients. The Tohoku Journal of Experimental Medicine. 1994;**174**:379-386. DOI: 10.1620/tjem.174.379

[30] Bando M, Ohno S, Hosono T, Yanase K, Sato Y, Sohara Y, et al. Risk of acute exacerbation after video-assisted Thoracoscopic lung biopsy for interstitial lung disease. J Bronchology Interv Pulmonol. 2009;**16**:229-235. DOI: 10.1097/LBR.0b013e3181b767cc

[31] Bando T, Date H. Surgical treatment of lung cancer in patients with pulmonary fibrosis. Kyobu Geka. 2012;**65**:714-719

[32] Ghatol A, Ruhl AP, Danoff SK. Exacerbations in idiopathic pulmonary fibrosis triggered by pulmonary and nonpulmonary surgery: A case series and comprehensive review of the literature. Lung. 2012;**190**:373-380. DOI: 10.1007/s00408-012-9389-5

[33] Malouf MA, Hopkins P, Snell G, Glanville AR. Everolimus in IPFSI: An investigator-driven study of everolimus in surgical lung biopsy confirmed idiopathic pulmonary fibrosis. Respirology. 2011;**16**:776-783. DOI: 10.1111/j.1440-1843.2011.01955.x

[34] Honore I, Nunes H, Groussard O, Kambouchner M, Chambellan A, Aubier M, et al. Acute respiratory failure after interferon-gamma therapy of end-stage pulmonary fibrosis. American Journal of Respiratory and Critical Care Medicine. 2003;**167**:953-957. DOI: 10.1164/rccm.200208-818CR

[35] Minegishi Y, Takenaka K, Mizutani H, Sudoh J, Noro R, Okano T,

et al. Exacerbation of idiopathic interstitial pneumonias associated with lung cancer therapy. Internal Medicine. 2009;**48**:665-672. DOI: 10.2169/internalmedicine.48.1650

[36] Collard HR, Calfee CS, Wolters PJ, Song JW, Hong SB, Brady S, et al. Plasma biomarker profiles in acute exacerbation of idiopathic pulmonary fibrosis. American Journal of Physiology. Lung Cellular and Molecular Physiology. 2010;**299**:L3-L7. DOI: 10.1152/ajplung.90637.2008

[37] Konishi K, Gibson KF, Lindell KO, Richards TJ, Zhang Y, Dhir R, et al. Gene expression profiles of acute exacerbations of idiopathic pulmonary fibrosis. American Journal of Respiratory and Critical Care Medicine. 2009;**180**:167-175. DOI: 10.1164/rccm.200810-1596OC

[38] Kurosu K, Takiguchi Y, Okada O, Yumoto N, Sakao S, Tada Y, et al. Identification of annexin 1 as a novel autoantigen in acute exacerbation of idiopathic pulmonary fibrosis. Journal of Immunology. 2008;**181**:756-767. DOI: 10.4049/jimmunol.181.1.756

[39] Kakugawa T, Yokota S-I, Ishimatsu Y, Hayashi T, Nakashima S, Hara S, et al. Serum heat shock protein 47 levels are elevated in acute exacerbation of idiopathic pulmonary fibrosis. Cell Stress & Chaperones. 2013;**18**:581-590. DOI: 10.1007/s12192-013-0411-5

[40] Kahloon RA, Xue J, Bhargava A, Csizmadia E, Otterbein L, Kass DJ, et al. Patients with idiopathic pulmonary fibrosis with antibodies to heat shock protein 70 have poor prognoses. American Journal of Respiratory and Critical Care Medicine. 2013;**187**:768-775. DOI: 10.1164/rccm.201203-0506OC

[41] Wells AU, Kelleher WP. Idiopathic pulmonary fibrosis pathogenesis and novel approaches to immunomodulation:

We must not be tyrannized by the PANTHER data. American Journal of Respiratory and Critical Care Medicine. 2013;**187**:677-679. DOI: 10.1164/rccm.201302-0336ed

[42] Antoniou KM, Wells AU. Acute exacerbations of idiopathic pulmonary fibrosis. Respiration. 2013;**86**:265-274. DOI: 10.1159/000355485

[43] Moeller A, Gilpin SE, Ask K, Cox G, Cook D, Gauldie J, et al. Circulating fibrocytes are an indicator of poor prognosis in idiopathic pulmonary fibrosis. American Journal of Respiratory and Critical Care Medicine. 2009;**179**:588-594. DOI: 10.1164/rccm.200810-1534OC

[44] Lynn M, Schnapp M, Timothy Whelan, MD: Acute exacerbations of idiopathic pulmonary fibrosis. Uptodate Inc. Kevin R, Flaherty M, Helen Hollingsworth MD, editors. 2022

[45] Ding J, Chen Z, Feng K. Procalcitonin-guided antibiotic use in acute exacerbations of idiopathic pulmonary fibrosis. International Journal of Medical Sciences. 2013;**10**:903-907. DOI: 10.7150/ijms.4972

[46] Hutchinson JP, Fogarty AW, TM MK, Hubbard RB. In-hospital mortality after surgical lung biopsy for interstitial lung disease in the United States. 2000 to 2011. American Journal of Respiratory and Critical Care Medicine. 2016;**193**:1161-1167. DOI: 10.1164/rccm.201508-1632OC

[47] Huie TJ, Olson AL, Cosgrove GP, Janssen WJ, Lara AR, Lynch DA, et al. A detailed evaluation of acute respiratory decline in patients with fibrotic lung disease: Aetiology and outcomes. Respirology. 2010;**15**:909-917. DOI: 10.1111/j.1440-1843.2010.01774.x

[48] Okamoto T, Ichiyasu H, Ichikado K, Muranaka H, Sato K, Okamoto S, et al. Clinical analysis of the acute exacerbation in patients with idiopathic pulmonary fibrosis. Nihon Kokyūki Gakkai Zasshi. 2006;**44**:359-367

[49] Natsuizaka M, Chiba H, Kuronuma K, Otsuka M, Kudo K, Mori M, et al. Epidemiologic survey of Japanese patients with idiopathic pulmonary fibrosis and investigation of ethnic differences. American Journal of Respiratory and Critical Care Medicine. 2014;**190**:773-779. DOI: 10.1164/rccm.201403-0566OC

[50] Mallick S. Outcome of patients with idiopathic pulmonary fibrosis (IPF) ventilated in intensive care unit. Respiratory Medicine. 2008;**102**:1355-1359. DOI: 10.1016/j.rmed.2008.06.003

[51] Rush B, Wiskar K, Berger L, Griesdale D. The use of mechanical ventilation in patients with idiopathic pulmonary fibrosis in the United States: A nationwide retrospective cohort analysis. Respiratory Medicine. 2016;**111**:72-76. DOI: 10.1016/j.rmed.2015.12.005

[52] Kondoh Y, Cottin V, Brown KK. Recent lessons learned in the management of acute exacerbation of idiopathic pulmonary fibrosis. European Respiratory Review. 2017;**26**. DOI: 10.1183/16000617.0050-2017

[53] Bozso S, Sidhu S, Garg M, Freed DH, Nagendran J. Canada's longest experience with extracorporeal membrane oxygenation as a bridge to lung transplantation: A case report. Transplantation Proceedings. 2015;**47**:186-189. DOI: 10.1016/j.transproceed.2014.10.039

[54] Umei N, Ichiba S, Sakamoto A. Idiopathic pulmonary fibrosis patient supported with extracorporeal membrane oxygenation for 403 days while waiting for a lung transplant: A case report. Respiratory Medicine Case Reports. 2018;**24**:86-88. DOI: 10.1016/j.rmcr.2018.04.015

[55] Marchioni A, Tonelli R, Ball L, Fantini R, Castaniere I, Cerri S, et al. Acute exacerbation of idiopathic pulmonary fibrosis: Lessons learned from acute respiratory distress syndrome? Critical Care. 2018;**22**:80. DOI: 10.1186/s13054-018-2002-4

[56] Fernandez-Perez ER, Yilmaz M, Jenad H, Daniels CE, Ryu JH, Hubmayr RD, et al. Ventilator settings and outcome of respiratory failure in chronic interstitial lung disease. Chest. 2008;**133**(5):1113-1119. DOI: 10.1378/chest.07-1481

[57] Kolb M, Bondue B, Pesci A, Miyazaki Y, Song JW, Bhatt NY, et al. Acute exacerbations of progressive-fibrosing interstitial lung diseases. European Respiratory Review. 2018;**27**. DOI: 10.1183/16000617.0071-2018

[58] Koyauchi T, Hasegawa H, Kanata K, Kakutani T, Amano Y, Ozawa Y, et al. Efficacy and tolerability of high-flow nasal cannula oxygen therapy for hypoxemic respiratory failure in patients with interstitial lung disease with do-not-intubate orders: A retrospective single-center study. Respiration. 2018;**96**:323-329. DOI: 10.1159/000489890

[59] Horio Y, Takihara T, Niimi K, Komatsu M, Sato M, Tanaka J, et al. High-flow nasal cannula oxygen therapy for acute exacerbation of interstitial pneumonia: A case series. Respiratory Investigation. 2016;**54**:125-129. DOI: 10.1016/j.resinv.2015.09.005

[60] Kondoh Y, Taniguchi H, Kitaichi M, et al. Acute exacerbation of interstitial pneumonia following surgical lung biopsy. Respiratory Medicine. 2006;**100**(10):1753-1759. DOI: 10.1016/j.rmed.2006.02.002

[61] Johannson K, Collard HR. Acute exacerbation of idiopathic pulmonary fibrosis: A proposal. Current Respiratory Care Reports. 2013;**2**. DOI: 10.1007/s13665-013-0065-x

[62] Juarez MM, Chan AL, Norris AG, Morrissey BM, Albertson TE. Acute exacerbation of idiopathic pulmonary fibrosis-a review of current and novel pharmacotherapies. Journal of Thoracic Disease. 2015;**7**:499-519. DOI: 10.3978/j.issn.2072-1439.2015.01.17

[63] Noth I, Anstrom KJ, Calvert SB, de Andrade J, Flaherty KR, Glazer C, et al. Idiopathic pulmonary fibrosis clinical research N: A placebo-controlled randomized trial of warfarin in idiopathic pulmonary fibrosis. American Journal of Respiratory and Critical Care Medicine. 2012;**186**:88-95. DOI: 10.1164/rccm.201202-0314OC

[64] Kondoh Y, Azuma A, Inoue Y, Ogura T, Sakamoto S, Tsushima K, et al. Thrombomodulin alfa for acute exacerbation of idiopathic pulmonary fibrosis. A randomized, double-blind placebo-controlled trial. American Journal of Respiratory and Critical Care Medicine. 2020;**201**:1110-1119. DOI: 10.1164/rccm.201909-1818OC

[65] Tomassetti S, Ruy JH, Gurioli C, Ravaglia C, Buccioli M, Tantalocco P, et al. The effect of anticoagulant therapy for idiopathic pulmonary fibrosis in real life practice. Sarcoidosis, Vasculitis, and Diffuse Lung Diseases. 2013;**30**:121-127

[66] Sprunger DB, Olson AL, Huie TJ, Fernandez-Perez ER, Fischer A, Solomon JJ, et al. Pulmonary fibrosis is associated with an elevated risk of thromboembolic disease. The European Respiratory Journal. 2012;**39**:125-132. DOI: 10.1183/09031936.00041411

[67] Boonpheng B, Ungprasert P. Risk of venous thromboembolism in patients with idiopathic pulmonary fibrosis: A systematic review and meta-analysis. Sarcoidosis, Vasculitis, and Diffuse Lung Diseases. 2018;**35**:109-114. DOI: 10.36141/svdld.v35i2.6213

[68] Jain NK, Khedr A, Mushtaq HA, Bartlett B, Lanz A, Zoesch G, et al. Gastroesophageal Reflux and Idiopathic Pulmonary Fibrosis. In: Idiopathic Pulmonary Fibrosis. London: IntechOpen; 2022. DOI: 10.5772/intechopen.102464

[69] Kreuter M, Spagnolo P, Wuyts W, Renzoni E, Koschel D, Bonella F, et al. Antacid therapy and disease progression in patients with idiopathic pulmonary fibrosis who received pirfenidone. Respiration. 2017;**93**:415-423

[70] Lee JS, Collard HR, Anstrom KJ, Martinez FJ, Noth I, Roberts RS, et al. Anti-acid treatment and disease progression in idiopathic pulmonary fibrosis: An analysis of data from three randomised controlled trials. The Lancet Respiratory Medicine. 2013;**1**:369-376. DOI: 10.1016/s2213-2600 (13)70105-x

[71] Raghu G, Wells AU, Nicholson AG, Richeldi L, Flaherty KR, Le Maulf F, et al. Effect of Nintedanib in subgroups of idiopathic pulmonary fibrosis by diagnostic criteria. American Journal of Respiratory and Critical Care Medicine. 2017;**195**:78-85. DOI: 10.1164/rccm.201602-0402OC

[72] Boyle AJ, Mac Sweeney R, McAuley DF. Pharmacological treatments in ARDS; a state-of-the-art update. BMC Medicine. 2013;**11**:166. DOI: 10.1186/1741-7015-11-166

[73] Meduri GU, Headley AS, Golden E, Carson SJ, Umberger RA, Kelso T, et al. Effect of prolonged methylprednisolone therapy in unresolving acute respiratory distress syndrome: A randomized controlled trial. Journal of the American Medical Association. 1998;**280**:159-165. DOI: 10.1001/jama.280.2.159

[74] Steinberg KP, Hudson LD, Goodman RB, Hough CL, Lanken PN, Hyzy R, et al. Efficacy and safety of corticosteroids for persistent acute respiratory distress syndrome. The New England Journal of Medicine. 2006;**354**:1671-1684. DOI: 10.1056/NEJMoa051693

[75] Naccache JM, Jouneau S, Didier M, Borie R, Cachanado M, Bourdin A, et al. Investigators E, the OrphaLung n: Cyclophosphamide added to glucocorticoids in acute exacerbation of idiopathic pulmonary fibrosis (EXAFIP): A randomised, double-blind, placebo-controlled, phase 3 trial. The Lancet Respiratory Medicine. 2022;**10**:26-34. DOI: 10.1016/S2213-2600 (21)00354-4

[76] Jang HJ, Yong SH, Leem AY, Lee SH, Kim SY, Lee SH, et al. Corticosteroid responsiveness in patients with acute exacerbation of interstitial lung disease admitted to the emergency department. Scientific Reports. 2021;**11**:5762. DOI: 10.1038/s41598-021-85539-1

[77] Yamazaki R, Nishiyama O, Saeki S, Sano H, Iwanaga T, Tohda Y. Initial therapeutic dose of corticosteroid for an acute exacerbation of IPF is associated with subsequent early recurrence of another exacerbation. Scientific Reports. 2021;**11**:5782. DOI: 10.1038/s41598-021-85234-1

[78] Sakamoto S, Homma S, Miyamoto A, Kurosaki A, Fujii T, Yoshimura K. Cyclosporin a in the treatment of acute exacerbation of idiopathic pulmonary fibrosis. Internal Medicine. 2010;**49**:109-115. DOI: 10.2169/internalmedicine.49.2359

[79] Aso S, Matsui H, Fushimi K, Yasunaga H. Effect of cyclosporine a on mortality after acute exacerbation of idiopathic pulmonary fibrosis. Journal of Thoracic Disease. 2018;**10**:5275-5282. DOI: 10.21037/jtd.2018.08.08

[80] Horita N, Akahane M, Okada Y, Kobayashi Y, Arai T, Amano I, et al. Tacrolimus and steroid treatment for acute exacerbation of idiopathic

pulmonary fibrosis. Internal Medicine. 2011;**50**:189-195. DOI: 10.2169/internalmedicine.50.4327

[81] Cruz DN, Antonelli M, Fumagalli R, Foltran F, Brienza N, Donati A, et al. Early use of polymyxin B hemoperfusion in abdominal septic shock: The EUPHAS randomized controlled trial. Journal of the American Medical Association. 2009;**301**:2445-2452. DOI: 10.1001/jama.2009.856

[82] Abe S, Azuma A, Mukae H, Ogura T, Taniguchi H, Bando M, et al. Polymyxin B-immobilized fiber column (PMX) treatment for idiopathic pulmonary fibrosis with acute exacerbation: A multicenter retrospective analysis. Internal Medicine. 2012;**51**:1487-1491. DOI: 10.2169/internalmedicine.51.6965

[83] Oishi K, Mimura-Kimura Y, Miyasho T, Aoe K, Ogata Y, Katayama H, et al. Association between cytokine removal by polymyxin B hemoperfusion and improved pulmonary oxygenation in patients with acute exacerbation of idiopathic pulmonary fibrosis. Cytokine. 2013;**61**:84-89. DOI: 10.1016/j.cyto.2012.08.032

[84] Tachibana K, Inoue Y, Nishiyama A, Sugimoto C, Matsumuro A, Hirose M, et al. Polymyxin-B hemoperfusion for acute exacerbation of idiopathic pulmonary fibrosis: Serum IL-7 as a prognostic marker. Sarcoidosis, Vasculitis, and Diffuse Lung Diseases. 2011;**28**:113-122

[85] Donahoe M, Valentine VG, Chien N, Gibson KF, Raval JS, Saul M, et al. Autoantibody-targeted treatments for acute exacerbations of idiopathic pulmonary fibrosis. PLoS One. 2015;**10**:e0127771. DOI: 10.1371/journal.pone.0127771

[86] Suzuki T, Hozumi H, Miyashita K, Kono M, Suzuki Y, Karayama M, et al. Prognostic classification in acute exacerbation of idiopathic pulmonary fibrosis: A multicentre retrospective cohort study. Scientific Reports. 2021;**11**:9120. DOI: 10.1038/s41598-021-88718-2

[87] Sakamoto S, Shimizu H, Isshiki T, Nakamura Y, Usui Y, Kurosaki A. Isobe K, Takai Y, Homma S: New risk scoring system for predicting 3-month mortality after acute exacerbation of idiopathic pulmonary fibrosis. Scientific Reports. 2022;**12**:1134. DOI: 10.1038/s41598-022-05138-6

[88] Kamiya H, Panlaqui OM. Systematic review and meta-analysis of prognostic factors of acute exacerbation of idiopathic pulmonary fibrosis. BMJ Open. 2020;**10**:e035420. DOI: 10.1136/bmjopen-2019-035420

[89] Azuma A, Nukiwa T, Tsuboi E, Suga M, Abe S, Nakata K, et al. Double-blind, placebo-controlled trial of pirfenidone in patients with idiopathic pulmonary fibrosis. American Journal of Respiratory and Critical Care Medicine. 2005;**171**:1040-1047. DOI: 10.1164/rccm.200404-571OC

[90] King TE Jr, Bradford WZ, Castro-Bernardini S, et al. A phase 3 trial of pirfenidone in patients with idiopathic pulmonary fibrosis. The New England Journal of Medicine. 2014;**370**:2083-2092. DOI: 10.1056/NEJMoa1402582

[91] Noble PW, Albera C, Bradford WZ, Costabel U, Glassberg MK, Kardatzke D, et al. Pirfenidone in patients with idiopathic pulmonary fibrosis (CAPACITY): Two randomised trials. Lancet. 2011;**377**:1760-1769. DOI: 10.1016/s0140-6736 (11)60405-4

[92] Ley B, Swigris J, Day BM, Stauffer JL, Raimundo K, Chou W, et al. Pirfenidone reduces respiratory-related hospitalizations in idiopathic pulmonary fibrosis. American Journal of Respiratory and Critical Care

Medicine. 2017;**196**:756-761.
DOI: 10.1164/rccm.201701-0091OC

[93] Iwata T, Yoshino I, Yoshida S, Ikeda N, Tsuboi M, Asato Y, et al. West Japan oncology G: A phase II trial evaluating the efficacy and safety of perioperative pirfenidone for prevention of acute exacerbation of idiopathic pulmonary fibrosis in lung cancer patients undergoing pulmonary resection: West Japan oncology group 6711 L (PEOPLE study). Respiratory Research. 2016;**17**:90-90. DOI: 10.1186/s12931-016-0398-4

[94] Iwata T, Yoshida S, Fujiwara T, Wada H, Nakajima T, Suzuki H, et al. Effect of perioperative Pirfenidone treatment in lung cancer patients with idiopathic pulmonary fibrosis. The Annals of Thoracic Surgery. 2016;**102**:1905-1910. DOI: 10.1016/j.athoracsur.2016.05.094

[95] Richeldi L, Costabel U, Selman M, Kim DS, Hansell DM, Nicholson AG, et al. Efficacy of a tyrosine kinase inhibitor in idiopathic pulmonary fibrosis. The New England Journal of Medicine. 2011;**365**:1079-1087. DOI: 10.1056/NEJMoa1103690

[96] Richeldi L, du Bois RM, Raghu G, Azuma A, Brown KK, Costabel U, et al. Efficacy and safety of Nintedanib in idiopathic pulmonary fibrosis. New England Journal of Medicine. 2014;**370**: 2071-2082. DOI: 10.1056/NEJMoa1402584

[97] Isshiki T, Sakamoto S, Yamasaki A, Shimizu H, Miyoshi S, Nakamura Y, et al. Incidence of acute exacerbation of idiopathic pulmonary fibrosis in patients receiving antifibrotic agents: Real-world experience. Respiratory Medicine. 2021;**187**. DOI: 10.1016/j.rmed.2021.106551

Section 5

Associated Diseases and Conditions

Chapter 6

Gastroesophageal Reflux and Idiopathic Pulmonary Fibrosis

Nitesh Kumar Jain, Anwar Khedr, Hisham Ahmed Mushtaq,
Brian Bartlett, April Lanz, Greta Zoesch, Stephanie Welle,
Sumeet Yadav, Thoyaja Koritala, Shikha Jain, Aysun Tekin,
Ramesh Adhikari, Aishwarya Reddy Korsapati, Mool Chand,
Vishwanath Pattan, Vikas Bansal, Ali Rabaan, Amos Lal,
Hasnain Saifee Bawaadam, Aman Sethi, Lavanya Dondapati,
Raghavendra Tirupathi, Mack Sheraton, Maureen Muigai,
David Rokser, Chetna Dengri, Kovid Trivedi,
Samir Chandra Gautam, Simon Zec, Ibtisam Rauf,
Mantravadi Srinivasa Chandramouli, Rahul Kashyap
and Syed Anjum Khan

Abstract

Idiopathic pulmonary fibrosis (IPF) and Gastroesophageal reflux disease (GERD) commonly co-exist. Pathophysiological mechanisms causing IPF are still not well understood, and GERD has been implicated in both as a probable causative and disease-promoting entity. Although not conclusively proven, this relationship has been the subject of several studies, including therapeutic interventions aimed at treating GERD and its resultant effect on IPF and related outcomes. Our review aims to present the current concepts and understanding of these two disease processes, which are multifaceted. Their complex interaction includes epidemiology, pathophysiology, diagnosis, treatment, review of research studies conducted to date, and future directions for research.

Keywords: idiopathic pulmonary fibrosis (IPF), gastro-esophageal reflux disease (GERD), microaspiration, proton pump inhibitor, risk factors

1. Introduction

Idiopathic Pulmonary Fibrosis (IPF) is the most common type of Idiopathic Interstitial Pneumonia. It is more prevalent in men, and its incidence increases with age, especially beyond the fifth decade [1]. Its incidence is estimated to be 3–9 cases per 100,000 per year in the western hemisphere [2]. As per a systematic review, the prevalence is estimated to be 0.5–27.9/100,000 [3]. Although newer therapies such as

Pirfenidone and Nintedanib are available to slow the progression of the disease, the mortality and prognosis remain dismal, comparable to that of certain malignancies [4]. A key consideration has been the lack of optimal understanding of the pathophysiological mechanisms underlying the disease process, as interventions can then be targeted to modify the disease process and achieve better outcomes for the patients [4]. In a genetically susceptible individual, many risk factors have been proposed [1]. One such factor that has been closely associated with IPF is Gastroesophageal reflux disease (GERD) [1]. Their association has been hypothesized, studied, and targeted therapeutically. However, its role as a causative and aggravating factor has not yet been crystallized. Our chapter aims to review the association of GERD with IPF, its alleged role in causing or promoting lung injury, the effect of GERD therapy on IPF, recommendations from clinical guidelines, and the direction for future research.

1.1 Gastroesophageal reflux disease (GERD) and its relevance to IPF

GERD is a disease caused by reflux of stomach contents into the esophagus and beyond, causing troublesome symptoms and complications [5]. It causes esophageal and stomach symptoms characterized by chest pain, nausea, bloating, heartburn, and regurgitation. It can also cause extraesophageal symptoms such as throat pain, burning, lump in the throat, the sensation of needing to clear the throat, hoarseness of voice, cough, wheezing, bronchospasm, etc. [5, 6]. Importantly not all reflux events are symptomatic as there could be non-acid reflux [5–7].

Prevalence of GERD is very common in the western world, with North American estimates being 18.1–27.8% [8]. Europe, similarly, has a prevalence of up to 25% [8]. In a United Kingdom general practice database, IPF was much more likely to be associated with a diagnosis of GERD (65%) or use of anti-reflux therapy (71%) when compared to controls [4, 7, 9]. The prevalence of erosive esophagitis and hiatal hernia, both of which are associated with increased reflux, is also much higher in pulmonary fibrosis patients when compared to the general population [8, 10]. Hence there is a strong epidemiological association between these two disease entities.

GERD occurs commonly as a result of increased frequency of transient lower esophageal sphincter relaxations (TLESRs), which are defined as brief moments of lower esophageal sphincter tone inhibition that are independent of a swallow [11]. Other pathophysiological mechanisms implicated in the causation of GERD are reduced lower esophageal sphincter (LES) pressure, reduced upper esophageal sphincter pressure, reduced esophageal motility, Hiatal hernias, which distorts the gastroesophageal junctional anatomy, impairment of esophageal clearance, and sluggish gastric emptying [4, 5, 7]. A combination of these factors leads to the reflux establishing contact with mucosa in the upper gastrointestinal tract, pharynx, tracheobronchial tree, and lungs, causing extra esophageal symptoms as previously described [4, 5, 7].

Evaluation of GERD can be made by direct visual examination by esophagogastroduodenoscopy (EGD). The chief advantage is that the mucosa can be visualized directly and is helpful in the diagnosis of possible complications of GERD, including Barret's esophagitis, esophagitis, gastritis, gastric and esophageal stricture, and malignancy. However, pH monitoring better evaluates reflux, wherein a pH measuring probe is placed in the esophagus [5]. The primary measurement is the amount of time spent with a pH less than 4.0 [5]. However, it has its inherent limitations, as non-acid reflux cannot be measured and can remain totally asymptomatic. This limitation has been overcome by the placement of channels that measure impedance. Liquid reflux has low impedance and high conductance, while gaseous reflux, such as belching, has high impedance with low conductance [12]. Combined 24-hr multichannel intraluminal impedance-pH monitoring (MII-pH) are available to determine the amount of refluxate, its proximal extent, and/or the presence of both acid and weakly acidic reflux [7, 13]. The chief metric when using MII-pH is the "Total number of refluxes" (Pathological when more than 80 and normal if less than 40 in a 24-hour period) and esophageal "Acid exposure time (AET)" as the percentage of time with pH less than 4.0 in the distal esophagus [14]. The use of MII-pH in GERD associated with extra esophageal disease, particularly in IPF, is rather novel and promising to help illuminate the pathophysiological mechanisms between the two diseases [15]. It is noteworthy that IPF belongs to a group of diseases that are only possibly or likely associated with GERD, and its role is only speculated [7]. The use and application of MII-pH for the study of extraesophageal diseases and symptoms has not been as productive as for typical GERD [7].

1.2 The pathophysiological relationship and co-existence between GERD and IPF

The relationship between IPF and GERD is quite intriguing. The epidemiological association suggests that there appear to be plausible biological and mechanical factors underlying this pathophysiology.

It is suggested that GERD is associated with decreased upper and lower esophageal sphincter tone (hypotensive esophagogastric junction) with or without increased frequency of transient lower esophageal sphincter relaxations (TLESRs), leading to increased refluxate with an associated micro-aspiration of the gastric contents into the trachea and lungs [16–18]. Contrary to this proposed theory, it has been proposed that lung fibrosis causes decreased lung compliance along with lower lung elasticity, resulting in increased negative intrathoracic pressure during inspiration that is transmitted to the mediastinal structures, including the esophagus and its sphincters [17]. This causes increased transient lower esophageal sphincter relaxations (TLESRs) with lower and upper esophageal sphincters [17]. There is also a pressure gradient across the diaphragm in respiratory diseases like IPF, which may promote these favorable refluxate mechanisms, especially during coughing, increased respiratory excursions during exacerbations, and may potentially be further aggravated by hypoxia/hypercapnia, medications like antacids, glucocorticoids, and obstructive sleep apnea/hypopnea syndromes [19]. Hiatal hernia alters the physical and physiologic function of the lower esophageal sphincter, thereby promoting reflux [20–22]. Furthermore, it has been proposed that esophageal dysmotility may contribute to reflux [23, 24]. Ultimately, the result of these phenomena is that the gastric refluxate, which contains both acidic and non-acidic contents, leads to delayed esophageal clearance and micro-aspiration in the tracheobronchial tree injure the pulmonary parenchyma consisting of both alveolar and interstitial components [4, 7, 19]. The healing of this injury eventually occurs by fibrosis, and the pulmonary remodeling that ensues culminates in a distorted fibrotic architecture [4, 7].

Many studies have been performed to provide evidence and study the relationship between GERD and IPF. Most of these studies have limitations and often conclude with contradictory results. Therefore, evidence has shown a co-existence and/or association between IPF and GERD. However, causality has yet to be determined [4, 7, 25].

Gao et al. conducted a study involving 69 IPF patients, 62 healthy volunteers, and 88 IPF negative GERD patients. The prevalence of GERD was high in patients with IPF, and in relation to their comparator group showed the variable presence of esophageal dysmotility and decreased lower and upper esophageal sphincter pressure. IPF patients also had increased reflux events proximally and impaired bolus transit time [16]. Raghu et al. studied 65 patients with IPF who were subjected to 24-h pH monitoring and esophageal manometry with a comparison group of 133 asthmatic patients and symptoms of GERD. The prevalence of abnormal gastroesophageal reflux in IPF patients was high at 87%, with 76% and 63% demonstrating abnormal distal and proximal esophageal acid exposures, respectively; a finding higher than within the comparison group [18]. The study also showed that the presence of GERD was not always symptomatic, and there was no correlation with IPF severity [18]. This was further confirmed in a study involving 28 patients with histologically confirmed IPF using hypopharyngeal multichannel intraluminal impedance (HMII) [26]. HMII used a specialized impedance catheter to directly measure laryngopharyngeal reflux (LPR) and full column reflux (reflux 2 cm distal to the upper esophageal sphincter). The study included 16 males and 12 females with a mean age of 60.4 years (range, 41–78) and a BMI of 28.4 (range, 21.1–38.1), respectively. Abnormal proximal exposure was present in 54% (15/28) of patients. This latter group was more likely to have a defective lower esophageal sphincter (LES) compared with those without (93% vs. 75%). Fourteen patients (56%) had abnormal esophageal motility, including aperistaltic esophagus (n = 9), suggesting that this may be common in this patient population [26]. GERD was noted to be highly prevalent at more than 70% in patients with IPF; abnormal proximal reflux events such as LPR and full column reflux were also quite common despite a frequently negative DeMeester score (It is a composite of six different parameters which measures acid exposure giving a pH score used to diagnose GERD), suggesting that nonacid reflux (25% of patients) is prevalent in this patient population [26]. A high rate of esophageal mucosal injury and a longer acid clearance time was also noted [26]. 67–76% of the systematic review demonstrated abnormal esophageal acid exposure off PPI treatment [27].

In another study conducted by Savarino et al. [28], 40 IPF patients were studied alongside 40 non-IPF ILD patients and 50 healthy volunteers, who served as controls. Patients were off reflux therapy and underwent a High-resolution Lung CT scan (HRCT) and pH-impedance monitoring. Patients with IPF had significantly increased esophageal acid exposure, the number of acidic, weakly acidic, and proximal reflux events relative to the comparison groups. Pulmonary fibrosis HRCT scores correlated well with reflux episodes in both the distal and proximal esophagus. Patients with IPF had more bile acids and pepsin (p < 0.03) in bronchoalveolar lavage fluid (62% and 67%, respectively) and saliva (61% and 68%, respectively) relative to the comparison groups [28]. Gavini et al. conducted an elegant study involving 45 pre-transplants patients with IPF who had received pulmonary function tests within the last 3 months. Patients were off reflux therapy and had no reflux surgery. They measured GER on multichannel intraluminal impedance and pH study (MII-pH). Six pH/acid reflux parameters with corresponding MII/bolus reflux measures were prespecified. Multivariate analyses were applied using forward stepwise logistic regression. Severe pulmonary dysfunction was defined using diffusion capacity for carbon monoxide (DLCO) ≤40%. Abnormal total reflux episodes and prolonged bolus clearance time (OR = 1.21 p = 0.05), but not the refluxate pH values, were significantly associated with pulmonary dysfunction severity on univariate and multivariate analyses [29]. Overall, it appears that esophageal dysmotility, the total number of acidic, weakly acidic, and non-acidic refluxes with prolonged bolus clearance time, appear to impact the underlying lung pathology.

Animal and human studies have shown that the presence of gastric contents (pepsin, bile acids, gastric acid) via microaspiration in bronchoalveolar lavage (BAL) fluid can cause tissue damage and inflammatory infiltrate [28, 30–35]. Histologically presence of thickened alveolar walls, collagen deposition in the interstitium, epithelial-mesenchymal transition, and presence of various fibrogenic factors has been found [28, 34, 35]. The latter consists of TGF-beta, NFκB, Farnesoid X receptor, and others. TGF-beta can be induced by gastric contents, leading to fibroblast proliferation and fibroproliferative changes [4, 7].

1.3 The role of proton pump inhibitor (PPI)/histamine-2 receptor blockers (H2RA) and anti-reflux surgery in IPF

There has been a long-standing interest in the use of anti-secretory therapy/ anti-reflux surgery in IPF patients, given that GERD has been thought of as having a relationship with IPF [4, 7]. While it is not unreasonable to give anti-secretory therapy to patients with symptomatic GERD patients, it has certainly been hard to objectively justify the use in all patients with IPF, some of whom may not have any reflux or reflux with non-acidic gastric contents [36]. This has indeed been a recommendation from international guidelines, albeit it was a week level of recommendation [37]. As per literature, PPIs are the most frequently used medications, and further discussion will relate henceforth to PPI.

PPIs are known for increasing the pH of gastric acid; a mechanism thought to prevent microaspiration of acidic contents into the lung and hence potentially protect against acid-induced pneumonitis [37]. In vitro studies show that PPIs like Esomeprazole have pleiotropic effects, can inhibit expression of pro-inflammatory molecules like vascular cell adhesion molecule-1, inducible nitric oxide synthase, tumor necrosis factor-alpha (TNF-α), and interleukins (IL-1β and IL-6), and exhibit antioxidant and anti-fibrotic properties by downregulation of profibrotic proteins including receptors for transforming growth factor β (TGFβ), fibronectin and matrix metalloproteinases (MMPs) [38, 39]. They may also inhibit apoptosis of pneumocytes expressing Surfactant (SP-C) [38, 39]. Retrospective studies have also demonstrated that PPIs may prolong transplant-free survival of IPF patients [38, 39].

However, PPIs are not without risks. They have been shown to alter the microbiome of the respiratory tract and increase the risk of pneumonia [17]. Furthermore, they increase the risk of micronutrient deficiencies like Vitamin B12, cause dementia, *Clostridium difficile* infection, decrease bone density and increase the risk of fractures. They may increase the risk of chronic kidney disease progressing to end-stage renal disease [40]. However, it is to be noted that most of the evidence for this comes from observational data and meta-analyses, which have their own inherent limitations [40].

Anti-reflux surgery is an important therapeutic option in patients with GERD. Nissen fundoplication and Laparoscopic anti-reflux surgery (LARS) are the two most performed surgeries, both of which are generally safe in IPF [4, 14]. Lee JS et al. reported a retrospective cohort of 204 IPF patients consisting of individuals with symptoms of GERD (34%), a history of GERD (45%), reported use of GERD medications (47%), and Nissen fundoplication (5%). After the multivariate adjustment, the use of GERD medication was associated with a lower radiologic fibrotic score. It was also an independent predictor of longer survival time in patients with IPF [41]. Lee JS et al. also reported the combined results of 3 prospectively collected randomized controlled trial data, including 242 patients only from the placebo arm. Although the data came from RCTs, this was not an RCT. Of the total 242 patients, 124 patients were taking PPI/H2RA, and 118 patients were not taking any antisecretory therapy. In IPF, a slower decline in Forced vital capacity (FVC) has shown a correlation with improved survival time in IPF [42]. The study showed that there was a slower decline in FVC in the PPI/H2RA group, which was statistically significant. Also, there were fewer acute exacerbations in the PPI/H2RA group, and this result did not contribute to the slower decline in FVC. However, there was no change in mortality, presumably due to the follow-up period not being sufficient. This study result generated an interesting hypothesis that the use of PPI/H2RA could slow disease progression [43].

Furthermore, Fidler et al. conducted a systematic review and meta-analysis, studying the effect of pharmacological therapy of GERD in IPF patients, which showed a significant improvement in IPF related survival (adjusted risk: HR 0.45) but no effect on all-cause mortality. There was a change in progression-free survival, FVC, acute exacerbation, and other Pulmonary function test parameters. In patients with FVC less than 70% of predicted, there was an increase in pulmonary infection, which was significant as this is a known side effect of PPI affecting patients with more advanced disease [44]. It follows from this discussion that the studies once again have small numbers, mostly observational, and hence have limitations providing poor or limited quality of evidence [44].

In a randomized controlled trial, Raghu et al. analyzed data from 27 patients who underwent Laparoscopic anti-reflux surgery (LARS) and 20 patients who did not undergo surgery with FVC measurement at 48 weeks as the endpoint in an intention to treat analysis. All patients had abnormal acid GER with a confirmed DeMeester score of ≥14·7; measured by 24-h pH monitoring and preserved forced vital capacity (FVC) of more than 50%. Patients were allowed to use Nintedanib and Pirfenidone. Patients in the surgery group had a slower decline in FVC, which was not statistically significant at 48 weeks in the non-surgery group (p = 0·28)}. Acute exacerbation of IPF, hospitalization for respiratory etiology, and mortality were also less in the surgical group, however not to statistical significance [45].

2. Discussion

GERD has been known to be co-existent with many Pulmonary disorders such as Systemic Sclerosis, Chronic obstructive pulmonary disease (COPD), Bronchial Asthma, IPF, Bronchiectasis, Aspiration Pneumonia, Lung transplant complications such as Bronchiolitis obliterans (BOS), etc. [6]. These plethora's of lung conditions being associated with GERD are likely due to the shared common genetic embryological and developmental origin of the two organ systems from the foregut [6, 46]. In addition, they share the intrathoracic cavity and also have the same vagal innervation [6, 46]. As such, two predominant theories are in vogue, the "Refluxate theory" and the "Reflux theory," which attempt to explain the disease mechanisms with their common origin and development as background. The "Refluxate theory," as previously described, implicates acid reflux from the GI tract and its micro-aspiration into the Respiratory tree, causing physicochemical damage to the latter culminating in fibrosis [6]. The "Reflex theory" pertains to the reflex increase in bronchoconstriction and airway resistance in response to the presence of acid in the esophagus and respiratory tree [6]. Furthermore, as discussed previously, the presence of pulmonary fibrosis may aggravate the gastroesophageal reflux due to decreased compliance, elasticity, and need for increased negative intrathoracic pressure generated during inspiration, causing increased gradient across thoracic and abdominal compartments [6]. Hence there is possibly a bidirectional relationship between the two organ systems, as depicted in **Figure 1.** A Summary of the studies that evaluated the role of antireflux therapy and surgery in the management of IPF is available in **Table 1**.

Studies designed to test the relationships between the two diseases entities have several limitations. They are mostly retrospective, have small sample sizes, with poorly defined inclusion and exclusion criteria, resulting in many confounders. While these limitations can be addressed partially by conducting prospective studies, randomized controlled data with a large sample size will remain elusive due to the prolonged time required for a disease process like IPF takes to evolve and manifest [25]. Besides, diseases like IPF are not clearly recognizable early, and GERD with non-acid reflux or poorly acidic reflux may not manifest with classic symptoms [6, 25], hence denying the opportunity for early recognition and follow up. Hence, our reliance on smaller case-controlled studies with a few well-conducted meta-analyses has only revealed an association between GERD and IPF, far from the nine causality criteria propounded by "Hill" [61, 62]. Although not ruling out causality, a weak association between the two diseases still needs to be viewed with an abundance of caution as the effects of residual confounding generate sufficient bias to prevent a robust causal inference from these types of studies [62]. Although such challenges will limit future studies, investigating

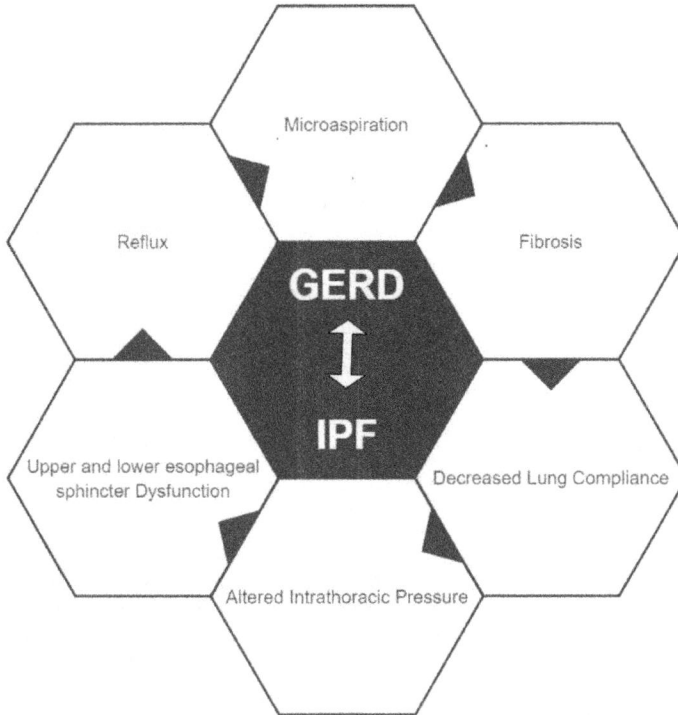

Figure 1.
The bidirectional relationship between IPF and GERD.

Authors	Year	Study type	Anti-reflux therapy type	Population size	Outcomes
Cantu et al. [47]	2004	Retrospective cohort study	Fundoplication	457	• Fourteen patients with early fundoplication had better survival when compared to those with reflux and no intervention. • As compared to patients with reflux who did not have early fundoplication, those who had early fundoplication had less incidence of BOS at 1 and 3 years.
Raghu et al. [18]	2006	Case series	PPIs	4	• In all four patients, PFTs stabilized or improved, and their status was maintained with proper PPI therapy. • At the latest follow-up, all of the patients were still alive, and none of them had an acute exacerbation of IPF or required therapy for respiratory difficulties during this time.

Authors	Year	Study type	Anti-reflux therapy type	Population size	Outcomes
Linden et al. [48]	2006	Retrospective cohort study	Fundoplication	45	• During the average 15-month follow-up, there were no perioperative complications or a reduction in lung function. • Patients with idiopathic pulmonary fibrosis treated with fundoplication had better oxygen levels, but the oxygen requirements of control patients with idiopathic pulmonary fibrosis who did not have the surgery increased significantly
Lee et al. [41]	2011	Retrospective cohort study	PPIs–H$_2$RAs	204	• The usage of anti-reflux medications was found to be an independent predictor of a prolonged life expectancy. • Using antacids for gastric reflux was linked to a reduced radiologic fibrosis score.
Fisichella et al. [49]	2011	Prospective study	LARS	39	• GERD patients with lung transplants had higher pepsin in their BALF than lung transplant patients who had LARS.
Noth et al. [10]	2012	Retrospective cohort study	PPIs–H$_2$RAs	74	• Compared to matched controls, IPF patients with hiatal hernia who used antacid medicines had substantially higher DLCO and better composite physiologic index scores.
Raghu et al. [50]	2016	Retrospective cohort study	LARS	27	• FVC measurements taken before and after LARS revealed no significant change over1 year but there was a trend towards stabilization of FVC
Lee et al. [43]	2013	Post hoc analysis of RCTs	PPIs–H$_2$RAs	242	• FVC loss is lower at 30 and 52 weeks with fewer acute exacerbations.
Ghebremariam et al. [38]	2015	A retrospective analysis from 2 databases	PPIs	215	• Patients with IPF who used PPIs lived longer than those who did not (median survival of 3.4 vs. 2 years).
Raghu et al. [37]	2015	Post hoc analysis of RCTs	PPIs–H$_2$RAs	1061	• The use of anti-acid medications at the start of the study had no effect on the therapeutic effect of Nintedanib on slowing FVC decrease in IPF patients.

Authors	Year	Study type	Anti-reflux therapy type	Population size	Outcomes
Kreuter et al. [51]	2016	*Post hoc analysis of RCTs*	PPIs–H2RAs	624	• Antacid therapy was not associated with disease progression, all-cause mortality, IPF-related mortality, absolute FVC decrease of 10% or more, mean observed change in FVC and FVC percent of predicted, hospital admission rate, 6 Minute walk distance(MWD) stratified by baseline FVC, and adverse events at 52 weeks.
Lee et al. [52]	2016	Retrospective cohort study	PPIs	786	• PPI usage for more than 4 months was linked with a lower IPF-related mortality rate than PPI use for less than 4 months.
Kreuter et al. [53]	2016	Retrospective cohort study	PPIs	272	• PPI use at the start was not linked to a longer median survival time.
Elkstrom et al. [54]	2016	Prospective population-based study	PPIs–H_2RAs	462	• The use of antacids was not linked to mortality.
Kulkarni et al. [55]	2016	Retrospective cohort study	PPIs–H2RAs	284	• Antireflux treatment was not linked to an increased risk of mortality or lung transplantation.
Raghu et al. [56]	2016	Retrospective cohort study	LARS	27	• There were no fatalities in the first 90 days after surgery, and 81.5 percent of the individuals were still alive two years later. • Over the course of a year, there were no statistically significant variations in FVC decreased rates pre- and post-LARS.
Kreuter et al. [57]	2017	Post hoc analysis of RCTs	PPIs–H_2Ras	632	• There were no significant differences in disease progression, all-cause mortality, IPF-related mortality, all-cause hospitalization rate, or mean change in % FVC at 52 weeks between the two groups (with or without antacid therapy).
Restivo et al. [58]	2017	Population-based study	PPIs–H_2RAs	6797	• PPI usage was linked to fewer high attenuation regions in CT scans of a large group of asymptomatic community-dwelling middle-aged and older people, suggesting a possible benefit in ILD.

Authors	Year	Study type	Anti-reflux therapy type	Population size	Outcomes
Raghu et al. [45]	2018	A prospective randomized controlled study	LARS	58	• LARS was linked to a reduced rate of FVC decrease, a longer duration until FVC decline or death, and fewer clinical events and fatalities.
Costabel et al. [59]	2018	*Post hoc analysis of RCTs*	PPIs–H$_2$RAs	406	• In both antisecretory therapy treated and nontreated individuals, the yearly decline rate of FVC was identical in both Nintedanib/placebo-treated patients. • Antisecretory medicine did not influence the therapeutic effect of Nintedanib and was not related to a better course of illness
Helen et al. [60]	2019	A retrospective analysis from 1 database	PPIs–H$_2$RAs	587	• There were no differences in survival or illness progression in patients on antacid therapy

Abbreviations: BOS: bronchitis obliterans syndrome; PPIs: proton pump inhibitors; PFT: pulmonary function tests; H$_2$RAs: H2 receptor antagonists; LARS: laparoscopic anti-reflux surgery; GERD: gastroesophageal reflux disease; IPF: idiopathic pulmonary fibrosis; DLCO: diffusion lung capacity for carbon monoxide; BALF: bronchoalveolar lavage fluid; RCTs: randomized controlled trials; FVC: forced vital capacity; ILD: interstitial lung disease; CI: confidence interval; HR: hazard ratio.

Table 1.
Summary of the studies that evaluated the role of antireflux therapy and surgery in the management of IPF.

therapeutic interventions like LARS and PPIs along with disease-modifying therapies like Nintedanib and Pirfenidone may improve outcomes for our IPF patients [25].

The large database-based clinical studies with robust timestamping of initiation of each disease entity will be helpful in establishing a temporal relationship. A machine learning model development is the need of the hour to answer this clinical question.

3. Conclusion

The co-existence of IPF and GERD is very common. There is likely a bidirectional pathophysiological relationship between the two disease entities. Although there is no causality established, current guidelines do recommend therapy with PPI in all patients with IPF. There remain many important challenges to the study of these coexisting conditions, and it may not be possible to obtain robust data establishing causality. Nevertheless, an attempt can be made to further conduct well-designed interventional studies to benefit patients in need.

Acknowledgements

Kristina Kardum Cvitan, Author Service Manager, IntechOpen.

Conflict of interest

The authors declare no conflict of interest.

Author details

Nitesh Kumar Jain[1*], Anwar Khedr[1], Hisham Ahmed Mushtaq[1], Brian Bartlett[1],
April Lanz[1], Greta Zoesch[1], Stephanie Welle[1], Sumeet Yadav[1], Thoyaja Koritala[1],
Shikha Jain[2], Aysun Tekin[3], Ramesh Adhikari[4], Aishwarya Reddy Korsapati[5],
Mool Chand[1], Vishwanath Pattan[6], Vikas Bansal[3], Ali Rabaan[7], Amos Lal[3],
Hasnain Saifee Bawaadam[8], Aman Sethi[9], Lavanya Dondapati[10],
Raghavendra Tirupathi[11], Mack Sheraton[12], Maureen Muigai[1], David Rokser[1],
Chetna Dengri[13], Kovid Trivedi[14], Samir Chandra Gautam[15], Simon Zec[3],
Ibtisam Rauf[16], Mantravadi Srinivasa Chandramouli[17], Rahul Kashyap[3]
and Syed Anjum Khan[1]

1 Mayo Clinic Health System, Mankato, USA

2 MVJ Medical College and Research Hospital, Bangalore, India

3 Mayo Clinic, Rochester, USA

4 Franciscan Health, Lafayette, USA

5 University of Buckingham Medical School, London, GBR

6 Wyoming Medical Center, Casper, USA

7 Johns Hopkins Aramco Healthcare, Dhahran, Saudi Arabia

8 Aurora Medical Center, Kenosha, Wisconsin, USA

9 Advocate Medical Group, Aurora, Illinois, USA

10 NTR University of Health Sciences, Vijayawada, India

11 Keystone Health, Chambersburg, USA

12 Johns Hopkins University, Baltimore, USA

13 Sir Gangaram Hospital, Delhi, India

14 Salem Pulmonary Associates, Salem, Oregon, USA

15 Johns Hopkins Bayview Medical Center, Baltimore, USA

16 St George's University, True Blue, Grenada

17 Trust Hospital, Kakinada, India

*Address all correspondence to: jain.nitesh@mayo.edu

IntechOpen

References

[1] Raghu G, Collard HR, Egan JJ, Martinez FJ, Behr J, Brown KK, et al. An official ATS/ERS/JRS/ALAT statement: Idiopathic pulmonary fibrosis: evidence-based guidelines for diagnosis and management. American Journal of Respiratory and Critical Care Medicine. 2011;**183**:788-824. DOI: 10.1164/rccm.2009-040GL

[2] Hutchinson J, Fogarty A, Hubbard R, McKeever T. Global incidence and mortality of idiopathic pulmonary fibrosis: A systematic review. The European Respiratory Journal. 2015;**46**:795-806. DOI: 10.1183/09031936.00185114

[3] Kaunisto J, Salomaa ER, Hodgson U, Kaarteenaho R, Myllärniemi M. Idiopathic pulmonary fibrosis--A systematic review on methodology for the collection of epidemiological data. BMC Pulmonary Medicine. 2013;**13**:53. DOI: 10.1186/1471-2466-13-53

[4] Wang Z, Bonella F, Li W, Boerner EB, Guo Q, Kong X, et al. Gastroesophageal reflux disease in idiopathic pulmonary fibrosis: uncertainties and controversies. Respiration. 2018;**96**:571-587. DOI: 10.1159/000492336

[5] Clarrett DM, Hachem C. Gastroesophageal reflux disease (GERD). Missouri Medicine. 2018;**115**:214-218

[6] Okwara NC, Chan WW. Sorting out the relationship between esophageal and pulmonary disease. Gastroenterology Clinics of North America. 2021;**50**:919-934. DOI: 10.1016/j.gtc.2021.08.006

[7] Ghisa M, Marinelli C, Savarino V, Savarino E. Idiopathic pulmonary fibrosis and GERD: Links and risks. Therapeutics and Clinical Risk Management. 2019;**15**:1081-1093. DOI: 10.2147/tcrm.S184291

[8] El-Serag HB, Sweet S, Winchester CC, Dent J. Update on the epidemiology of gastro-oesophageal reflux disease: A systematic review. Gut. 2014;**63**:871-880. DOI: 10.1136/gutjnl-2012-304269

[9] Gribbin J, Hubbard R, Smith C. Role of diabetes mellitus and gastro-oesophageal reflux in the aetiology of idiopathic pulmonary fibrosis. Respiratory Medicine. 2009;**103**:927-931. DOI: 10.1016/j.rmed.2008.11.001

[10] Noth I, Zangan SM, Soares RV, Forsythe A, Demchuk C, Takahashi SM, et al. Prevalence of hiatal hernia by blinded multidetector CT in patients with idiopathic pulmonary fibrosis. The European Respiratory Journal. 2012;**39**:344-351. DOI: 10.1183/09031936.00099910

[11] Herregods TV, Bredenoord AJ, Smout AJ. Pathophysiology of gastroesophageal reflux disease: New understanding in a new era. Neurogastroenterology and Motility. 2015;**27**:1202-1213. DOI: 10.1111/nmo.12611

[12] Pritchett JM, Aslam M, Slaughter JC, Ness RM, Garrett CG, Vaezi MF. Efficacy of esophageal impedance/pH monitoring in patients with refractory gastroesophageal reflux disease, on and off therapy. Clinical Gastroenterology and Hepatology. 2009;**7**:743-748. DOI: 10.1016/j.cgh.2009.02.022

[13] Zentilin P, Dulbecco P, Savarino E, Giannini E, Savarino V. Combined multichannel intraluminal impedance and pH-metry: A novel technique to improve detection of gastro-oesophageal reflux literature review. Digestive and Liver Disease. 2004;**36**:565-569. DOI: 10.1016/j.dld.2004.03.019

[14] Gyawali CP, Kahrilas PJ, Savarino E, Zerbib F, Mion F, Smout A, et al.

Modern diagnosis of GERD: The Lyon Consensus. Gut. 2018;**67**:1351-1362. DOI: 10.1136/gutjnl-2017-314722

[15] Cheah R, Chirnaksorn S, Abdelrahim AH, Horgan L, Capstick T, Casey J, et al. The perils and pitfalls of esophageal dysmotility in idiopathic pulmonary fibrosis. The American Journal of Gastroenterology. 2021;**116**:1189-1200. DOI: 10.14309/ajg.0000000000001202

[16] Gao F, Hobson AR, Shang ZM, Pei YX, Gao Y, Wang JX, et al. The prevalence of gastro-esophageal reflux disease and esophageal dysmotility in Chinese patients with idiopathic pulmonary fibrosis. BMC Gastroenterology. 2015;**15**:26. DOI: 10.1186/s12876-015-0253-y

[17] Johannson KA, Strâmbu I, Ravaglia C, Grutters JC, Valenzuela C, Mogulkoc N, et al. Antacid therapy in idiopathic pulmonary fibrosis: more questions than answers? The Lancet Respiratory Medicine. 2017;**5**:591-598. DOI: 10.1016/s2213-2600(17)30219-9

[18] Raghu G, Freudenberger TD, Yang S, Curtis JR, Spada C, Hayes J, et al. High prevalence of abnormal acid gastro-oesophageal reflux in idiopathic pulmonary fibrosis. The European Respiratory Journal. 2006;**27**:136-142. DOI: 10.1183/09031936.06.00037005

[19] Houghton LA, Lee AS, Badri H, DeVault KR, Smith JA. Respiratory disease and the oesophagus: Reflux, reflexes and microaspiration. Nature Reviews. Gastroenterology & Hepatology. 2016;**13**:445-460. DOI: 10.1038/nrgastro.2016.91

[20] Tolone S, de Cassan C, de Bortoli N, Roman S, Galeazzi F, Salvador R, et al. Esophagogastric junction morphology is associated with a positive impedance-pH monitoring in patients with GERD. Neuro gastroenterology and Motility.

2015;**27**:1175-1182. DOI: 10.1111/nmo.12606

[21] Tossier C, Dupin C, Plantier L, Leger J, Flament T, Favelle O, et al. Hiatal hernia on thoracic computed tomography in pulmonary fibrosis. The European Respiratory Journal. 2016;**48**:833-842. DOI: 10.1183/13993003.01796-2015

[22] Mays EE, Dubois JJ, Hamilton GB. Pulmonary fibrosis associated with tracheobronchial aspiration. A study of the frequency of hiatal hernia and gastroesophageal reflux in interstitial pulmonary fibrosis of obscure etiology. Chest. 1976;**69**:512-515. DOI: 10.1378/chest.69.4.512

[23] Allaix ME, Rebecchi F, Morino M, Schlottmann F, Patti MG. Gastroesophageal reflux and idiopathic pulmonary fibrosis. World Journal of Surgery. 2017;**41**:1691-1697. DOI: 10.1007/s00268-017-3956-0

[24] Fouad YM, Katz PO, Hatlebakk JG, Castell DO. Ineffective esophageal motility: the most common motility abnormality in patients with GERD-associated respiratory symptoms. The American Journal of Gastroenterology. 1999;**94**:1464-1467. DOI: 10.1111/j.1572-0241.1999.1127_e.x

[25] Bédard Méthot D, Leblanc É, Lacasse Y. Meta-analysis of Gastroesophageal Reflux Disease and Idiopathic Pulmonary Fibrosis. Chest. 2019;**155**:33-43. DOI: 10.1016/j.chest.2018.07.038

[26] Hoppo T, Komatsu Y, Jobe BA. Gastroesophageal reflux disease and patterns of reflux in patients with idiopathic pulmonary fibrosis using hypopharyngeal multichannel intraluminal impedance. Diseases of the Esophagus. 2014;**27**:530-537. DOI: 10.1111/j.1442-2050.2012.01446.x

[27] Hershcovici T, Jha LK, Johnson T, Gerson L, Stave C, Malo J, et al.

Systematic review: The relationship between interstitial lung diseases and gastro-oesophageal reflux disease. Alimentary Pharmacology & Therapeutics. 2011;**34**:1295-1305. DOI: 10.1111/j.1365-2036.2011.04870.x

[28] Savarino E, Carbone R, Marabotto E, Furnari M, Sconfienza L, Ghio M, et al. Gastro-oesophageal reflux and gastric aspiration in idiopathic pulmonary fibrosis patients. The European Respiratory Journal. 2013;**42**:1322-1331. DOI: 10.1183/09031936.00101212

[29] Gavini S, Finn RT, Lo WK, Goldberg HJ, Burakoff R, Feldman N, et al. Idiopathic pulmonary fibrosis is associated with increased impedance measures of reflux compared to non-fibrotic disease among pre-lung transplant patients. Neurogastro enterology and Motility. 2015;**27**:1326-1332. DOI: 10.1111/nmo.12627

[30] Appel JZ 3rd, Lee SM, Hartwig MG, Li B, Hsieh CC, Cantu E 3rd, et al. Characterization of the innate immune response to chronic aspiration in a novel rodent model. Respiratory Research. 2007;**8**:87. DOI: 10.1186/1465-9921-8-87

[31] Chen B, You WJ, Liu XQ, Xue S, Qin H, Jiang HD. Chronic microaspiration of bile acids induces lung fibrosis through multiple mechanisms in rats. Clinical Science (London, England). 2017;**131**:951-963. DOI: 10.1042/cs20160926

[32] Downing TE, Sporn TA, Bollinger RR, Davis RD, Parker W, Lin SS. Pulmonary histopathology in an experimental model of chronic aspiration is independent of acidity. Experimental Biology and Medicine (Maywood, N.J.). 2008;**233**:1202-1212. DOI: 10.3181/0801-rm-17

[33] Lozo Vukovac E, Lozo M, Mise K, Gudelj I, Puljiz Z, Jurcev-Savicevic A, et al. Bronchoalveolar pH and inflammatory biomarkers in newly diagnosed IPF and GERD patients: A case-control study. Medical Science Monitor. 2014;**20**:255-261. DOI: 10.12659/MSM.889800

[34] Davis CS, Mendez BM, Flint DV, Pelletiere K, Lowery E, Ramirez L, et al. Pepsin concentrations are elevated in the bronchoalveolar lavage fluid of patients with idiopathic pulmonary fibrosis after lung transplantation. The Journal of Surgical Research. 2013;**185**:e101-e108. DOI: 10.1016/j.jss.2013.06.011

[35] Lee JS, Song JW, Wolters PJ, Elicker BM, King TE, Kim DS, et al. Bronchoalveolar lavage pepsin in acute exacerbation of idiopathic pulmonary fibrosis. European Respiratory Journal. 2012;**39**:352-358. DOI: 10.1183/09031936.00050911

[36] Richeldi L, Collard HR, Jones MG. Idiopathic pulmonary fibrosis. Lancet. 2017;**389**:1941-1952. DOI: 10.1016/s0140-6736(17)30866-8

[37] Raghu G, Crestani B, Bailes Z, Schlenker-Herceg R, Costabel U. Effect of anti-acid medication on reduction in FVC decline with nintedanib. European Respiratory Journal. 2015;**46**:OA4502. DOI: 10.1183/13993003.congress-2015.OA4502

[38] Ghebremariam YT, Cooke JP, Gerhart W, Griego C, Brower JB, Doyle-Eisele M, et al. Pleiotropic effect of the proton pump inhibitor esomeprazole leading to suppression of lung inflammation and fibrosis. Journal of Translational Medicine. 2015;**13**:249. DOI: 10.1186/s12967-015-0614-x

[39] Ghebre YT, Raghu G. Idiopathic pulmonary fibrosis: Novel concepts of proton pump inhibitors as antifibrotic drugs. American Journal of Respiratory and Critical Care Medicine. 2016; **193**:1345-1352. DOI: 10.1164/rccm.201512-2316PP

[40] Jaynes M, Kumar AB. The risks of long-term use of proton pump inhibitors: A critical review. Therapeutic Advances in Drug Safety. 2019; **10**:2042098618809927. DOI: 10.1177/ 2042098618809927

[41] Lee JS, Ryu JH, Elicker BM, Lydell CP, Jones KD, Wolters PJ, et al. Gastroesophageal reflux therapy is associated with longer survival in patients with idiopathic pulmonary fibrosis. American Journal of Respiratory and Critical Care Medicine. 2011;**184**:1390-1394. DOI: 10.1164/ rccm.201101-0138OC

[42] Paterniti MO, Bi Y, Rekic D, Wang Y, Karimi-Shah BA, Chowdhury BA. Acute exacerbation and decline in forced vital capacity are associated with increased mortality in idiopathic pulmonary fibrosis. Annals of the American Thoracic Society. 2017;**14**:1395-1402. DOI: 10.1513/AnnalsATS.201606-458OC

[43] Lee JS, Collard HR, Anstrom KJ, Martinez FJ, Noth I, Roberts RS, et al. Anti-acid treatment and disease progression in idiopathic pulmonary fibrosis: An analysis of data from three randomised controlled trials. The Lancet Respiratory Medicine. 2013;**1**:369-376. DOI: 10.1016/ s2213-2600(13)70105-x

[44] Fidler L, Sitzer N, Shapera S, Shah PS. Treatment of gastroesophageal reflux in patients with idiopathic pulmonary fibrosis: A systematic review and meta-analysis. Chest. 2018;**153**:1405-1415. DOI: 10.1016/j. chest.2018.03.008

[45] Raghu G, Pellegrini CA, Yow E, Flaherty KR, Meyer K, Noth I, et al. Laparoscopic anti-reflux surgery for the treatment of idiopathic pulmonary fibrosis (WRAP-IPF): A multicentre, randomised, controlled phase 2 trial. The Lancet Respiratory Medicine. 2018;**6**:707-714. DOI: 10.1016/ S2213-2600(18)30301-1

[46] Mansfield LE. Embryonic origins of the relation of gastroesophageal reflux disease and airway disease. The American Journal of Medicine. 2001;**111**(Suppl 8A):3S-7S. DOI: 10.1016/s0002-9343(01)00846-4

[47] Cantu E, Appel JZ, Hartwig M, Woreta H, Green CL, Messier RH, et al. Early fundoplication prevents chronic allograft dysfunction in patients with gastroesophageal reflux disease. The Annals of Thoracic Surgery. 2004; **78**:1142-1151

[48] Linden PA, Gilbert RJ, Yeap BY, Boyle K, Deykin A, Jaklitsch MT, et al. Laparoscopic fundoplication in patients with end-stage lung disease awaiting transplantation. The Journal of Thoracic and Cardiovascular Surgery. 2006; **131**:438-446. DOI: 10.1016/j.jtcvs. 2005.10.014

[49] Fisichella PM, Davis CS, Lundberg PW, Lowery E, Burnham EL, Alex CG, et al. The protective role of laparoscopic antireflux surgery against aspiration of pepsin after lung transplantation. Surgery. 2011;**150**:598-606. DOI: 10.1016/j.surg.2011.07.053

[50] Raghu G, Morrow E, Collins BF, Ho LA, Hinojosa MW, Hayes JM, et al. Laparoscopic anti-reflux surgery for idiopathic pulmonary fibrosis at a single center. European Respiratory Journal. 2016 Sep;**48**(3):826-832. DOI: 10.1183/ 13993003.00488-2016. Epub 2016 Aug 4. PMID: 27492835

[51] Kreuter M, Wuyts W, Renzoni E, Koschel D, Maher TM, Kolb M, et al. Antacid therapy and disease outcomes in idiopathic pulmonary fibrosis: A pooled analysis. The Lancet Respiratory Medicine. 2016;**4**:381-389. DOI: 10.1016/ s2213-2600(16)00067-9

[52] Lee CM, Lee DH, Ahn BK, Hwang JJ, Yoon H, Shin CM, et al. Protective effect of proton pump inhibitor for survival in patients with gastroesophageal reflux

disease and idiopathic pulmonary fibrosis. Journal of Neurogastro enterology and Motility. 2016;**22**: 444-451. DOI: 10.5056/jnm15192

[53] Kreuter M, Ehlers-Tenenbaum S, Palmowski K, Bruhwyler J, Oltmanns U, Muley T, et al. Impact of comorbidities on mortality in patients with idiopathic pulmonary fibrosis. PLoS One. 2016;**11**:e0151425. DOI: 10.1371/journal. pone.0151425

[54] Ekström M, Bornefalk-Hermansson A. Cardiovascular and antacid treatment and mortality in oxygen-dependent pulmonary fibrosis: A population-based longitudinal study. Respirology. 2016;**21**: 705-711. DOI: 10.1111/resp.12781

[55] Kulkarni T, Willoughby J, Acosta Lara Mdel P, Kim YI, Ramachandran R, Alexander CB, et al. A bundled care approach to patients with idiopathic pulmonary fibrosis improves transplant-free survival. Respiratory Medicine. 2016;**115**:33-38. DOI: 10.1016/j. rmed.2016.04.010

[56] Raghu G, Morrow E, Collins BF, Ho LAT, Hinojosa MW, Hayes JM, et al. Laparoscopic anti-reflux surgery for idiopathic pulmonary fibrosis at a single centre. European Respiratory Journal. 2016;**48**:826-832. DOI: 10.1183/ 13993003.00488-2016

[57] Kreuter M, Spagnolo P, Wuyts W, Renzoni E, Koschel D, Bonella F, et al. Antacid therapy and disease progression in patients with idiopathic pulmonary fibrosis who received pirfenidone. Respiration. 2017;**93**:415-423. DOI: 10.1159/000468546

[58] Restivo MD, Podolanczuk A, Kawut SM, Raghu G, Leary P, Barr RG, et al. Antacid use and subclinical interstitial lung disease: The MESA study. The European Respiratory Journal. 2017;**49**:1602566. DOI: 10.1183/ 13993003.02566-2016. Available from: ersjournals.com. PMID: 28526800

[59] Costabel U, Behr J, Crestani B, Stansen W, Schlenker-Herceg R, Stowasser S, et al. Anti-acid therapy in idiopathic pulmonary fibrosis: Insights from the INPULSIS® trials. Respiratory Research. 2018;**19**:167. DOI: 10.1186/ s12931-018-0866-0

[60] Jo HE, Corte TJ, Glaspole I, Grainge C, Hopkins PMA, Moodley Y, et al. Gastroesophageal reflux and antacid therapy in IPF: Analysis from the Australia IPF Registry. BMC Pulmonary Medicine. 2019;**19**:84. DOI: 10.1186/s12890-019-0846-2

[61] Hill AB. The environment and disease: association or causation? Proceedings of the Royal Society of Medicine. 1965;**58**:295-300

[62] Vaezi MF, Yang YX, Howden CW. Complications of proton pump inhibitor therapy. Gastroenterology. 2017;**153**:35-48. DOI: 10.1053/j.gastro.2017.04.047

Chapter 7

Perspective Chapter: Pulmonary System and Sjogren's Syndrome

Moiz Ehtesham, Anupama Tiwari, Rose Sneha George and Ruben A. Peredo

Abstract

Sjogren's syndrome (SS) is a connective tissue disease targeting the exocrine glands with subsequent sicca symptoms mainly in eyes and mouth. Respiratory symptoms may be the most frequent extraglandular manifestation following fatigue and pain. Mucosal dysfunction may affect the upper and lower airways, being the small airways more frequently involved. Parenchymal disease carries most of the morbidity and mortality. Nonspecific interstitial pneumonia (NSIP) is the most common radiographic feature, whereas the fibrotic NSIP type is the most reported finding in biopsies. Pulmonary lymphoma may arise from bronchial-associated lymphoid tissue lesions, and although rare, it is prevalent in SS. Chronic hypertrophic bronchial wall changes may ascribe to the various cystic lesions. Under their presence, possible lymphocytic interstitial pneumonia, amyloidosis, and lymphoma should be explored. Pulmonary arterial hypertension may present as frequently as in lupus, especially in Asian populations. Advanced knowledge in the pathogenesis has helped in understanding the various presentations within the respiratory system, contrasting with the scarce therapeutic options to treat both the airway and parenchymal disease. Anti-fibrotic parenchymal lung therapy offers promising outcomes. The pulmonary involvement in SS may associate with a decline in quality of life and reduced life expectancy. Subsequently, clinicians should know these facts for a timely intervention.

Keywords: Sjogren's syndrome, interstitial lung disease, airway disease, lymphoma, cystic lung disease

1. Introduction

Sjogren's syndrome (SS) is a chronic, progressive, and systemic autoinflammatory disease, with exocrine (mainly salivary and lacrimal) glands as the main target organs, leading to the development of sicca symptoms [1, 2]. They are the main clinical feature of the disease. Fatigue, diffuse pain, cognitive dysfunction, and arthralgias follow, constituting common findings [3, 4]. A subset of patients may express disease in extraglandular organs/systems, reflecting the systemic nature of the disease [5–7]. This pattern is more prevalent in the pediatric population [8]. Articular, peripheral neurological and pulmonary manifestations are described often [5], followed by other disease features: hematologic, gastrointestinal, renal, cutaneous, and endocrine [5, 9]. A subset of patients may progress to develop lymphoproliferative diseases, mainly stemming from mucosal-associated lymphoid tissue but also presenting as other types of non-Hodgkin (mainly B-cell) lymphomas [10]. Pulmonary manifestations are reported with various frequencies, depending on the criteria and methodology used to define them averaging an estimate of 9–24% in most of the studies [9, 11, 12]. Sjogren's syndrome when presenting alone is labeled as primary SS (pSS), while if it associates with another autoimmune (and mainly connective tissue) disease [13].

2. Epidemiology of Sjogren's syndrome

The disease affects more women than men in a proportion of 9:1 [14, 15] and peaks in the fourth to sixth decade of life [16]. The pooled incidence ratio for primary SS (pSS) is 6.92 per 100,000 person-years, and has a prevalence ranging from 0.05% to 0.23% [15, 17–19]. It is considered the second (if not first) most common connective tissue disorder, with an estimate of 1–3% of the population being affected [20].

3. Pathogenesis

3.1 Histopathology

The cellular [21] and humoral [22] components participate actively in the gland dysfunction and eventual destruction. Invasion of mononuclear cellular infiltrate, mainly composed of lymphocytes, tends to localize around the salivary ducts, vessels, and adjacent to the intact mucous acini [23]. This infiltrate tends to aggregate forming clusters, and if they count ≥50 cells, they are named as focal lymphocytic sialadenitis (FLS) (**Figure 1**). Quantifying the number of FLS within 4 mm^2 and dividing it by the area of normal glandular tissue will give an outcome. If this result is ≥1, it is reported as a *focus score* [24]. Focus scoring constitutes the main histopathological definition of SS [23, 25] and may range from 1 to 12. Higher values are obviated as they will be difficult to interpret due to the confluency of lymphocytic aggregates. Presence of a *focus score* helps the expert to define SS and to differentiate it from other inflammatory sialadenitides, including nonspecific chronic sialadenitis, sclerosing chronic sialadenitis, and others (**Figure 1**) [23].

3.2 Serology

Specific serology in SS associates with characteristic disease phenotypes and helps defining the disease [26]. The most characteristic and specific antibody is anti-SSA/Ro [27], and it is included in the 2016 classification criteria of SS [28]. Other serology, although less specific or not so prevalent, associates with SS as well, but is excluded from the currently accepted European-American classification criteria for Sjogren's syndrome. For instance, in a large multicenter cohort study of 10,500 patients, serology at the time of diagnosis of SS showed the following frequencies in decreasing order: antinuclear antibody (ANA) (79.3%), anti-SSA/Ro (73.2%), rheumatoid factor (48.6%), and anti-SSB/La antibodies (45.1%) [26]. Despite this distribution, anti-SSA/Ro and anti-SSB/La antibodies have been specifically identified to participate in SS's pathogenesis. They are also present in other connective tissue diseases (CTDs), lowering their specificity [29]. Cryoglobulins and low complements, mainly low C4, may reveal disease activity and define prognosis [27, 30, 31]. Their presence is additionally predictive of lymphoma [32]. Presence of circulating autoantibodies in patients with SS prior to the diagnosis

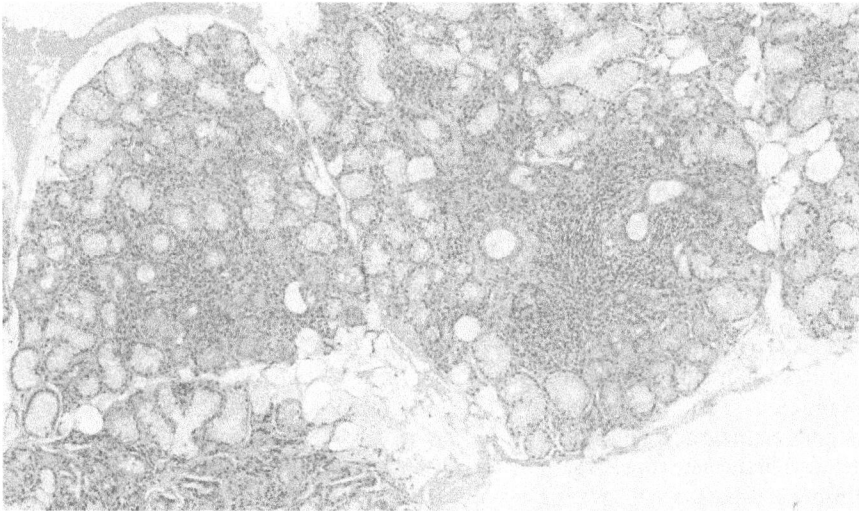

(a)

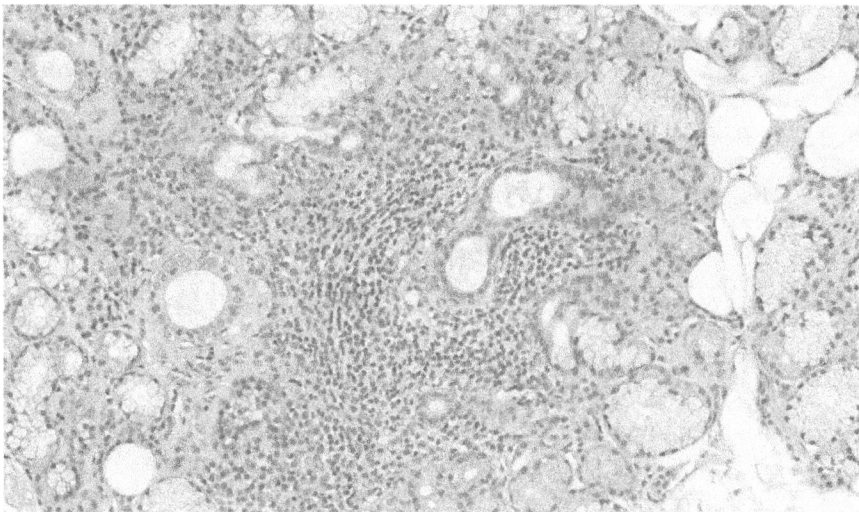

(b)

Figure 1.
a (10×), b (20×): H&E section of this excisional biopsy of minor salivary gland tissue reveals periductular lymphoplasmacytic infiltrate. Multiple foci of periductular nodular lymphoplasmacytic infiltrates are identified. The number of mononuclear cell infiltrate per nodular focus is estimated to be greater than 50 lymphocytes per 4 mm^2 of tissue examined, and each lobule examined contains at least one focus of inflammation. Thus, the focus score for the above biopsy was estimated to be ≥1. Therefore, this picture of chronic sialadenitis with a focus score ≥ 1 in the right clinical context is consistent with Sjögren's syndrome.

suggests that the immune activation has been previously triggered by an unknown antigen, and it may take months or years to progress onto a phenotypical expression [33]. A two-hit hypothesis, in this scenario, may possibly be the most likely explanation for this phenomenon. Sensitization and priming of the immune system by a prior insult (first hit) may define and determine the fate of the upcoming a programmed immune response following the exposure of a second stressor (second hit). During this second insult the immune tolerance seems to be breached, with which the sequence of autoimmune events activate the disease [34, 35]. Presence of other circulating antibodies reported in SS may be the result of the polygenic nature of the disease and possibly due to different antigens activating the immune system, and hitting specific targets [26, 36–39]. Novel autoantibodies linked with sicca eyes reveal our still limited knowledge in SS's pathogenesis [40, 41].

4. Symptoms and disease definition

Symptoms associated with dry mucosae in the eyes and mouth (sicca) are complains the clinicians should explore to consider the disease [42, 43]. To define the dry eyes and mouth, several techniques objectively measure their quantity [2, 44]. In addition, recommendations on to elaborate questions regarding sicca symptoms, fatigue, arthralgia, Raynaud's, and other remarkable features common in SS, are detailed in the new consensus guidelines for the evaluation and management of pulmonary disease in Sjogren's syndrome [45]. Sicca symptoms constitute the core finding in SS and have always been included in any classification criteria. The composite of sicca eyes, mouth, positive serology (anti-SSA/Ro antibodies) and abnormal findings in the histopathology (a *focus score* of ≥1), constitute the current four pivotal components to fulfill the SS classification criteria [28]. Along the last five or more decades, the classification criteria have been modified more than 15 times [46–49]. These changes reveal the difficulties met on agreements to define the disease, and mainly due to variability in the cohorts used, the protean disease manifestations, variability in the serology on different populations, and the need for more than one expert (specialist) to define each one of the criteria components. In addition, the continuous changes in the classification criteria mirror the difficulties to understand the intricate and still poorly understood immunopathogenesis [12, 50].

The initial descriptions of pulmonary manifestations are detailed in accurate observations almost a century ago, and are described ahead.

5. History

5.1 Sjogren's syndrome as a systemic illness

The initial description of Sjogren's syndrome (SS) included the dry eye, and Leber [51] described filamentary keratitis (FK) [51], a finding that years later was linked with the lacrimal gland dysfunction (described by Stock in 1925). Around the same time, descriptions of a combination of dry eyes and mouth, detailed by Hadden [52], was followed by further clinical associations of deforming arthritis, and detailed by several authors in case series [53–55]. In his doctoral thesis in 1933, Henrik Sjogren, a Swedish ophthalmologist, accurately detailed what we know as the syndrome that carries his name. In his treaty, he accurately depicted the disease as we currently know, "...ocular changes because of dry eyes and hypofunction of salivary secretion, along with the arthritis and other systemic symptoms deals with a generalized disease and is not purely a coincidence" [56]. Ever since we know the concept of SS and its extent. Dr. Sjogren's pristine and sharp description made it possible to link all the clinical manifestations within a syndrome. This concept of a systemic illness manifesting in various organs was already familiar facilitating him to launch it as a unique disease. Decades prior, Dr. William Osler described systemic lupus on several patients (in 1895 and 1903) who presented with multiorgan involvement, other than the skin [57]. During the postwar era, in the 1950s, several scientists uncovered thyroid antibodies, and following Dr. Hashimoto's hypothesis from 1912, in which he sustained the thyroid gland to be the target of specific auto-antibodies. Dr. Jones applied this knowledge in SS. In this case, the salivary/lacrimal glands were the main target rather than the thyroid gland [58]. And indeed, the collaborative group of scientists from the National Institutes of Health in Maryland, USA, were able to identify them [53]. Two other concepts evolved as well: primary SS (pSS), when the disease presented alone; and secondary SS (sSS), when it was associated with other CTDs [13, 59].

5.2 Sjogren's syndrome and the respiratory system in history

The pulmonary involvement was documented in the 1950s. In a registry of pSS, pulmonary infiltrates were reported in 7/40 cases [60]. In the original case series, Dr. Sjogren early on (in the 1930s and 1940s) described diverse respiratory findings including rhinitis sicca, pharyngitis sicca, and laryngitis sicca, and considered them to be components of the whole dryness spectrum added to keratoconjunctivitis sicca and xerostomia. In the mid-1940s, Dr. Weber extended this concept to other tissues, proposing that the exocrine gland's dysfunction and destruction might precede sicca manifestations with an inflammatory continuum in the nasal, pharyngeal, and laryngeal mucosa, and other distant organs: the skin, vagina, gastric mucosa (this later with subsequent achlorydia) [61]. Management was mostly symptomatic. Further progression of several discoveries made it possible to elaborate definitions of lung compromise within SS's disease spectrum. Baruch and coauthors launched the concept of SS to be classified in two types: (1) those related to major CTD, and (2) sicca complex in the lungs that encompassed the following: chronic bronchitis, subsegmental atelectasis, bronchiectasis, pneumonia, lymphoproliferative pulmonary infiltrates, and chronic interstitial pneumonia, later leading to fibrosis [62]. Bloch published a series of 62 SS cases 37 (60%) who complained of nasal dryness and adherent crusts. One of them had sudden hearing loss linked to otitis, and chronic sinusitis was present in 4 (6%), throat dryness in 28 (45%), hoarseness in 20 (32%), and chronic dry cough in 5 (24%) [49]. In the lower respiratory tract, Bloch and coauthors reported: pleurisy, pleural adhesions, focal and lipoid pneumonia, pulmonary atelectasis, and fibrosis [49].

5.3 Pathology in history

Histopathological findings of most cases revealed submucous gland atrophy and lymphocytic infiltration intermixed with plasma cells at all levels of the respiratory tract [49, 63, 64]. The descriptions of pulmonary disease detailed different scenarios, from asymptomatic to severely ill patients. In this latter group, authors described two cases of acute parenchymal infiltrates in the setting of recurrent bronchitis and pneumonia. These cases presented with pneumonia composed of different cellular types with lymphocytic predominance and nodular lesions without evidence of an underlying infection or malignancy [49]. Brown attributed the cellular clustering to the diminished secretion of mucus, poor bronchial drainage, and secondary infection. Poor cellular immune response was considered [65], but it was also linked secondarily to a phenomenon known as pseudolymphoma [66, 67]. The latter consisted of marked cervical lymphadenopathy, pulmonary infiltrates of lymphocytes without enough atypia or monoclonality to label it as lymphoma [49]. Years later (1972), a full description further reinforced the diversity on pulmonary presentations, ranging from asymptomatic cases to overwhelming lymphoproliferation. Examples within this process were considered, such as pseudolymphoma, Waldenstrom's macroglobulinemia, reticulum-cell sarcoma within the lymph nodes and other types [68]. Similar findings were described in lymphoproliferative processes arisen in other autoimmune diseases (e.g., lupus), certain immune deficiency states, and hydantoin and use of other anticonvulsant drugs [68]. Finally, knowledge of SS in the respiratory system was expanded. Cases of amyloid in the lungs in patients with SS were reported in the 1970s [69], and other lower airway manifestations such as bronchiolitis, asthma, bronchiectasis, bronchiolitis obliterans with organizing pneumonia and also parenchymal disease, such as the interstitial pneumonia with potential to lead to diffuse interstitial pulmonary fibrosis, were linked with SS [62, 70, 71].

6. Prevalence and patterns of pulmonary disease in Sjogren's syndrome

As described in the history, respiratory symptoms exhibit a plethora of manifestations with variable ranges of severity of different areas within the respiratory system. The airways and the lung parenchyma, or an admixture of both, may present alone and combined. Rarely the pleura may show inflammatory changes [72, 73], and pulmonary hypertension, although rare, has been more frequently recognized in East Asian populations [74]. Each one of the compartments may present with a range of different pathologies expanding the disease variety. For instance, in the lung parenchyma, NSIP may prevail [75, 76], but other manifestations have been reported [77].

The prevalence of lung and respiratory manifestations fluctuates from 9 to 24% [9, 11, 12] that include symptoms and abnormal pulmonary function tests or abnormal radiographic findings. Prevalence can go up to [78] 43%-75% [79] if patients are followed prospectively and analyzed based on a composite of multiple studies [80–83]. Symptoms may represent an estimate of an average of 40–66% [84–86], with an increase in sensitivity if radiographic images are included. The involvement of lower airways seem to be the most common respiratory presentation in SS [84, 87, 88]. The cumulative incidence of interstitial lung disease (ILD) at 1 year of pSS diagnosis was found to be of 10%, and went up to 20% after 5 years and 47% at 15 years, a fact that becomes relevant as SS patients age, making an impact on the prevalence [89]. The high prevalence of SS and the respiratory system involvement are a concern for the clinician, alerting her/him to have a full evaluation consisting of obtaining a detailed medical history, at the onset and during the follow-up appointments [45].

7. Morbidity, mortality, and prognostic factors in Sjogren's syndrome and pulmonary compromise

Many of patients with SS and respiratory manifestations, and mainly interstitial lung disease associated with SS (ILD-SS), experience a decline in their quality of life [90, 91]. This seems to be tightly associated with increased morbidity that ultimately will decrease their life expectancy [89]. Mortality risk increases fourfold in a 10-year timeframe [90], making lung involvement one of the most common causes of death [92] and a predictor for mortality [89]. In a meta-analysis of large cohorts of patients with pSS, the overall mortality risk was 1.46-fold higher than that of the general population, and patient profiles with this higher risk revealed to be in the European group, older age, males, presence of ILD, cryoglobulinemia, positive serology (anti-SSB/La), and low complement) [93]. This coincided with another meta-analysis, in which results of mortality risk showed the same, plus additional factors, such as the parotid enlargement, abnormal parotid scintigraphy, and extraglandular involvement [94]. The hazard ratio (HR) for death in pSS and ILD is between 2.1 and 3.2 [89, 95]. Among patients with pSS and already established ILD, respiratory failure accounted for the most common cause of death, and risk factors for mortality were older patients, with smoking habit, and carriers of severe ILD [96], either based on the number of reticulations on the chest HRCT and lymphoblastic foci in the biopsy [97].

8. Radiographic features in Sjogren's syndrome and respiratory involvement

The chest X-ray may disclose features of both the airway, parenchymal and pleural involvement, but has a lower sensitivity than the chest HRCT [98]. The high-resolution chest computed tomography (HRCT) represents the most sensitive technique to uncover pulmonary features even in asymptomatic patients, followed by the pulmonary function tests (including plethysmography) [82]. Computed tomography (CT) changes have been reported in 34–50% [98]. In a cohort of 527 patients with pSS, prevalence of ILD was identified in 39.1% (206/527) based on abnormal chest HRCT. In this large cohort, the most common characteristics in the HRCT reported were associated with parenchymal disease in decreasing order: reticular pattern in 92.7%, ground-glass attenuation in 87.4%, and bronchovascular bundle thickening in 82% [99].

9. Pulmonary function testing in SS and respiratory involvement

The pulmonary function tests are of relevant utility since they will describe patterns of either obstructive, restrictive or a combination of both diseases. Prevailing features in pSS are seen in a pattern of obstruction in most patients and is mainly observed in the maximal expiratory flows (MEFs) 25–50% that test the small airway disease [84, 100]. Decreases in DLco have been reported in several studies [99, 101–104], but the significance of such findings is still unclear. Usually, they precede the FVC decline. Correlations of DLco and higher Schurawitzki score on the chest HRCT have been made, representing a prognostic factor for mortality [104]. Disproportionally low DLco in equivalence to the FVC might represent alveolitis in ILD cases, or pulmonary arterial hypertension (PAH), seen in pSS more than thought in the past. The decline in FVC is more prominent once ILD is established [105, 106].

10. Bronchoalveolar lavage in Sjogren's syndrome and respiratory involvement

Bronchioalveolar lavage in patients with SS may represent an extraordinary tool to define on whether the respiratory system is involved, especially in patients who would present with symptoms and negative changes on PFTs or chest HRCT [100, 107]. Results may disclose prevailing specific CD4(+) T lymphocytes in the cellular differential [108]. Thus, it may improve the sensitivity to detect disturbances in the respiratory system [84], especially for patients with unexplained respiratory symptoms with normal HRCT and PFTs. Furthermore, BAL will reveal an inflammatory pattern on cases with alveolitis, showing the T lymphocyte predominance [108].

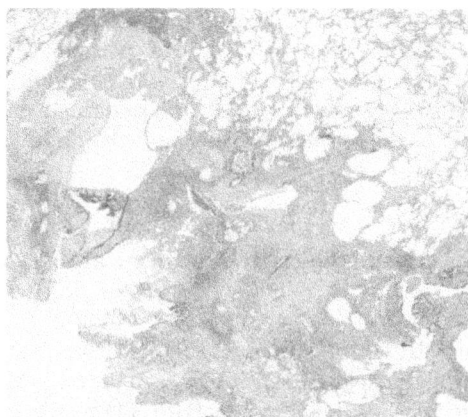

(a)

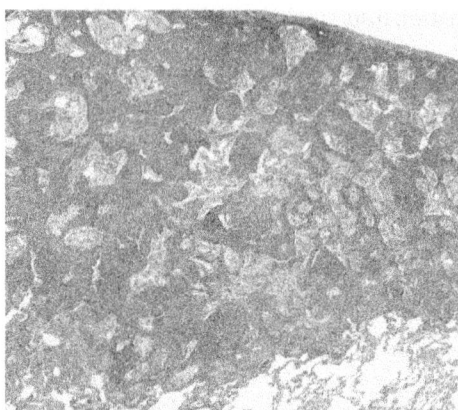

(b)

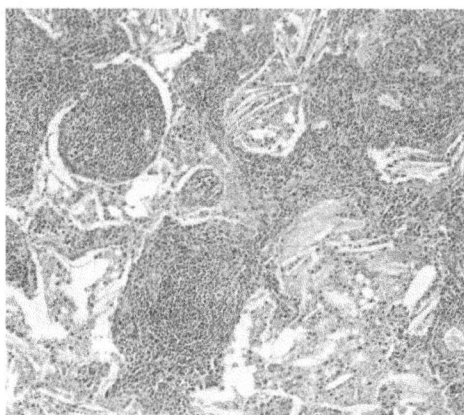

(c)

Figure 2.
H&E sections from a right upper lobe of lung wedge resection reveal focal areas of subpleural scar and fibrosis admixed with cystic airway distention (image a). These areas are associated with an adjacent prominent lymphoplasmacytic inflammation with lymphoid follicular hyperplasia (images b and c). The lymphoid expansion is associated with frequent airspace cholesterol clefts, histiocytes, eosinophilic debris, and sparse neutrophils (image A), mostly resembling changes secondary to localized airspace obstruction possibly secondary to the degree of hyperplastic lymphoplasmacytic reaction. Subpleural cysts and lymphoid hyperplasia are seen in Sjogren's syndrome.

11. Biopsy utility in Sjogren's syndrome and respiratory involvement

Biopsy is currently limited to specific scenarios to (1) determine a clear etiology of the disease, (2) define fibrotic non-interstitial pneumonia (NSIP) vs. usual interstitial pneumonia (UIP), or admixed patterns (3), and establish underlying malignancy, especially in cases with lymphocytic interstitial pneumonia (LIP). In the biopsy, most of results may disclose a fibrotic NSIP pattern (**Figures 2** and **3**) [97]. Furthermore, many of the biopsies will reveal presence of small airway inflammatory changes in association with ILD. Amyloidosis will be identified in association with SS and nodular lung disease, and UIP will increase a yield to up to 33% with the biopsy [97, 103, 109, 110].

The significance of SS exhibiting extraglandular manifestations represents a higher inflammatory state. This is remarkably noticed when the respiratory system is affected. Hypergammaglobulinemia reflects this notion [81, 107]. Additionally, positive anti-SSA/Ro and anti-SSA/La antibodies may associate with the respiratory system [78, 111], so were other acknowledged makers: ANA and the rheumatoid factor (RF) [81, 83]; in addition, some authors consider the evidence of serology as a predictor for lung disease in SS conflicting [80].

12. European league against rheumatism and measurers of disease activity in Sjogren's syndrome

The European League Against Rheumatism (EULAR) task force on SS has created the EULAR-SS Disease Activity Index (ESSDAI) to determine specific organ expression [112, 113]. It is used now as an index to quantify the disease activity in pSS, and applied in randomized control trials [114]. This index includes 12 domains, and representing the target organs and systems affected by the disease (organ systems that are explored are: cutaneous, respiratory, renal, articular, muscular, peripheral nervous system (PNS), central nervous system (CNS), hematological, glandular, constitutional, lymphatic, and immunological). For each domain, the scoring assigns the disease activity in 3–4 levels depending on the severity. Low activity is the ESSDAI of < 5 points; moderate-activity falls between $5 \leq ESSDAI \leq 13$; and high activity scores the $ESSDAI \geq 14$ [115]. A minimal clinically important improvement (MCII) is established as a decrease of at least three points in follow-up visits, when the prior scoring showed moderate activity [115]. The pulmonary domain is divided into four categories, based on the activity level, and range from no activity equivalent to 0, or to symptoms unrelated to pSS, to high activity level or scored as 4 (**Table 1**). The range between low and high activity levels will define the severity based on symptoms (the magnitude of dyspnea will be determined and scored by using the NYHA stratification) and progression of the respiratory symptoms analyzed with ancillary tests (PFTs) or alternatively with the chest HRCT. Patients who fall in the high-activity group may have a worse outcome. In a large cohort of 921 pSS patients, the pulmonary domain of ESSDAI scoring at the time of the diagnosis revealed any pulmonary activity in 6.1% of them, 94% of patients had no pulmonary symptoms. At the end of 75 months, 15% had any pulmonary activity, and sixty percent of the cumulated score corresponded to a new activity [5]. The pulmonary activity had the highest mean cumulated score at the last visit along with the renal and muscular domains, revealing the higher incidence as longer the disease progresses in these three domains [5].

Sjogren's syndrome may selectively affect different compartments within the respiratory system, but it seems it affects almost all and frequently simultaneously.

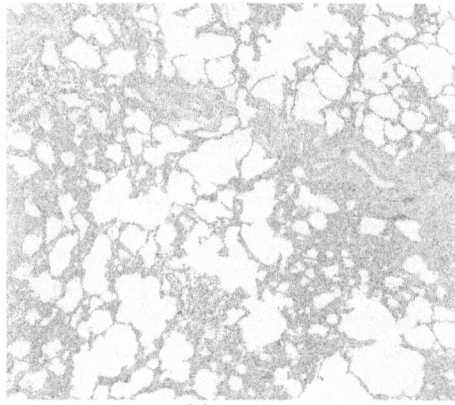

(a)

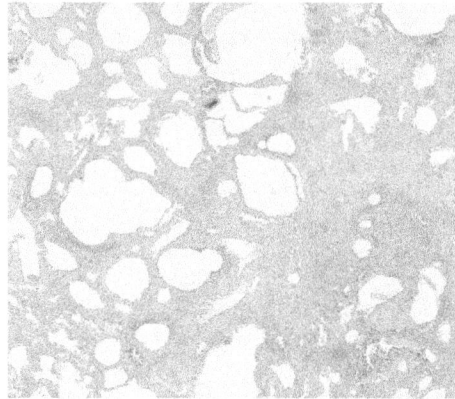

(b)

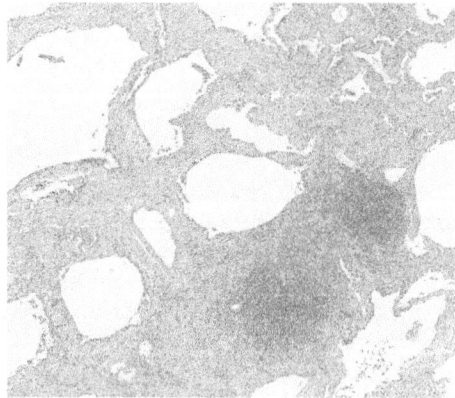

(c)

Figure 3.
H&E sections from this right upper lobe lung wedge biopsy (image a) reveal a cellular interstitial inflammatory infiltrate predominantly composed of lymphocytes admixed with interstitial fibrosis, which is mostly centrilobular. These constellations of findings are consistent with a cellular interstitial pneumonitis with fibrosis. Sections from the right lower lobe wedge biopsy (images b and c) reveal a more markedly altered lung parenchyma compared with the right upper lobe. There is extensive panlobular collagen fibrosis with multifocal areas demonstrating cystic spaces lined by bronchiolar epithelium and fibrotic walls (honeycomb changes). The findings identified in the lower lobe biopsy are not specific to an interstitial lung process but points toward the differential diagnosis of lesions that can have a nonspecific interstitial pneumonia (NSIP) pattern with temporal heterogeneity and extensive honeycombing, which would include connective tissue disorders such as Sjögren's syndrome.

Domain	Activity level	Description
Pulmonary Rate as 'No activity' stable long-lasting features related to damage, or respiratory involvement not related to the disease (tobacco use, etc.)	No = 0	Absence of currently active pulmonary involvement
	Low = 5	Persistent cough due to bronchial involvement with no radiographic abnormalities on radiography or radiological or HRCT evidence of interstitial lung disease with no breathlessness and normal lung function test
	Moderate = 10	Moderately active pulmonary involvement, such as interstitial lung disease shown by HRCT with shortness of breath on exercise (NHYA II) or abnormal lung function tests restricted to: 70% > DLCO ≥ 40% or 80% > FVC ≥ 60%
	High = 15	Highly active pulmonary involvement, such as interstitial lung disease shown by HRCT with shortness of breath at rest (NHYA III, IV) or with abnormal lung function tests: DLCO <40% or FVC <60%

FVC, forced vital capacity; HRCT, high-resolution CT; NYHA, New York Heart Association. *The pulmonary domain is subdivided into four category levels based on the severity of symptoms (NYHA scoring system) and findings in the HRCT and the pulmonary function tests. Cough should be part of the disease and not related with tobacco use. Persistent dry cough and long-lasting cough due to damage should be scored as 0. Interpretation of HRCT should be linked to the activity to ground-glass and not honeycombing aspects. Shortness of breath should be attributable to the disease, and confounders (tobacco use, cardiac insufficiency, arterial pulmonary embolism, or infection) should be excluded.*

Table 1.
EULAR Sjogren's syndrome disease activity index (ESSDAI). Pulmonary domain [114]. *

They may present in an overlap complicating their identification for the subsequent therapeutic intervention. For a better understanding, however, the following compartments should be studied separately.

13. The upper airways

The upper airways seem to be a continuity of the mucosal invasion of inflammatory mononuclear cells, or sialadenitis, affecting the mucosal surfaces in the sinuses, larynx, and ears. The cumulative incidence of chronic rhinosinusitis in pSS has a HR of 2.5 as compared to controls [116].

Dysfunction of salivary glands with the resultant dry mucosa changes the microenvironment in the oral and distant mucosae and thus, promotes a chronic inflammatory state. One good example highlights that pSS patients are at 2.5 times higher risk of developing chronic rhinosinusitis [116]. In addition, the consequent dryness alters or sets off the mucociliary clearance, as seen in the tracheobronchial tree [117]. Furthermore, the histopathology of mucosal surfaces shows infiltrates, similar to what it is seen in the minor salivary glands, where lymphocytic cells surround the mucosal acini configuring the focal lymphocytic sialadenitis [24]. In a study comparing bronchial biopsies of patients with pSS vs. controls, the former showed higher number of infiltrating neutrophils, mast cells, and T lymphocytes. The epithelial damage and structural changes in the subepithelium resembled changes seen in atopic asthma [118]. Moreover, lymphocytic infiltrates are present in BAL of both symptomatic and even asymptomatic patients, representing the continuous and silent inflammatory state along the airways [84, 107, 108, 119].

14. Oral microbiome and Sjogren's syndrome

Sicca mouth in SS has an impact on the oral microbiome, favoring the growth of a dysbiotic environment that replaces the normal flora compared with controls [120]. It is unclear if this hostile environment predisposes this microbiome shifting, favoring its growth. Also, it is unclear if the dysbiosis may impact on the disease establishment and/or progression. Supporting possible impact on glands by the microbiome, experiments on animal models, revealed an association of dysbiotic oral microbiota with the development of lymphocytic sialadenitis [121]. This hypothesis was evaluated in a recent study that demonstrated the immunomodulatory properties of commensal bacteria (*Haemophilus Parainfluenzae*). This bacterium keeps the regulatory immune homeostasis, explored at the cellular level. In a study of salivary microbiome, patients with pSS had lower amounts of *H. Parainfluenzae*. The analized A253 cells, once primed with *H. Parainfluenzae* exposure, induced suppression of CD4 T cell proliferation and induction of PD-L1 expression [122]. Moreover, treatment with low-dose doxycycline normalized the levels of some salivary metabolites associated with the dysbiotic microenvironment in patients with pSS to levels comparable with healthy controls [123]. These findings support the role of the microbiome on pSS pathogenesis and mucosal dysfunction.

15. Dry mucosae in the mouth and upper respiratory airways and SS

Sicca mucosae in SS may impact on dental and periodontal health. It is common to see gum retraction in most of the teeth and specific dental caries at the neck of them. The sicca environment predisposes patients to develop the growth of opportinistic infections, like candida growth. Candida colonization presents in various forms, ranging from asymptomatic, including leukoplakia, and even as burning mouth syndrome [124]. Many patients may lose their teeth and have a significant decrease in their quality of life. This later is in part attributable to the dysphagia and dysphonia, both related with xerostomia [125]. Hoarseness presents in a frequency between 26% and 33% [125, 126]. The laryngeal mucus and vocal folds will harden causing morphological revealing distinctive vessels and/or edema on the exam. In the video-assisted swallowing test abnormal motility will be seen [125]. Gastric reflux may account for this finding predisposing the dysfunctional esophageal motility [127]. The *bamboo node* represents a chronic inflammatory state of vocal cords reported in SS and other CTDs [126]. Although not fully recognized as a common finding in pSS, hearing dysfunction and loss were reported in 80% of patients (24/30), with severe hearing loss in 10% of them. However, most of the pathology seemed to be linked with vestibulocochlear (cranial) neuropathy [128].

Cough is common in pSS, and especially dry cough is representative of, mainly but not only, airway inflammation. The term xerotrachea defines dry tracheal mucosa with the inflammatory background that extends distally, causing significant morbidity [84]. Again, difficulties in clearance will prolong inflammation and promote further functional and anatomic changes such as atelectasis, bronchiectasis, bronchitis, peribronchial and peribronchiolar scarring and airway narrowing [70, 83, 119, 129–131].

16. Lower airways: epidemiology

Patients with SS have a frequent hyperreactive tracheobronchial response in 42–60% [132, 133], and sustained and extended cough following persistent stimuli (dust, tobacco, etc.). They will have abnormally bronchial hyperreaction to the methacholine challenge test, but become inert to the adenosine monophosphate, cold, or hyperventilation. Under the chronic inflammatory state, the pulmonary function test will reveal a decline in the different lung volumes [134, 135]. The pathogenic background of bronchial hyperreaction is unclear, making it difficult to interpret and treat [132]. As previously described, the mucosal chronic inflammation will interfere with clearance, perpetuating and aggravating the dysfunctional hyperresponsiveness [117]. The chest HRCT will be of utility to identify lower airway disease. Findings will be: peripheral bronchiectasis in 5-46%, bronchial wall thickening in 68-85%, nodules in 6-29%, and air trapping in 32%. Together with ground-glass attenuation as the representative parenchymal disease, these are the most common features identified with this modality [87, 107, 136].

16.1 Bronchiolitis

Inflammation in bronchioles has predilection for SS and presenting in different types, such as obliterative bronchiolitis, chronic bronchiolitis, lymphocytic bronchiolitis, constrictive bronchiolitis, and panbronchiolitis [11]. However, the most representative type in SS is follicular bronchiolitis. In biopsies, it may associate with interstitial pneumonia (especially NSIP) [97, 109], and in some cases, along LIP, they may form a continuum, the former limited to peribronchiolar area while the latter to the alveolar septa [119, 137]. Frequencies increase from 12% to 24% when radiographic images accompany the pathological interpretation [109]. Follicular bronchiolitis has a bronchovascular distribution, and the hyperplastic lymphoid follicles with reactive germinal centers run along the bronchovascular bundles [117, 138, 139]. The CT scan will define changes of bronchial thickening in 8–22%, and bronchiolar nodules in 6–24% [82, 84, 133, 140]. Many studies have shown a decline in the DLco that is attributable to bronchiolitis, a fact that needs to be fully proven [99]. Symptoms are represented by dry cough, wheezing, dyspnea, and overlapping infection. Treatment for bronchiolitis challenges the clinician since most of the therapies only seem to be partially responsive. Starting with antibiotic therapy aimed at preventing infectious overlap and especially with use of macrolides, given their anti-inflammatory properties, the mainstream therapy remains on inhaler and/or systemic glucocorticoids, if the disease progresses or becomes seriously symptomatic [141, 142]. Applied disease-modifying drug therapies include azathioprine (AZA), mycophenolate mofetil (MMF), and even rituximab [142]. In the presence of comorbid immune deficiencies (i.e., immune globulin deficiencies, mainly IgG), replacement therapy is recommended [143]. Overall, the treatment intensity should correspond the severity of each case. In complex cases combination of therapies might show better outcomes.

17. Bronchus-associated lymphoid tissue (BALT)

The chronic antigenic stimulus will drive the follicular bronchiolitis to conform a bronchus-associated lymphoid tissue (BALT), which is a benign inflammatory state of polyclonal lymphoid hyperplasia [144], and dense cluster of lymphocytes with follicular structures. These cells follow an antigen-driven stimulus. Well-defined aggregation within a network will separate B from T cells. The B cell compartment encloses follicular dendritic cells (FDCs), which is related with the vascular structures (venules and lymphatics) [142]. BALT is equivalent to the gastric mucosal-associated lymphoid tissue (MALT). In addition, the perivascular compartments are encased by lymphocytic aggregates, labeled as *perivascular cuffing*. They may extend to the small airways and run parallel to the vessels. This organized lymphocytic aggregation is known as induced BALT that is a chronic inflammatory state ready to get reactivated after a second insult [145].

18. Chronic obstructive pulmonary disease

Patients with SS have significantly decreased PFTs showing a composite of decreased VC, TLC, FEV1, FEV1/VC, and DLco but high RV. This pattern fulfills criteria for COPD even in nonsmokers, a fact that may be explained by the presence of chronic tracheobronchitis [146].

18.1 Bronchiectasis

Structural damage with dilatation in distal bronchi and bronchioles may associate with dry mucosa, poor clearance, and superimposed infectious processes [147, 148]. In SS, the cylindrical pattern seen on the HRCT seems to be the prevailing finding [149]. Frequencies vary depending on the cohorts, from 7% to 54% [11]. The clinical presentation is frequently seen in women with chronic sinusitis, with age at the time of diagnosis, and comorbid gastroesophageal reflux. Antismooth muscle but unfrequent anti-SSA/Ro antibodies were detected in this group. The HRCT will describe cylindrical bronchiectasis localized preferentially in the lower lobes (**Figure 4**) [11]. A plethora of symptoms may ensue, especially chronic cough, dyspnea, and even recurrent remitting hemoptysis. The concomitant recurrent superimposed infections worsens the prognosis, reported in 10–35% [70, 71, 150]. Multifactorial etiologies play a role, such as gastroesophageal reflux, dysfunction in the tracheobronchial mucociliary clearance, chronic sinusitis, immune suppressor drug therapy, climate, and presence of bronchiectasis [148, 151, 152]. Combination of bronchodilators, secretagogues, chronic antibiotic use as preventative means for flares seem to be the mainstay of therapy [11]. The use of immune suppressor therapy favors higher

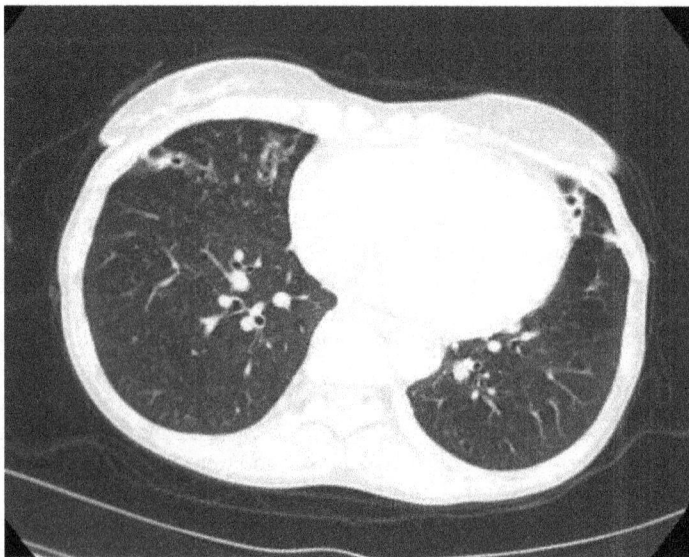

Figure 4.
HRCT. Scattered, ectatic airways more visible in right middle lung and lingula where there is also bronchiectasis and scarring/volume loss. They represent airway-related disease (bronchiectasis).

risks for infections as bronchi may already be chronically colonized with abnormal and pathogenic flora [153].

As described previously, follicular bronchiolitis may be seen in association with parenchymal disease, mainly interstitial pneumonia. The following sections will display the various types of parenchymal disease in SS.

19. Parenchymal lung disease: epidemiology and patterns

Most of the studies report a prevalence of interstitial lung disease associated with primary Sjogren's syndrome (ILD-pSS) of around 20% [85, 89, 95, 101, 102, 151, 154–158]. Other cohorts report variable frequency, ranging from 3% up to 60% [99, 152]. Furthermore, the EULAR task force reported a prevalence of 49% in 526 group of patients with SS, and based on chest HRCT [9], which appears a real-life frequency. Incident cases range between 8% and 17% [85, 101]. Lymphocytic interstitial pneumonia (LIP) was thought to be the most common ILD type [159], but recent large cohorts reveal the following patterns in decreasing order of frequency, based on the HRCT: NSIP in 41.7%, UIP in 10.7%, OP in 3.9%, and LIP in 3.9% of cases out of a total of 124 patients [99]. Other large cohorts with similar frequencies of the various ILD types include amyloidosis in 11%. Admixed patterns were also present in 82 cases reviewed, with combinations of NISP/OP (43.9%), NSIP/UIP (35.4%), and NSIP/ LIP (19.5%). Biopsies confirm NSIP to be the most frequent pathology. Symptoms and findings associated with ILD were found to be dry cough, clubbing, elevated lactate dehydrogenase, and positive anti-SSA/Ro antibodies [99, 103, 160]. Interstitial lung disease associates with older age at the disease onset, longer SS duration, fever, xerostomia, xerophthalmia, and neuropathy [161]. It may be the first presentation in a third to a half of patients [162]. Subsequently, not aware of SS's features, the disease may run undetected. The contribution of lip biopsy in such cases is crucial for this goal especially in cases with negative serology [163]. Laboratories might help and are important for a full evaluation. Hypergammaglobulinemia, lymphopenia, low C4, and high acute-phase reactants are common findings [160]. The PFTs will disclose a restrictive pattern, and low DLco is frequently reported (even up to 64%) [101, 102, 162]. It is common to see an admixture with an obstructive pattern (25%), as a reflection of the association with lower airway disease [162]. The chest X-ray will be of great utility to determine any possible finding in the lung parenchyma, such as linear and reticular patterns, but it has the limitations in sensitivity to detect fine changes [98, 103, 109]. In the chest HRCT, up to 90% of findings will be disclosed [11]. Frequent findings are bilateral infiltrates in almost 99% of cases and predominance in lower lobes and subpleural spaces. Also, lesions distribute in perihilar areas in 9% [99]. Other common findings are the reticular pattern, ground-glass attenuation (92%), non-septal linear opacities (75%), interlobular septal thickening (55%), cystic formation (30%), reticulation, and fibrosis [109, 164]. Honeycombing and features of UIP are unusual [165] (**Figure 4**). Cystic lesions may present at different sizes and distributed along and imbibed withing the parenchyma. They have thin-walled demarcations and may be a consequence of a valve phenomenon [166]. They are associated with LIP, lymphoma, and even amyloidosis [167].

19.1 Nonspecific interstitial pneumonia

This subtype is the most frequent form of ILD-pSS and presents with variable degrees of symptoms, including cough, dyspnea or, rarely, may run asymptomatic [9]. Alveolitis may correlate with NSIP, and one way to identify it is with the BAL. This later study will disclose lymphocytic cells [108]. Frequencies vary depending on the cohorts and methodology used. In a series of 33 cases of ILD, the lung biopsy yielded NSIP pattern in 20/33 61% with the fibrotic type in 19 (57%) [109]. In a cohort of 263 patients with pSS, 8% were identified with ILD with a third of them having NISP pattern [85]. In another study, 19.3% had ILD-pSS, and almost half to them had NSIP pattern based on on HRCT [96]. On the chest HRCT, relevant features in this subtype are the ground-glass opacities, mainly in lower lung fields and subpleural predominance. Other findings are reticular abnormalities, traction bronchiectasis, peri-bronchovascular extension, and pulmonary consolidation. Sparing between pleura-parenchyma interface is a hallmark along with tracking of opacities along lower-zone bronchovascular bundles (**Figure 5**) [168]. The biopsy will reveal preservation of architecture and a composite of inflammatory cells. The distribution characterizes by the lymphocytic expansion of alveolar septa. Fibrosis is also seen and associates with traction bronchiectasis (**Figure 3A**). Honeycombing is rarely seen. Depending on the cellular/fibrotic predominance, NSIP is subdivided into the cellular or fibrotic types. As said, this later is the most frequent presentation in pSS [97].

The 5-year survival rate was of 83–87.4% [97, 109]. Low PaO2 and presence of microscopic honeycombing were associated with worse survival [109]. In another study, worse survival was associated with PaCo2, extent of reticular abnormality on HRCT, and severity of fibroblastic foci on the biopsy [97]. No differences between the NSIP and UIP patterns in terms of prognosis were identified [97], although this is controversial. The clinical course will vary, but this pattern usually is responsive to the immune modulation.

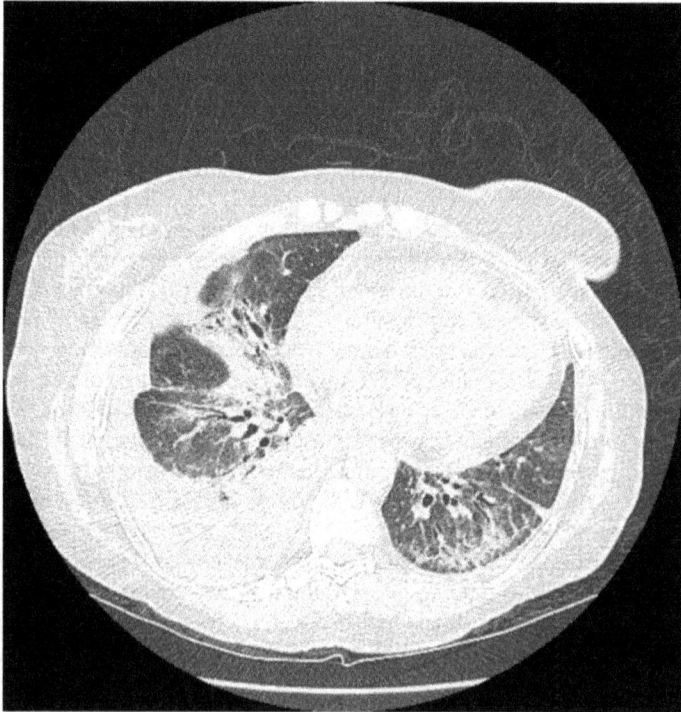

Figure 5.
Parenchyma with reticulation, ground-glass attenuation, and traction bronchiectasis in the lower lobes, middle lobe, and lingula. This process is peribronchial in distribution and extends into peripheral portions of the lung parenchyma. Portions of the subpleural lung parenchyma in these regions are spared. There is no honeycombing. Bilateral pleural effusions larger in right than left lower lobes. Findings are consistent with nonspecific interstitial pneumonia.

19.2 Usual interstitial pneumonia

This subtype is infrequent in SS, but prevalence varies between 10% and 17% [9, 99, 102]. Main differences between UIP and NSIP patterns are based on the HRCT features and interpretation. Intralobular reticulation, honeycombing, traction bronchiectasis, cystic lesions, and temporal heterogeneity may prevail as patterns. The hallmark for UIP is the honeycombing appearance (**Figures 2A, 3B and C and 6**) [168]. Although rare, UIP needs to be recognized as treatment usually is unresponsive to the therapy [103].

19.3 Lymphocytic interstitial pneumonia

Main histopathologic feature is the polymorphous lymphoid infiltrate involving diffusely the alveolar septa of lymphocytes (T and B cells), plasma cells, and histiocytes [169]. Plasma cells show a polyclonal pattern [170]. As described, lesions may present with follicular bronchiolitis along the bronchovascular structures [171], and occasionally will present with foci of BALT hyperplasia (**Figure 5**) [144]. Also amyloid deposits may overlap [159]. Lymphocytic Interstitial pneumonia (LIP) is a benign lymphoproliferative disease. Frequencies range between 3% and 15% [9, 99]. Cough, dyspnea, and inspiratory crackles are common. The CT studies will disclose a diffuse ground-glass opacity and consolidation as the most common features. Thin-walled cysts can be present, along with combination of thickened bronchovascular bundles and nodularity in association with follicular bronchiolitis [168]. Frequently, the biopsy is necessary to differentiate from lymphoma. In the

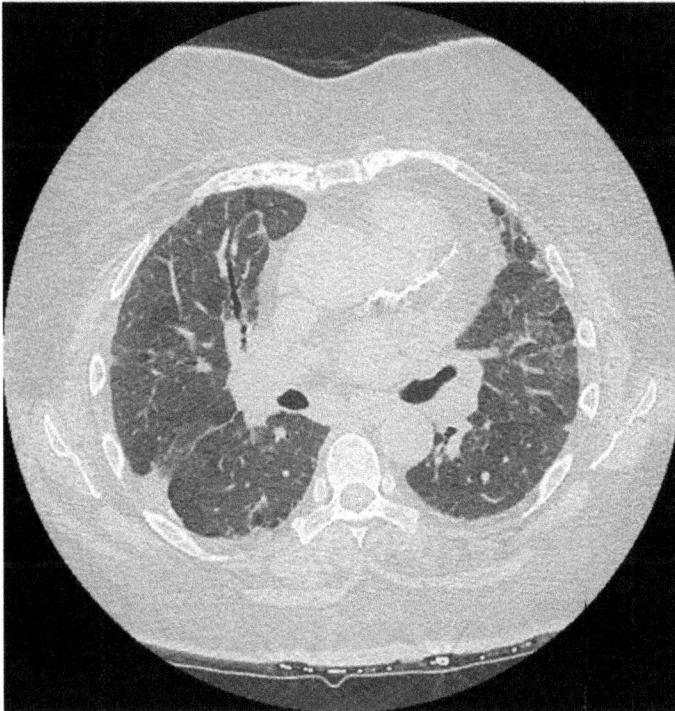

Figure 6.
There is extensive subpleural reticulation, honeycombing, and traction bronchiectasis/bronchiolectasis that predominate in the posterior basal lower lobes. There is no normal lung parenchyma between the fibrotic lung and the adjacent pleural surfaces. There are scattered foci of mild mosaicism indicative of air trapping. Findings are consistent with usual interstitial pneumonia.

presence of germinal centers (GC), this differential has a more relevant importance since both LIP and lymphoma can portray this distinction (**Figure 2B** and **C**). B-cell lymphoma arising from BALT lesions presents with monomorphous B-cell infiltrates with invasion of lymphatics, vessel walls, pleura, and subsequent destruction of alveolar architecture. Monoclonal plasma cells, Immunohistochemistry and gene rearrangements will help define this differential from LIP [172–174]. Differential from NSIP relies on the more intense lymphocyte density seen in LIP [173]. Early and aggressive pharmacologic approach with high-dose glucocorticoids, followed by immune modulators/suppressors, seems to halt the disease progression [11].

19.4 Organizing pneumonia

It is an unusual presentation more common in rheumatoid arthritis, with a frequency of 3.9–11% [9, 75, 160]. Symptoms reveal severe dyspnea, cough, and oxygen dependency. A restrictive pattern will prevail, but a mixed combination is seen. HRCT features consist of diffuse or multifocal patchy bilateral ground-glass opacities and/or consolidation without extensive reticulation or honeycombing [175, 176]. Other features are the reversed halo opacity and bronchial wall thickening [177, 178]. Histopathology will reveal plugs of granulation tissue within small airways (Masson bodies) and chronic inflammatory cell infiltration in alveolar walls [179, 180]. Case reports document the favorable response to glucocorticoids [180, 181], but others may be fatal [182]. Differences of OP with cryptogenic OP are the more frequency in women, positive serology, and relapse presentations. Mortality is linked with progressive dyspnea [183].

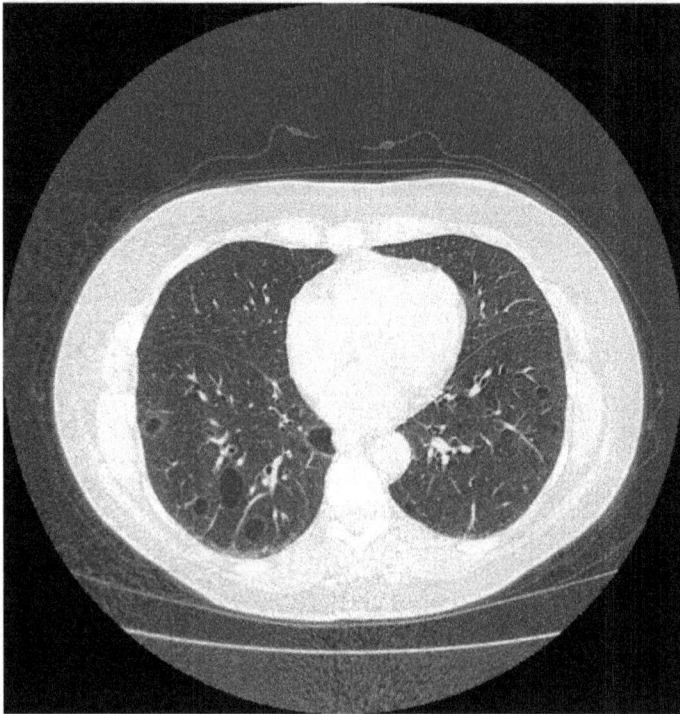

Figure 7.
Multiple thin-walled cysts noted on CT imaging-central predominance. Surrounding lung appears otherwise grossly unremarkable.

20. Cystic lung disease

Cystic lesions may have different dimensions ranging from 0.5 cm to 7 cm, in internal structure within cysts, and frequently associate with ground-glass opacities and nodules [167]. They typically tend to localize in lower lobes, but distribution may be diffuse. Underlying amyloidosis, LIP and lymphomas should be explored [167, 184]. Thin-walled cysts can also occur in the absence of other parenchymal lesions (**Figure 7**). Frequently, they have peribronchovascular distribution [167].

20.1 Lymphoma

Sjogren's syndrome has a higher risk for lymphoma as compared with other CTDs, with a standardized incidence ratio of 37.5, 95%,CI 20.7–67.6 [185]. An estimate of 5% of all SS patients may develop lymphoma with the low-grade extranodal marginal zone B-cell lymphoma (MZL) type being the most relevant histological type [186]. Chronic inflammation adjacent to epithelial cells may predispose to the generation of mucosal-associated lymphocyte tissue (MALT) hyperplasia and in the lungs labeled as bronchial-associated lymphocyte tissue, BALT [144]. The ongoing, relentless, and uncontrolled antigenic stimulus may promote activation of pro-oncogenic genes within lymph nodes or in extranodal lymphocytic aggregates (such as in the lungs), particularly under presence of germinal centers, driving them to endure a monoclonal transformation [187, 188]. MALT lymphomas surge from the marginal zone of B-cells that are localized surrounding the mantle zone and germinal centers, with the denomination of non-Hodgkin's lymphoma, arising from the extranodal marginal zone B-cell. Other types of B-cell lymphomas are present as well. Frequency of pulmonary lymphomas is of 1%–2% [189], and predictors are difficult to define due to the scarcity of cases. Symptoms reveal a dry, chronic cough, and slowly progressive dyspnea or may run undetected [190]. Few patients may have constitutional symptoms (B-symptoms, lymphadenopathy, fever, weight loss, sweats, malaise, etc.) [191]. Findings on the chest HRCT are bronchial wall thickening and bronchiectasis, preferably in lower lobes. Lung parenchyma surrounding the abnormal airways may associate with confluent alveolar opacifications or ground-glass changes. Nodular densities are common [191]. The biopsies will disclose lymphoepithelial lesions involving the bronchial and bronchiolar epithelium, positive CD20 stain, clonal kappa/lambda distribution, Ki-67 proliferation, and abnormal gene rearrangement. Prominent plasma cell proliferation was observed on flow cytometry [191]. Therapy is based on use of alkylating agents and a combination of chemotherapy drugs. Rituximab seems to be the current standard of care as most of plasma cells express CD20 marker [191]. Most of the combination therapies set lymphoma in remission.

21. Amyloidosis in pulmonary Sjogren's syndrome

This is a disorder caused by fibrillary plasma protein deposits on different tissues [192]. Rare cases of amyloidosis in SS are present, mainly in the skin and lungs, and very unusual, systemic amyloidosis. Other sites are reported including the tracheobronchial walls, kidneys, lacrimal glands, tongue, and mammary glands. When it affects the lungs or the tracheobronchial wall, symptoms may ensue, such as cough, dyspnea, pleuritic pain, and hemoptysis [193–203]. Amyloid composition in SS is usually of AL type (lambda or kappa) light chains, or less commonly, AA amyloid type [192]. Women are more frequently affected [195]. Radiographic images will reveal nodules, either calcified or not, and of different heterogeneity. They associate with cystic lesions. Histopathology will reveal infiltration of lymphocytes, plasma cells and amyloid deposits. Amorphous eosinophilic material and Congo red staining will reveal apple-green birefringence. MALT lymphoma should be explored as both associate frequently. Lymphocytic interstitial pneumonia is also frequently present with related cystic formation. The epithelium of cystic lesions may contain amyloid deposits [167]. Symptomatic therapy and glucocorticoids may be of help [192].

22. Pulmonary arterial hypertension, PAH

This is a rare condition in SS; however, the epidemiology reveals new data. Studies in East Asian ethnic group demonstrated a high frequency, such as systemic lupus erythematosus, in nearly half of a large group of 129 patients with confirmed PAH [204]. Women of ages between 30 and 40 are the most affected group [205]. Serology might be of great utility, as well as the biopsy of minor salivary glands. Prognosis at 1, 3, and 5 years is 80.2%, 74.8%, and 67.4%, respectively [206], being the anti-SSB/La antibodies poor predictors [207]. Of course, anti-phospholipid antibody syndrome always should be ruled out among other hypercoagulable risk factors to cause PAH [208].

23. Treatment of Sjogren syndrome and its pulmonary manifestations

23.1 Brief history

Therapy initially relied on symptom management, based on cholinergic pharmacologic drugs (e.g., Pilocarpine), mucolytics, but also radiation therapy (mostly targeting the parotid glands) [61]. The pivotal management, however, and since the 1950s, was based on glucocorticoids [209, 210]. Introduction of hydroxychloroquine in SS was not until the late 1980s and 1990s, and immune modulators have been extensively tried in case reports and case series [211, 212]. In 1998, Schnabel introduced IV cyclophosphamide for pulmonary disease and reported in cases of pseudolymphoma and associated lymphoma with pulmonary compromise [213–215]. Other immune modulators have been used, mainly on cases with advanced disease. Among the therapy, azathioprine [79, 216] and mycophenolate mofetil [217, 218] have been reported. Biologic therapy, such as rituximab, a humanized monoclonal antibody targeting mature B-cells (CD20+), was tried in case series and reports with promising results [219], in reparatory cases [220] and also associated with lymphoproliferative diseases [221–223], in special cases, such as in shrinking lung syndrome associated with SS [224]. Off-the-label cases reported other biologicals, such as tocilizumab [225] and abatacept [226].

24. The overall approach

Pulmonary complications of SS primarily comprise airway mucosal dryness (Xerotrachea), a range of interstitial lung diseases (ILDs), non-Hodgkin lymphomas, pleural effusion and/or thickening, and very rarely it can also cause pulmonary hypertension and/or thromboembolic phenomenon [12, 227].

We will layout an overview of symptomatic treatment of SS and sicca symptoms before discussing treatment of SS-associated pulmonary pathologies. Sicca symptoms are a common feature in most patients with SS, and its treatment can lead to dramatic symptomatic improvement in patients' health and understanding of the disease. Basic measures for prevention of dry eyes and dry mouth should be advised in all patients [228]. These include maintenance of good oral hygiene [229], avoidance of coffee, alcohol, and sugar-filled liquids [230]. Use of artificial tears and avoidance of medications with anticholinergic properties should be stressed, especially drugs used for urinary incontinence such as oxybutynin [231]. Furthermore, this strategy can be compounded with addition of muscarinic agonists such as cevimeline and pilocarpine. These medications are collectively called sialagogues and have been shown to increase salivary flow and improvement in xerostomia in several randomized trials [232–234].

There have been investigative developments in oral electrostimulators, which induce salivary production and flow [235, 236]. However, their usage is vastly limited due to lack of larger trials, greater efficacy of medications, and cumbersome device management.

Dry eyes (Xerophthalmia) can often be the main feature of SS presentation and is usually the most frustrating symptom faced by most patients. Daily use of artificial tears and nightly use of oral lubricant are highly advised. In patients who still complain of dry and itchy eyes after these measures, topical cyclosporine and/or lifitegrast can be utilized [237]. Topical cyclosporine emulsions can be used with daily use of artificial tears, its efficacy is shown to increase with more frequent daily applications [238–240].

Managing nasal dryness is an important consideration as nasal congestion can lead to mouth breathing and worsening of xerostomia. Nasal dryness can be effectively managed with intermittent nasal saline sprays and room humidifiers. Laryngopharyngeal reflux (LPR) is a known manifestation of SS affecting aerodigestive tract. This should be treated with anti-GERD therapy to mitigate the erosive effects of gastric acid on laryngeal structures [241].

25. Treatment of interstitial lung disease

Management of most SS-related ILDs is based on empiric treatment options as no randomized controlled trials (RCTs) have yet been performed. It is also important to understand that treatment of SS-ILD is based on longitudinal worsening in HRCT/PFT results and overall symptomatic nature of the disease. Asymptomatic patients with mild ILD based on HRCT/PFT may not need a lung biopsy for confirmation of exact ILD type and may be monitored with HRCT/PFT every 6–12 months to assess disease progression. NSIP is often the most common histopathology found with SS-ILD, with UIP being second most common. LIP is rarely observed, but it is classically associated with SS-ILD [85].

Patients with symptomatic SS-related NSIP need treatment and are usually started on prednisone 1 mg/kg up to a total of 60 mg per day [75]. Patients should be assessed in 4–6 weeks with a PFT and symptom evaluation. If improvement is observed, low-dose prednisone is usually continued for at least 6 months with subsequent PFT/HRCT and symptom evaluations. Specific details on caution to use glucocorticoids overall are highlighted on the recently published consensus guidelines for the evaluation and management of pulmonary disease in Sjogren's syndrome [45].

Immunosuppressive regimen with azathioprine (AZA) or mycophenolate mofetil (MMF) should be considered for patients as a glucocorticoid sparing therapy to prevent developing side effects to it. Both AZA and MMF have been shown to stabilize FVC decline in patients with CTD-ILDs (these cohorts had patients with SS-ILD as well) [79, 242]. In a recently published retrospective study, patients with pSS-ILD (19 cases) had a modest FVC% and DLco% slope improvement over time with use of both AZA and more favorably MMF, revealing the efficacy of both immune modulators on this condition [243]. In the same study, utility of rituximab was controversial.

Rituximab is left as an emerging option for patients who have refractory lung disease after use of above mentioned strategies. The benefit to target CD20 receptors in mature B-cell lineage has the advantage to blockade any antibody-mediated autoimmune disease. Its usage has been demonstrated in few case reports and case series in SS [244, 245]; however, there is still need of larger controlled trials to formally evaluate its efficacy. Experiences on rituximab in systemic sclerosis and ILD (SSc-ILD) added to the conventional treatment (methotrexate, AZA, or MMF), showed improvement in FVC after 2 years of use [246], and it may not only be a drug as a rescue strategy over MMF [247], but also possibly a line of standard of care therapy in the future when used upfront of other immune modulators (MMF) [248].

Cyclophosphamide has been used in few cases of SS-related ILD. Experiences from cyclophosphamide use in patients with SSc-ILD show efficacy to prevent FCV decline [249, 250]; however, their usage is markedly limited due to toxic effects and loss of efficacy once the drug is stopped [250]. Substitutes for cyclophosphamide after the induction phase were proposed. During the maintenance phase, azathioprine [251] and MMF [252] have been shown to preserve FVC. In the later study, comparing MMF vs. cyclophosphamide during the induction phase, MMF showed similar results in efficacy but lower toxic drug effects, encouraging providers to consider MMF as the drug of choice [252].

Other conventional drugs, including cyclosporine, have shown to prevent the progression of ILD in SS, but owing to their systemic side effects, their use is limited [110].

Tocilizumab, an IL-6 receptor inhibitor, has been tested in patients with SSc-ILD. Results are promising, especially in those individuals with active disease (alveolitis, high Rodnan skin score, high acute-phase reactants, and early stages of the disease) [253]. The decrease in the FVC slope at 24 and 48 weeks comparing with the placebo group that did worse contrasted the positive findings not described on the primary goal as was the prevention of further cutaneous fibrosis. The following trials of this drug confirmed the efficacy to preserve FVC [254], prompting for its FDA approval for SSc-ILD in early 2021. The utility in SS-ILD has not been systemically explored; yet the evidence reveals good outcomes in SS patients presenting with arthritis [255]. It seems tocilizumab to be a promising therapy for active inflammatory lung disease in SS. As an example, in a case report of refractory organizing pneumonia associated with SS, the use of tocilizumab showed to be very effective [225]. Contrasting with IL-6 blockers, TNF-alpha blocker therapy did not seem to be effective in SS overall [256, 257].

Abatacept is another biological therapy. It encompasses the fusion of a cytotoxic T-lymphocyte-associated protein 4 to the FC portion of an IgG1, with high binding affinity to the CD80 and CD86 receptors of the antigen-presenting cell (APC). This way it blocks costimulatory interaction of CD80/CD86 receptors with the T cell receptor (CD28) necessary for T cell activation and proliferation [258]. Approved for rheumatoid arthritis, the experience reveals stabilization of RA-ILD based on HRCT and FVC prospective evaluations [259–265]. Most of the impact was seen in carriers of the NSIP subtype [263], a finding that follows UIP in frequency in RA. Despite the subtype, the overall evidence reveals benefits of abatacept in this disease [261, 264, 266]. The impact of methotrexate on patients on abatacept seemed not to cause any worse pulmonary function deterioration; however, methotrexate's use in ILD raises questions on safety. The same may be considered with other medication class, such as the TNF-alpha blockers with frequent reports of worse ILD in the setting of CTDs [267]. In SS, the efficacy of abatacept has shown in salivary gland inflammatory findings and extraglandular manifestations [268]. A case report revealed improvement in pneumonitis while combining abatacept and tacrolimus [226], suggesting that synergy among both drugs potentiates efficacy on ILD settings.

Belimumab, a specific monoclonal antibody targeting the B-cell activating factor (BlyS), restores circulating B cell numbers, composition, and activity in patients with SS [269]. The BELISS open-label trial of 30 patients with pSS revealed a decline in ESSDAI at 28 weeks, with main improvement in fatigue, but not in sicca symptoms [270]. However, this study did not mention effects on the respiratory system. Main changes in extraglandular manifestations are expected to be observed when its application is sequentially combined with rituximab therapy [271]. Current data regarding the impact of such therapy on the respiratory system are awaited.

Even the backbone in the pathogenesis of SS has a cytokine signature orchestrated by interferon I and II [272, 273], trials on SS of anti-interferon therapies are missing. As compared with lupus trials with this type of treatment modality [274], results of several trials in SS are still pending.

26. Future treatment perspectives for SS-ILD

Two promising antifibrotic drugs, pirfenidone and nintedanib, initially indicated and approved for idiopathic pulmonary fibrosis (IPF), with clear benefits in retarding the annual FVC decline and stabilization, have been recently explored in non-IPF pulmonary fibrotic progressive phenotype. This latter group encompasses different diseases that include sarcoidosis, interstitial pneumonitis, idiopathic NSIP, and unclassifiable idiopathic interstitial pneumonia [275]. Considering this group to share similar pathogenic pathways as in IPF, in that the pulmonary function declines in time along with ominous outcomes, the application of these drugs in this group is reasonable.

Nintedanib, an indolione derivate, has tyrosine kinase inhibitory activity and initially tested as an anticancer drug [276], blocks different profibrotic pathways: fibroblast growth factor receptors, vascular endothelial growth factor receptors, platelet-derived growth factors, and other tyrosine kinases, cytokines and chemokines (CCL18) [277]. With properties to reduce the proliferation and migration of lung fibrocytes and few adverse effects, it has been an effective drug in IPF. Likewise, pirfenidone, a small molecule, a pyridine derivate, inhibits PDGF, transforming growth factor β1 (TGFβ1) [278, 279] and promotes the balance between profibrotic and antifibrotic metalloproteinases [280], in addition to inhibiting proinflammatory cytokines [281].

In the INBUILD trial, 633 patients who had non-IPF progressive fibrosing ILD and that included CTD-ILD patients (i.e., RA patients 89/633, 13%) [282] were tested either with nintedanib or conventional therapy (placebo). Annual FVC showed decreased slope decline in the nintedanib group across all etiologies, including the CTD-ILD group, and without differences even in the UIP-like subgroup [283]. Patients with CTD-ILD group stopped their immune suppressor drugs prior to enrolling in the trial, to avoid confounders [282]. These findings were the ground to establish evidence for nintedanib efficacy in non-IPF progressive fibrosing ILDs independently of the diagnosis, enabling the FDA approval for its use. Even most of the experience falls into patients with SSc-ILD and RA-ILD, based on this evidence, SS-ILD may benefit from nintedanib as well. It is worth to mention the phase III SENSCIS trial on 576 patients with SSc-ILD testing nintedanib vs. placebo. Results showed a lower annual rate of decline in FVC (primary endpoint) with nintedanib than with placebo, but with more gastrointestinal adverse events in the nintedanib group [284]. Safety on the use of pirfenidone in SSc-ILD showed similar adverse events as in the placebo group, and moreover, combination of pirfenidone and MMF showed adequate tolerability and safety (LOTUSS trial) [285]. Further ongoing trials will reveal more information regarding safety and efficacy. Similarly, data are pending for RA-ILD and on pirfenidone (TRAIL-1, on phase II trial).

An anecdotal report on SS-ILD with UIP subtype showed promising experience in FVC preservation [286] as single evidence of the experience in SS patients. In this case series, pirfenidone was the applied drug to treat ILD. Again, further studies will reveal much more information on these promising drugs [287].

Until more trials show documented efficacy of the abovementioned regimens, treatment for SS-ILD will be subjected to individual clinical scenarios and physician preferences.

27. Conclusions

Extraglandular expression of SS may encompass many organs, with the respiratory system as one of the most frequently affected systems, carrying significant morbidity. With the lower airways being the most common manifestations in SS, the upper airways may associate with multiple presentations, including sinusitis. The airway disease should be acknowledged to be part of the syndrome, particularly when patients have poor response to therapy and behave differently to bronchial asthma. Airway disease treatment may challenge conventional strategies offered. Although less frequent, ILD may carry most of the main problems. Mortality associates with severe parenchymal disease, shortening life expectations in vulnerable groups (older age, smokers, males, and longer disease duration). Many other parenchymal manifestations are associated with SS such as LIP, amyloidosis, cystic lesions, lymphoma, and pulmonary hypertension and should be contemplated in the differentials. Clinicians should follow up patients with SS keeping in mind that the manifestations of the respiratory system may present at any point in time. Conventional therapies are available with variable results such as mycophenolate mofetil, azathioprine, cyclophosphamide, cyclosporine, and biological therapy. Among the latter, IL-6 inhibitors, costimulatory receptor antagonists, B-cell antagonist therapy, and other cytokine blocker therapy, including interferon blockers, seem to offer promising and safe profiles for the treatment of SS-ILD. New promising antifibrotic therapy (e.g., nintedanib and pirfenidone) will probably change the outcome panorama in SS-ILD. Combination of therapies seems to be an excellent modality to treat difficult cases.

Author details

Moiz Ehtesham[1], Anupama Tiwari[2], Rose Sneha George[3] and Ruben A. Peredo[4*]

1 Internal Medicine, Albany Medical College, Albany, NY, USA

2 Division of Pulmonary, Albany Medical College, Albany, NY, USA

3 Department of Pathology, Albany Medical College, Albany, NY, USA

4 Division of Rheumatology, Stratton VA Medical Center, Albany, NY, USA

*Address all correspondence to: peredor@amc.edu

IntechOpen

References

[1] Parke AL, Buchanan WW. Sjogren's syndrome: History, clinical and pathological features. Inflammopharmacology. 1998;**6**(4): 271-287

[2] Fox RI, Howell FV, Bone RC, Michelson P. Primary Sjogren syndrome: Clinical and immunopathologic features. Seminars in Arthritis and Rheumatism. 1984;**14**(2):77-105

[3] Haldorsen K, Bjelland I, Bolstad AI, Jonsson R, Brun JG. A five-year prospective study of fatigue in primary Sjogren's syndrome. Arthritis Research & Therapy. 2011;**13**(5):R167

[4] Arends S, Meiners PM, Moerman RV, Kroese FG, Brouwer E, Spijkervet FK, et al. Physical fatigue characterises patient experience of primary Sjogren's syndrome. Clinical and Experimental Rheumatology. 2017;**35**(2):255-261

[5] Ramos-Casals M, Brito-Zeron P, Solans R, Camps MT, Casanovas A, Sopena B, et al. Systemic involvement in primary Sjogren's syndrome evaluated by the EULAR-SS disease activity index: Analysis of 921 Spanish patients (GEAS-SS registry). Rheumatology (Oxford, England). 2014;**53**(2):321-331

[6] Retamozo S, Acar-Denizli N, Rasmussen A, Horvath IF, Baldini C, Priori R, et al. Systemic manifestations of primary Sjogren's syndrome out of the ESSDAI classification: Prevalence and clinical relevance in a large international, multi-ethnic cohort of patients. Clinical and Experimental Rheumatology. 2019;**118**(3):97-106

[7] Asmussen K, Andersen V, Bendixen G, Schiodt M, Oxholm P. A new model for classification of disease manifestations in primary Sjogren's syndrome: Evaluation in a retrospective long-term study. Journal of Internal Medicine. 1996;**239**(6):475-482

[8] Ramos-Casals M, Acar-Denizli N, Vissink A, Brito-Zeron P, Li X, Carubbi F, et al. Childhood-onset of primary Sjogren's syndrome: Phenotypic characterization at diagnosis of 158 children. Rheumatology (Oxford, England). 2021;**60**(10):4558-4567

[9] Ramos-Casals M, Brito-Zeron P, Seror R, Bootsma H, Bowman SJ, Dorner T, et al. Characterization of systemic disease in primary Sjogren's syndrome: EULAR-SS task force recommendations for articular, cutaneous, pulmonary and renal involvements. Rheumatology (Oxford, England). 2015;**54**(12):2230-2238

[10] Dias C, Isenberg DA. Susceptibility of patients with rheumatic diseases to B-cell non-Hodgkin lymphoma. Nature Reviews Rheumatology. 2011;7(6): 360-368

[11] Flament T, Bigot A, Chaigne B, Henique H, Diot E, Marchand-Adam S. Pulmonary manifestations of Sjogren's syndrome. European Respiratory Review: An Official Journal of the European Respiratory Society. 2016;**25**(140):110-123

[12] Gupta S, Ferrada MA, Hasni SA. Pulmonary manifestations of primary Sjögren's syndrome: Underlying immunological mechanisms, clinical presentation, and management. Frontiers in Immunology. 2019;**10**:1327

[13] Fox RI. Sjogren's syndrome. Lancet. 2005;**366**(9482):321-331

[14] Mavragani CP, Moutsopoulos HM. The geoepidemiology of Sjogren's syndrome. Autoimmunity Reviews. 2010;**9**(5):A305-A310

[15] Qin B, Wang J, Yang Z, Yang M, Ma N, Huang F, et al. Epidemiology of primary Sjogren's syndrome: A systematic review and meta-analysis.

Annals of the Rheumatic Diseases. 2015;**74**(11):1983-1989

[16] Patel R, Shahane A. The epidemiology of Sjogren's syndrome. Clinical Epidemiology. 2014;**6**:247-255

[17] Birlik M, Akar S, Gurler O, Sari I, Birlik B, Sarioglu S, et al. Prevalence of primary Sjogren's syndrome in Turkey: A population-based epidemiological study. International Journal of Clinical Practice. 2009;**63**(6):954-961

[18] Anagnostopoulos I, Zinzaras E, Alexiou I, Papathanasiou AA, Davas E, Koutroumpas A, et al. The prevalence of rheumatic diseases in Central Greece: A population survey. BMC Musculoskeletal Disorders. 2010;**11**:98

[19] Goransson LG, Haldorsen K, Brun JG, Harboe E, Jonsson MV, Skarstein K, et al. The point prevalence of clinically relevant primary Sjogren's syndrome in two Norwegian counties. Scandinavian Journal of Rheumatology. 2011;**40**(3):221-224

[20] Peri Y, Agmon-Levin N, Theodor E, Shoenfeld Y. Sjögren's syndrome, the old and the new. Best Practice & Research. Clinical Rheumatology. 2012;**26**(1): 105-117

[21] Cornec D, Devauchelle-Pensec V, Tobon GJ, Pers JO, Jousse-Joulin S, Saraux A. B cells in Sjogren's syndrome: From pathophysiology to diagnosis and treatment. Journal of Autoimmunity. 2012;**39**(3):161-167

[22] Fayyaz A, Kurien BT, Scofield RH. Autoantibodies in Sjogren's Syndrome. Rheumatic Diseases Clinics of North America. 2016;**42**(3):419-434

[23] Daniels TE, Cox D, Shiboski CH, Schiodt M, Wu A, Lanfranchi H, et al. Associations between salivary gland histopathologic diagnoses and phenotypic features of Sjogren's syndrome among 1,726 registry participants. Arthritis and Rheumatism. 2011;**63**(7):2021-2030

[24] Greenspan JS, Daniels TE, Talal N, Sylvester RA. The histopathology of Sjogren's syndrome in labial salivary gland biopsies. Oral Surgery, Oral Medicine, and Oral Pathology. 1974;**37**(2):217-229

[25] Fisher BA, Jonsson R, Daniels T, Bombardieri M, Brown RM, Morgan P, et al. Standardisation of labial salivary gland histopathology in clinical trials in primary Sjogren's syndrome. Annals of the Rheumatic Diseases. 2017;**76**(7):1161-1168

[26] Brito-Zeron P, Acar-Denizli N, Ng WF, Zeher M, Rasmussen A, Mandl T, et al. How immunological profile drives clinical phenotype of primary Sjogren's syndrome at diagnosis: Analysis of 10,500 patients (Sjogren big data project). Clinical and Experimental Rheumatology. 2018;**112**(3):102-112

[27] Ramos-Casals M, Brito-Zeron P, Siso-Almirall A, Bosch X. Primary Sjogren syndrome. BMJ. 2012;**344**:e3821

[28] Shiboski CH, Shiboski SC, Seror R, Criswell LA, Labetoulle M, Lietman TM, et al. 2016 American College of Rheumatology/European league against rheumatism classification criteria for primary Sjogren's syndrome: A consensus and data-driven methodology involving three international patient cohorts. Arthritis & Rheumatology. 2017;**69**(1):35-45

[29] Defendenti C, Atzeni F, Spina MF, Grosso S, Cereda A, Guercilena G, et al. Clinical and laboratory aspects of Ro/SSA-52 autoantibodies. Autoimmunity Reviews. 2011;**10**(3):150-154

[30] Jordan-Gonzalez P, Gago-Pinero R, Varela-Rosario N, Perez-Rios N, Vila LM. Characterization of a subset of patients with primary Sjogren's

syndrome initially presenting with C3 or C4 hypocomplementemia. European Journal of Rheumatology. 2020;7(3):112-117

[31] Baldini C, Pepe P, Quartuccio L, Priori R, Bartoloni E, Alunno A, et al. Primary Sjogren's syndrome as a multi-organ disease: Impact of the serological profile on the clinical presentation of the disease in a large cohort of Italian patients. Rheumatology (Oxford, England). 2014;53(5):839-844

[32] Retamozo S, Brito-Zeron P, Ramos-Casals M. Prognostic markers of lymphoma development in primary Sjogren syndrome. Lupus. 2019;28(8): 923-936

[33] Theander E, Jonsson R, Sjostrom B, Brokstad K, Olsson P, Henriksson G. Prediction of Sjogren's syndrome years before diagnosis and identification of patients with early onset and severe disease course by autoantibody profiling. Arthritis & Rheumatology. 2015;67(9):2427-2436

[34] Arbuckle MR, McClain MT, Rubertone MV, Scofield RH, Dennis GJ, James JA, et al. Development of autoantibodies before the clinical onset of systemic lupus erythematosus. The New England Journal of Medicine. 2003;349(16):1526-1533

[35] Aoshiba K, Tsuji T, Yamaguchi K, Itoh M, Nakamura H. The danger signal plus DNA damage two-hit hypothesis for chronic inflammation in COPD. The European Respiratory Journal. 2013;42(6):1689-1695

[36] Beckman KA, Luchs J, Milner MS. Making the diagnosis of Sjogren's syndrome in patients with dry eye. Clinical Ophthalmology. 2016;10:43-53

[37] Hernandez-Molina G, Nunez-Alvarez C, Avila-Casado C, Llorente L, Hernandez-Hernandez C, Calderillo ML, et al. Usefulness of IgA anti-alpha-fodrin antibodies in combination with rheumatoid factor and/or antinuclear antibodies as substitute immunological criterion in Sjogren syndrome with negative anti-SSA/SSB antibodies. The Journal of Rheumatology. 2016;43(10):1852-1857

[38] He J, Guo JP, Ding Y, Li YN, Pan SS, Liu Y, et al. Diagnostic significance of measuring antibodies to cyclic type 3 muscarinic acetylcholine receptor peptides in primary Sjogren's syndrome. Rheumatology (Oxford, England). 2011;50(5):879-884

[39] Routsias JG, Tzioufas AG. Sjogren's syndrome—Study of autoantigens and autoantibodies. Clinical Reviews in Allergy & Immunology. 2007;32(3): 238-251

[40] Karakus S, Baer AN, Akpek EK. Clinical correlations of novel autoantibodies in patients with dry eye. Journal of Immunology Research. 2019;2019:7935451

[41] Shen L, Suresh L, Lindemann M, Xuan J, Kowal P, Malyavantham K, et al. Novel autoantibodies in Sjogren's syndrome. Clinical Immunology. 2012;145(3):251-255

[42] Brito-Zeron P, Acar-Denizli N, Zeher M, Rasmussen A, Seror R, Theander E, et al. Influence of geolocation and ethnicity on the phenotypic expression of primary Sjogren's syndrome at diagnosis in 8310 patients: A cross-sectional study from the big data Sjogren project consortium. Annals of the Rheumatic Diseases. 2017;76(6):1042-1050

[43] Kassan SS, Moutsopoulos HM. Clinical manifestations and early diagnosis of Sjogren syndrome. Archives of Internal Medicine. 2004;164(12): 1275-1284

[44] Vitali C, Bombardieri S, Jonsson R, Moutsopoulos HM, Alexander EL,

Carsons SE, et al. Classification criteria for Sjogren's syndrome: A revised version of the European criteria proposed by the American-European consensus group. Annals of the Rheumatic Diseases. 2002;**61**(6): 554-558

[45] Lee AS, Scofield RH, Hammitt KM, Gupta N, Thomas DE, Moua T, et al. Consensus guidelines for evaluation and management of pulmonary disease in Sjogren's. Chest. 2021;**159**(2):683-698

[46] Rasmussen A, Ice JA, Li H, Grundahl K, Kelly JA, Radfar L, et al. Comparison of the American-European consensus group Sjogren's syndrome classification criteria to newly proposed American College of Rheumatology criteria in a large, carefully characterised sicca cohort. Annals of the Rheumatic Diseases. 2014;**73**(1):31-38

[47] Fox RI, Robinson CA, Curd JG, Kozin F, Howell FV. Sjogren's syndrome. Proposed criteria for classification. Arthritis and Rheumatism. 1986;**29**(5): 577-585

[48] Vitali C, Bombardieri S, Moutsopoulos HM, Balestrieri G, Bencivelli W, Bernstein RM, et al. Preliminary criteria for the classification of Sjogren's syndrome. Results of a prospective concerted action supported by the European Community. Arthritis and Rheumatism. 1993;**36**(3):340-347

[49] Bloch KJ, Buchanan WW, Wohl MJ, Bunim JJ. Sjoegren's syndrome. A clinical, pathological, and serological study of sixty-two cases. Medicine (Baltimore). 1965;**44**:187-231

[50] Bombardieri M, Argyropoulou OD, Ferro F, Coleby R, Pontarini E, Governato G, et al. One year in review 2020: Pathogenesis of primary Sjogren's syndrome. Clinical and Experimental Rheumatology. 2020;**38 Suppl 126**(4): 3-9

[51] Leber T. Praparate zu dem Vortag uber Entstnhung der Netzhautablosung und uber verschiedene Hornhautaffecttionen. Ber Ophthalmol Ges Heidelberg. 1882;**14**:165-166

[52] Hadden WB. On "dry mouth," or suppression of the salivary and buccal secretions. Transactions of the Clinical Society of London. 1888;**21**: 176-179

[53] Bloch KJ, Wohl MJ, Ship II, Oglesby BB, Bunim JJ, Sjogren's syndrome. 1. Serologic reactions in patients with Sjogren's syndrome with and without rheumatoid arthritis. Arthritis and Rheumatism. 1960;**3**: 287-297

[54] Fischer E. Uber Fadchenkeratitis. Graefe's Archive. 1889;**35**:201

[55] Houwer AM. Keratitis filamentosa and chronic arthritis. Transactions of the Ophthalmological Societies of the United Kingdom. 1927;**47**:88-96

[56] Holm S, Sjogren H, et al. Studies on keratoconjunctivitis sicca, based on examination of 500 subjects affected with rheumatism and an equally large control material. Acta Ophthalmologica. 1948;**26**(2):269-273

[57] Hill LC. Systemic lupus erythematosus. British Medical Journal. 1957;**2**(5047):726-732

[58] Jones BR. Lacrimal and salivary precipitating antibodies in Sjogren's syndrome. Lancet. 1958;**2**(7050): 773-776

[59] Delaleu N, Jonsson R, Koller MM. Sjogren's syndrome. European Journal of Oral Sciences. 2005;**113**(2): 101-113

[60] Bunim JJ. A broader spectrum of Sjogren's syndrome and its pathogenetic implications. Annals of the Rheumatic Diseases. 1961;**20**:1-10

[61] Weber FP. Sjogren's syndrome, especially its non-ocular features. The British Journal of Ophthalmology. 1945;**29**(6):299-312

[62] Baruch HH, Firooznia H, Sackler JP, Genieser NB, Rafii M, Golimbu C. Pulmonary disorders associated with Sjogren's syndrome. Revista Interamericana de Radiología. 1977;**2**(2):77-81

[63] Bucher UG, Reid L. Sjogren's syndrome: Report of a fatal case with pulmonary and renal lesions. British Journal of Diseases of the Chest. 1959;**53**:237-252

[64] Ellman P, Weber FP, Goodier TE. A contribution to the pathology of Sjogren's disease. The Quarterly Journal of Medicine. 1951;**20**(77):33-42

[65] Leventhal BG, Waldorf DS, Talal N. Impaired lymphocyte transformation and delayed hypersensitivity in Sjogren's syndrome. The Journal of Clinical Investigation. 1967;**46**(8):1338-1345

[66] Talal N, Bunim JJ. The development of malignant lymphoma in the course of Sjoegren's syndrome. The American Journal of Medicine. 1964;**36**:529-540

[67] Talal N, Sokoloff L, Barth WF. Extrasalivary lymphoid abnormalities in Sjogren's syndrome (reticulum cell sarcoma, "pseudolymphoma," macroglobulinemia). The American Journal of Medicine. 1967;**43**(1):50-65

[68] Anderson LG, Talal N. The spectrum of benign to malignant lymphoproliferation in Sjogren's syndrome. Clinical and Experimental Immunology. 1972;**10**(2):199-221

[69] Bonner H Jr, Ennis RS, Geelhoed GW, Tarpley TM Jr. Lymphoid infiltration and amyloidosis of lung in Sjogren's syndrome. Archives of Pathology. 1973;**95**(1):42-44

[70] Fairfax AJ, Haslam PL, Pavia D, Sheahan NF, Bateman JR, Agnew JE, et al. Pulmonary disorders associated with Sjogren's syndrome. The Quarterly Journal of Medicine. 1981;**50**(199):279-295

[71] Strimlan CV, Rosenow EC 3rd, Weiland LH, Brown LR. Lymphocytic interstitial pneumonitis. Review of 13 cases. Annals of Internal Medicine. 1978;**88**(5):616-621

[72] Yamamoto Y, Otsuka Y, Katsuyama T, Nishimura Y, Oka K, Hasegawa K, et al. An elderly male with primary Sjogren's syndrome presenting Pleuritis as the initial manifestation. Acta Medica Okayama. 2021;**75**(4):539-542

[73] Teshigawara K, Kakizaki S, Horiya M, Kikuchi Y, Hashida T, Tomizawa Y, et al. Primary Sjogren's syndrome complicated by bilateral pleural effusion. Respirology. 2008;**13**(1):155-158

[74] Sato T, Hatano M, Iwasaki Y, Maki H, Saito A, Minatsuki S, et al. Prevalence of primary Sjogren's syndrome in patients undergoing evaluation for pulmonary arterial hypertension. PLoS One. 2018;**13**(5):e0197297

[75] Parambil JG, Myers JL, Lindell RM, Matteson EL, Ryu JH. Interstitial lung disease in primary Sjögren syndrome. Chest. 2006;**130**(5):1489-1495

[76] Sambataro G, Ferro F, Orlandi M, Sambataro D, Torrisi SE, Quartuccio L, et al. Clinical, morphological features and prognostic factors associated with interstitial lung disease in primary Sjgren's syndrome: A systematic review from the Italian Society of Rheumatology. Autoimmunity Reviews. 2020;**19**(2):102447

[77] Natalini JG, Johr C, Kreider M. Pulmonary involvement in Sjogren

syndrome. Clinics in Chest Medicine. 2019;**40**(3):531-544

[78] Davidson BK, Kelly CA, Griffiths ID. Ten year follow up of pulmonary function in patients with primary Sjogren's syndrome. Annals of the Rheumatic Diseases. 2000;**59**(9): 709-712

[79] Deheinzelin D, Capelozzi VL, Kairalla RA, Barbas Filho JV, Saldiva PH, de Carvalho CR. Interstitial lung disease in primary Sjögren's syndrome. Clinical-pathological evaluation and response to treatment. American Journal of Respiratory and Critical Care Medicine. 1996;**154** (3 Pt 1):794-799

[80] Yazisiz V, Arslan G, Ozbudak IH, Turker S, Erbasan F, Avci AB, et al. Lung involvement in patients with primary Sjogren's syndrome: What are the predictors? Rheumatology International. 2010;**30**(10):1317-1324

[81] Garcia-Carrasco M, Ramos-Casals M, Rosas J, Pallares L, Calvo-Alen J, Cervera R, et al. Primary Sjogren syndrome: Clinical and immunologic disease patterns in a cohort of 400 patients. Medicine (Baltimore). 2002;**81**(4):270-280

[82] Uffmann M, Kiener HP, Bankier AA, Baldt MM, Zontsich T, Herold CJ. Lung manifestation in asymptomatic patients with primary Sjogren syndrome: Assessment with high resolution CT and pulmonary function tests. Journal of Thoracic Imaging. 2001;**16**(4):282-289

[83] Strimlan CV, Rosenow EC 3rd, Divertie MB, Harrison EG Jr. Pulmonary manifestations of Sjogren's syndrome. Chest. 1976;**70**(03):354-361

[84] Papiris SA, Maniati M, Constantopoulos SH, Roussos C, Moutsopoulos HM, Skopouli FN. Lung involvement in primary Sjogren's

syndrome is mainly related to the small airway disease. Annals of the Rheumatic Diseases. 1999;**58**(1):61-64

[85] Roca F, Dominique S, Schmidt J, Smail A, Duhaut P, Levesque H, et al. Interstitial lung disease in primary Sjogren's syndrome. Autoimmunity Reviews. 2017;**16**(1):48-54

[86] Kurumagawa T, Kobayashi H, Motoyoshi K. Potential involvement of subclinical Sjogren's syndrome in various lung diseases. Respirology. 2005;**10**(1):86-91

[87] Egashira R, Kondo T, Hirai T, Kamochi N, Yakushiji M, Yamasaki F, et al. CT findings of thoracic manifestations of primary Sjogren syndrome: Radiologic-pathologic correlation. Radiographics: A review publication of the Radiological Society of North America. Inc. 2013;**33**(7): 1933-1949

[88] Nakanishi M, Fukuoka J, Tanaka T, Demura Y, Umeda Y, Ameshima S, et al. Small airway disease associated with Sjogren's syndrome: Clinico-pathological correlations. Respiratory Medicine. 2011;**105**(12):1931-1938

[89] Nannini C, Jebakumar AJ, Crowson CS, Ryu JH, Matteson EL. Primary Sjogren's syndrome 1976-2005 and associated interstitial lung disease: A population-based study of incidence and mortality. BMJ Open. 2013;**3**(11): e003569

[90] Palm O, Garen T, Berge Enger T, Jensen JL, Lund MB, Aalokken TM, et al. Clinical pulmonary involvement in primary Sjogren's syndrome: Prevalence, quality of life and mortality—A retrospective study based on registry data. Rheumatology (Oxford, England). 2013;**52**(1):173-179

[91] Belenguer R, Ramos-Casals M, Brito-Zeron P, del Pino J, Sentis J, Aguilo S, et al. Influence of clinical and

immunological parameters on the health-related quality of life of patients with primary Sjogren's syndrome. Clinical and Experimental Rheumatology. 2005;**23**(3):351-356

[92] Kim HJ, Kim KH, Hann HJ, Han S, Kim Y, Lee SH, et al. Incidence, mortality, and causes of death in physician-diagnosed primary Sjogren's syndrome in Korea: A nationwide, population-based study. Seminars in Arthritis and Rheumatism. 2017;**47**(2): 222-227

[93] Huang H, Xie W, Geng Y, Fan Y, Zhang Z. Mortality in patients with primary Sjogren's syndrome: A systematic review and meta-analysis. Rheumatology (Oxford, England). 2021;**60**(9):4029-4038

[94] Singh AG, Singh S, Matteson EL. Rate, risk factors and causes of mortality in patients with Sjogren's syndrome: A systematic review and meta-analysis of cohort studies. Rheumatology (Oxford, England). 2016;**55**(3):450-460

[95] Lin DF, Yan SM, Zhao Y, Zhang W, Li MT, Zeng XF, et al. Clinical and prognostic characteristics of 573 cases of primary Sjogren's syndrome. Chinese Medical Journal. 2010;**123**(22):3252-3257

[96] Gao H, Sun Y, Zhang XY, Xie L, Zhang XW, Zhong YC, et al. Characteristics and mortality in primary Sjogren syndrome-related interstitial lung disease. Medicine (Baltimore). 2021;**100**(35):e26777

[97] Enomoto Y, Takemura T, Hagiwara E, Iwasawa T, Fukuda Y, Yanagawa N, et al. Prognostic factors in interstitial lung disease associated with primary Sjogren's syndrome: A retrospective analysis of 33 pathologically-proven cases. PLoS One. 2013;**8**(9):e73774

[98] Matsuyama N, Ashizawa K, Okimoto T, Kadota J, Amano H,

Hayashi K. Pulmonary lesions associated with Sjogren's syndrome: Radiographic and CT findings. The British Journal of Radiology. 2003;**76**(912):880-884

[99] Dong X, Zhou J, Guo X, Li Y, Xu Y, Fu Q, et al. A retrospective analysis of distinguishing features of chest HRCT and clinical manifestation in primary Sjogren's syndrome-related interstitial lung disease in a Chinese population. Clinical Rheumatology. 2018;**37**(11): 2981-2988

[100] Kampolis CF, Fragkioudaki S, Mavragani CP, Zormpala A, Samakovli A, Moutsopoulos HM. Prevalence and spectrum of symptomatic pulmonary involvement in primary Sjogren's syndrome. Clinical and Experimental Rheumatology. 2018;**112**(3):94-101

[101] Manfredi A, Sebastiani M, Cerri S, Cassone G, Bellini P, Casa GD, et al. Prevalence and characterization of non-sicca onset primary Sjogren syndrome with interstitial lung involvement. Clinical Rheumatology. 2017;**36**(6):1261-1268

[102] Wang Y, Hou Z, Qiu M, Ye Q. Risk factors for primary Sjogren syndrome-associated interstitial lung disease. Journal of Thoracic Disease. 2018;**10**(4):2108-2117

[103] Parambil JG, Myers JL, Lindell RM, Matteson EL, Ryu JH. Interstitial lung disease in primary Sjogren syndrome. Chest. 2006;**130**(5):1489-1495

[104] Chen MH, Chou HP, Lai CC, Chen YD, Chen MH, Lin HY, et al. Lung involvement in primary Sjogren's syndrome: Correlation between high-resolution computed tomography score and mortality. Journal of the Chinese Medical Association. 2014;**77**(2):75-82

[105] Yan S, Li M, Wang H, Yang X, Zhao J, Wang Q, et al. Characteristics

and risk factors of pulmonary arterial hypertension in patients with primary Sjogren's syndrome. International Journal of Rheumatic Diseases. 2018;**21**(5):1068-1075

[106] Fox RI. The incidence of pulmonary hypertension is higher in systemic lupus and Sjogren's patients than in scleroderma patients in China. Lupus. 2018;**27**(7):1051-1052

[107] Hatron PY, Wallaert B, Gosset D, Tonnel AB, Gosselin B, Voisin C, et al. Subclinical lung inflammation in primary Sjogren's syndrome. Relationship between bronchoalveolar lavage cellular analysis findings and characteristics of the disease. Arthritis and Rheumatism. 1987;**30**(11):1226-1231

[108] Papiris SA, Saetta M, Turato G, La Corte R, Trevisani L, Mapp CE, et al. CD4-positive T-lymphocytes infiltrate the bronchial mucosa of patients with Sjogren's syndrome. American Journal of Respiratory and Critical Care Medicine. 1997;**156**(2 Pt 1):637-641

[109] Ito I, Nagai S, Kitaichi M, Nicholson AG, Johkoh T, Noma S, et al. Pulmonary manifestations of primary Sjogren's syndrome: A clinical, radiologic, and pathologic study. American Journal of Respiratory and Critical Care Medicine. 2005;**171**(6):632-638

[110] Shi JH, Liu HR, Xu WB, Feng RE, Zhang ZH, Tian XL, et al. Pulmonary manifestations of Sjogren's syndrome. Respiration; International Review of Thoracic Diseases. 2009;**78**(4):377-386

[111] Kelly C, Gardiner P, Pal B, Griffiths I. Lung function in primary Sjogren's syndrome: A cross sectional and longitudinal study. Thorax. 1991;**46**(3):180-183

[112] Seror R, Ravaud P, Bowman SJ, Baron G, Tzioufas A, Theander E, et al. EULAR Sjogren's syndrome disease activity index: Development of a consensus systemic disease activity index for primary Sjogren's syndrome. Annals of the Rheumatic Diseases. 2010;**69**(6):1103-1109

[113] Seror R, Bootsma H, Bowman SJ, Dorner T, Gottenberg JE, Mariette X, et al. Outcome measures for primary Sjogren's syndrome. Journal of Autoimmunity. 2012;**39**(1-2, 102):97

[114] Seror R, Bowman SJ, Brito-Zeron P, Theander E, Bootsma H, Tzioufas A, et al. EULAR Sjogren's syndrome disease activity index (ESSDAI): A user guide. RMD Open. 2015;**1**(1):e000022

[115] Seror R, Bootsma H, Saraux A, Bowman SJ, Theander E, Brun JG, et al. Defining disease activity states and clinically meaningful improvement in primary Sjogren's syndrome with EULAR primary Sjogren's syndrome disease activity (ESSDAI) and patient-reported indexes (ESSPRI). Annals of the Rheumatic Diseases. 2016;**75**(2):382-389

[116] Chang GH, Chen YC, Lin KM, Yang YH, Liu CY, Lin MH, et al. Real-world database examining the association between Sjogren's syndrome and chronic rhinosinusitis. Journal of Clinical Medicine. 2019;**8**(2):155-166

[117] Mathieu A, Cauli A, Pala R, Satta L, Nurchis P, Loi GL, et al. Tracheo-bronchial mucociliary clearance in patients with primary and secondary Sjogren's syndrome. Scandinavian Journal of Rheumatology. 1995;**24**(5):300-304

[118] Amin K, Ludviksdottir D, Janson C, Nettelbladt O, Gudbjornsson B, Valtysdottir S, et al. Inflammation and structural changes in the airways of patients with primary Sjogren's syndrome. Respiratory Medicine. 2001;**95**(11):904-910

[119] Gardiner P, Ward C, Allison A, Ashcroft T, Simpson W, Walters H, et al.

Pleuropulmonary abnormalities in primary Sjogren's syndrome. The Journal of Rheumatology. 1993;**20**(5):831-837

[120] Rusthen S, Kristoffersen AK, Young A, Galtung HK, Petrovski BE, Palm O, et al. Dysbiotic salivary microbiota in dry mouth and primary Sjogren's syndrome patients. PLoS One. 2019;**14**(6):e0218319

[121] Lee J, Alam J, Choi E, Ko YK, Lee A, Choi Y. Association of a dysbiotic oral microbiota with the development of focal lymphocytic sialadenitis in IkappaB-zeta-deficient mice. NPJ Biofilms Microbiomes. 2020;**6**(1):49

[122] Tseng YC, Yang HY, Lin WT, Chang CB, Chien HC, Wang HP, et al. Salivary dysbiosis in Sjogren's syndrome and a commensal-mediated immunomodulatory effect of salivary gland epithelial cells. NPJ Biofilms Microbiomes. 2021;7(1):21

[123] Herrala M, Turunen S, Hanhineva K, Lehtonen M, Mikkonen JJW, Seitsalo H, et al. Low-dose doxycycline treatment normalizes levels of some salivary metabolites associated with oral microbiota in patients with primary Sjogren's syndrome. Metabolites. 2021;**11**(9):595-608

[124] Aljanobi H, Sabharwal A, Krishnakumar B, Kramer JM. Is it Sjogren's syndrome or burning mouth syndrome? Distinct pathoses with similar oral symptoms. Oral Surgery, Oral Medicine, Oral Pathology and Oral Radiology. 2017;**123**(4):482-495

[125] Graf S, Kirschstein L, Knopf A, Mansour N, Jeleff-Wolfler O, Buchberger AMS, et al. Systematic evaluation of laryngeal impairment in Sjogren's syndrome. European Archives of Oto-Rhino-Laryngology. 2021;**278**(7): 2421-2428

[126] Stojan G, Baer AN, Danoff SK. Pulmonary manifestations of Sjogren's

syndrome. Current Allergy and Asthma Reports. 2013;**13**(4):354-360

[127] Volter F, Fain O, Mathieu E, Thomas M. Esophageal function and Sjogren's syndrome. Digestive Diseases and Sciences. 2004;**49**(2):248-253

[128] Seeliger T, Bonig L, Witte T, Thiele T, Lesinski-Schiedat A, Stangel M, et al. Hearing dysfunction in patients with neuro-Sjogren: A cross-sectional study. Annals of Translational Medicine. 2020;**8**(17):1069

[129] Quismorio FP Jr. Pulmonary involvement in primary Sjogren's syndrome. Current Opinion in Pulmonary Medicine. 1996;**2**(5): 424-428

[130] Papathanasiou MP, Constantopoulos SH, Tsampoulas C, Drosos AA, Moutsopoulos HM. Reappraisal of respiratory abnormalities in primary and secondary Sjogren's syndrome. A controlled study. Chest. 1986;**90**(3):370-374

[131] Constantopoulos SH, Tsianos EV, Moutsopoulos HM. Pulmonary and gastrointestinal manifestations of Sjogren's syndrome. Rheumatic Diseases Clinics of North America. 1992;**18**(3): 617-635

[132] Gudbjornsson B, Hedenstrom H, Stalenheim G, Hallgren R. Bronchial hyperresponsiveness to methacholine in patients with primary Sjogren's syndrome. Annals of the Rheumatic Diseases. 1991;**50**(1):36-40

[133] La Corte R, Potena A, Bajocchi G, Fabbri L, Trotta F. Increased bronchial responsiveness in primary Sjogren's syndrome. A sign of tracheobronchial involvement. Clinical and Experimental Rheumatology. 1991;**9**(2):125-130

[134] Stalenheim G, Gudbjornsson B. Anti-inflammatory drugs do not alleviate bronchial hyperreactivity in

Sjogren's syndrome. Allergy. 1997;**52**(4):423-427

[135] Ludviksdottir D, Valtysdottir ST, Hedenstrom H, Hallgren R, Gudbjornsson B. Eight-year follow-up of airway hyperresponsiveness in patients with primary Sjogren's syndrome. Upsala Journal of Medical Sciences. 2017;**122**(1):51-55

[136] Bellido-Casado J, Plaza V, Diaz C, Geli C, Dominguez J, Margarit G, et al. Bronchial inflammation, respiratory symptoms and lung function in primary Sjogren's syndrome. Archivos de Bronconeumología. 2011;**47**(7): 330-334

[137] Fortoul TI, Cano-Valle F, Oliva E, Barrios R. Follicular bronchiolitis in association with connective tissue diseases. Lung. 1985;**163**(5):305-314

[138] Yousem SA, Colby TV, Carrington CB. Follicular bronchitis/bronchiolitis. Human Pathology. 1985;**16**(7):700-706

[139] Ryu JH, Myers JL, Swensen SJ. Bronchiolar disorders. American Journal of Respiratory and Critical Care Medicine. 2003;**168**(11):1277-1292

[140] Franquet T, Gimenez A, Monill JM, Diaz C, Geli C. Primary Sjogren's syndrome and associated lung disease: CT findings in 50 patients. AJR American Journal of Roentgenology. 1997;**169**(3):655-658

[141] Borie R, Schneider S, Debray MP, Adle-Biasssette H, Danel C, Bergeron A, et al. Severe chronic bronchiolitis as the presenting feature of primary Sjogren's syndrome. Respiratory Medicine. 2011;**105**(1):130-136

[142] Tashtoush B, Okafor NC, Ramirez JF, Smolley L. Follicular bronchiolitis: A literature review. Journal of Clinical and Diagnostic Research. 2015;**9**(9):OE01-OE05

[143] Camarasa Escrig A, Amat Humaran B, Sapia S, Leon Ramirez JM. Follicular bronchiolitis associated with common variable immunodeficiency. Archivos de Bronconeumología. 2013;**49**(4):166-168

[144] Travis WD, Galvin JR. Non-neoplastic pulmonary lymphoid lesions. Thorax. 2001;**56**(12):964-971

[145] Halle S, Dujardin HC, Bakocevic N, Fleige H, Danzer H, Willenzon S, et al. Induced bronchus-associated lymphoid tissue serves as a general priming site for T cells and is maintained by dendritic cells. The Journal of Experimental Medicine. 2009;**206**(12):2593-2601

[146] Mandl T, Diaz S, Ekberg O, Hesselstrand R, Piitulainen E, Wollmer P, et al. Frequent development of chronic obstructive pulmonary disease in primary SS—Results of a longitudinal follow-up. Rheumatology (Oxford, England). 2012;**51**(5):941-946

[147] Takenaka S, Ogura T, Oshima H, Izumi K, Hirata A, Ito H, et al. Development and exacerbation of pulmonary nontuberculous mycobacterial infection in patients with systemic autoimmune rheumatic diseases. Modern Rheumatology. 2020;**30**(3):558-563

[148] Chung A, Wilgus ML, Fishbein G, Lynch JP 3rd. Pulmonary and bronchiolar involvement in Sjogren's syndrome. Seminars in Respiratory and Critical Care Medicine. 2019;**40**(2):235-254

[149] Stenmark KR, Fagan KA, Frid MG. Hypoxia-induced pulmonary vascular remodeling: Cellular and molecular mechanisms. Circulation Research. 2006;**99**(7):675-691

[150] Newball HH, Brahim SA. Chronic obstructive airway disease in patients with Sjogren's syndrome. The American Review of Respiratory Disease. 1977;**115**(2):295-304

[151] Kakugawa T, Sakamoto N, Ishimoto H, Shimizu T, Nakamura H, Nawata A, et al. Lymphocytic focus score is positively related to airway and interstitial lung diseases in primary Sjogren's syndrome. Respiratory Medicine. 2018;**137**:95-102

[152] Soto-Cardenas MJ, Perez-De-Lis M, Bove A, Navarro C, Brito-Zeron P, Diaz-Lagares C, et al. Bronchiectasis in primary Sjogren's syndrome: Prevalence and clinical significance. Clinical and Experimental Rheumatology. 2010;**28**(5):647-653

[153] Di Pasquale M, Aliberti S, Mantero M, Gramegna A, Blasi F. Pharmacotherapeutic management of bronchial infections in adults: Non-cystic fibrosis bronchiectasis and chronic obstructive pulmonary disease. Expert Opinion on Pharmacotherapy. 2020;**21**(16):1975-1990

[154] Li X, Xu B, Ma Y, Li X, Cheng Q, Wang X, et al. Clinical and laboratory profiles of primary Sjogren's syndrome in a Chinese population: A retrospective analysis of 315 patients. International Journal of Rheumatic Diseases. 2015;**18**(4):439-446

[155] Liu C, Zhang H, Yao G, Hu Y, Qi J, Wang Y, et al. Characteristics of primary Sjogren's syndrome patients with IgG4 positive plasma cells infiltration in the labial salivary glands. Clinical Rheumatology. 2017;**36**(1):83-88

[156] Strevens Bolmgren V, Olsson P, Wollmer P, Hesselstrand R, Mandl T. Respiratory symptoms are poor predictors of concomitant chronic obstructive pulmonary disease in patients with primary Sjogren's syndrome. Rheumatology International. 2017;**37**(5):813-818

[157] Taouli B, Brauner MW, Mourey I, Lemouchi D, Grenier PA. Thin-section chest CT findings of primary Sjogren's syndrome: Correlation with pulmonary function. European Radiology. 2002;**12**(6):1504-1511

[158] Ter Borg EJ, Kelder JC. Development of new extra-glandular manifestations or associated auto-immune diseases after establishing the diagnosis of primary Sjogren's syndrome: A long-term study of the Antonius Nieuwegein Sjogren (ANS) cohort. Rheumatology International. 2017;**37**(7):1153-1158

[159] Liebow AA, Carrington CB. Diffuse pulmonary lymphoreticular infiltrations associated with dysproteinemia. The Medical Clinics of North America. 1973;**57**(3):809-843

[160] Lopez Velazquez M, Highland KB. Pulmonary manifestations of systemic lupus erythematosus and Sjogren's syndrome. Current Opinion in Rheumatology. 2018;**30**(5):449-464

[161] Zhang T, Yuan F, Xu L, Sun W, Liu L, Xue J. Characteristics of patients with primary Sjogren's syndrome associated interstitial lung disease and relevant features of disease progression. Clinical Rheumatology. 2020;**39**(5):1561-1568

[162] Reina D, Roig Vilaseca D, Torrente-Segarra V, Cerda D, Castellvi I, Diaz Torne C, et al. Sjogren's syndrome-associated interstitial lung disease: A multicenter study. Reumatologia Clinica. 2016;**12**(4):201-205

[163] Fischer A, Swigris JJ, du Bois RM, Groshong SD, Cool CD, Sahin H, et al. Minor salivary gland biopsy to detect primary Sjogren syndrome in patients with interstitial lung disease. Chest. 2009;**136**(4):1072-1078

[164] Aerni MR, Vassallo R, Myers JL, Lindell RM, Ryu JH. Follicular bronchiolitis in surgical lung biopsies: Clinical implications in 12 patients. Respiratory Medicine. 2008;**102**(2):307-312

[165] Desai SR, Veeraraghavan S, Hansell DM, Nikolakopolou A, Goh NS, Nicholson AG, et al. CT features of lung disease in patients with systemic sclerosis: Comparison with idiopathic pulmonary fibrosis and nonspecific interstitial pneumonia. Radiology. 2004;**232**(2):560-567

[166] Gupta N, Wikenheiser-Brokamp KA, Fischer A, McCormack FX. Diffuse cystic lung disease as the presenting manifestation of Sjogren syndrome. Annals of the American Thoracic Society. 2016;**13**(3):371-375

[167] Gupta N, Vassallo R, Wikenheiser-Brokamp KA, McCormack FX. Diffuse cystic lung disease. Part I. American Journal of Respiratory and Critical Care Medicine. 2015;**191**(12):1354-1366

[168] Elicker B, Pereira CA, Webb R, Leslie KO. High-resolution computed tomography patterns of diffuse interstitial lung disease with clinical and pathological correlation. Jornal Brasileiro de Pneumologia: Publicacao Oficial da Sociedade Brasileira de Pneumologia e Tisilogia. 2008;**34**(9): 715-744

[169] Arcadu A, Moua T, Yi ES, Ryu JH. Lymphoid interstitial pneumonia and other benign lymphoid disorders. Seminars in Respiratory and Critical Care Medicine. 2016;**37**(3):406-420

[170] Tashiro K, Ohshima K, Suzumiya J, Yoneda S, Yahiro M, Sugihara M, et al. Clonality of primary pulmonary lymphoproliferative disorders; using in situ hybridization and polymerase chain reaction for immunoglobulin. Leukemia & Lymphoma. 1999;**36**(1-2):157-167

[171] Guinee DG Jr. Update on nonneoplastic pulmonary lymphoproliferative disorders and related entities. Archives of Pathology & Laboratory Medicine. 2010;**134**(5): 691-701

[172] Katzenstein AL, Doxtader E, Narendra S. Lymphomatoid granulomatosis: Insights gained over 4 decades. The American Journal of Surgical Pathology. 2010;**34**(12): e35-e48

[173] Swigris JJ, Berry GJ, Raffin TA, Kuschner WG. Lymphoid interstitial pneumonia: A narrative review. Chest. 2002;**122**(6):2150-2164

[174] Nicholson AG. Lymphocytic interstitial pneumonia and other lymphoproliferative disorders in the lung. Seminars in Respiratory and Critical Care Medicine. 2001;**22**(4): 409-422

[175] American Thoracic S, European Respiratory S. American Thoracic Society/European Respiratory Society International Multidisciplinary Consensus Classification of the Idiopathic Interstitial Pneumonias. This joint statement of the American Thoracic Society (ATS), and the European Respiratory Society (ERS) was adopted by the ATS board of directors, June 2001 and by the ERS Executive Committee, June 2001. American Journal of Respiratory and Critical Care Medicine. 2002;**165**(2): 277-304

[176] Nicholson AG. Classification of idiopathic interstitial pneumonias: Making sense of the alphabet soup. Histopathology. 2002;**41**(5):381-391

[177] Baque-Juston M, Pellegrin A, Leroy S, Marquette CH, Padovani B. Organizing pneumonia: What is it? A conceptual approach and pictorial review. Diagnostic and Interventional Imaging. 2014;**95**(9):771-777

[178] Bouchardy LM, Kuhlman JE, Ball WC Jr, Hruban RH, Askin FB, Siegelman SS. CT findings in bronchiolitis obliterans organizing pneumonia (BOOP) with radiographic, clinical, and histologic correlation.

Journal of Computer Assisted Tomography. 1993;**17**(3):352-357

[179] Lazor R, Vandevenne A, Pelletier A, Leclerc P, Court-Fortune I, Cordier JF. Cryptogenic organizing pneumonia. Characteristics of relapses in a series of 48 patients. The Groupe d'Etudes et de Recherche sur les Maladles "Orphelines" Pulmonaires (GERM"O"P). American Journal of Respiratory and Critical Care Medicine. 2000;**162**(2 Pt 1):571-577

[180] Cordier JF, Cottin V, Lazor R, Thivolet-Bejui F. Many faces of bronchiolitis and organizing pneumonia. Seminars in Respiratory and Critical Care Medicine. 2016;**37**(3):421-440

[181] Matteson EL, Ike RW. Bronchiolitis obliterans organizing pneumonia and Sjogren's syndrome. The Journal of Rheumatology. 1990;**17**(5):676-679

[182] Vourlekis JS, Brown KK, Cool CD, Young DA, Cherniack RM, King TE, et al. Acute interstitial pneumonitis. Case series and review of the literature. Medicine (Baltimore). 2000;**79**(6): 369-378

[183] Yoo JW, Song JW, Jang SJ, Lee CK, Kim MY, Lee HK, et al. Comparison between cryptogenic organizing pneumonia and connective tissue disease-related organizing pneumonia. Rheumatology (Oxford, England). 2011;**50**(5):932-938

[184] Takahashi H, Tsuboi H, Yokosawa M, Asashima H, Hirota T, Kondo Y, et al. Diffusion-weighted magnetic resonance imaging of parotid glands before and after abatacept therapy in patients with Sjogren's syndrome associated with rheumatoid arthritis: Utility to evaluate and predict response to treatment. Modern Rheumatology. 2018;**28**(2):300-307

[185] Lazarus MN, Robinson D, Mak V, Moller H, Isenberg DA. Incidence of cancer in a cohort of patients with primary Sjogren's syndrome. Rheumatology (Oxford, England). 2006;**45**(8):1012-1015

[186] Kovacs L, Szodoray P, Kiss E. Secondary tumours in Sjogren's syndrome. Autoimmunity Reviews. 2010;**9**(4):203-206

[187] Papageorgiou A, Voulgarelis M, Tzioufas AG. Clinical picture, outcome and predictive factors of lymphoma in Sjgren syndrome. Autoimmunity Reviews. 2015;**14**(7):641-649

[188] Ramos-Casals M, De Vita S, Tzioufas AG. Hepatitis C virus, Sjogren's syndrome and B-cell lymphoma: Linking infection, autoimmunity and cancer. Autoimmunity Reviews. 2005;**4**(1):8-15

[189] Hansen LA, Prakash UB, Colby TV. Pulmonary lymphoma in Sjogren's syndrome. Mayo Clinic Proceedings. 1989;**64**(8):920-931

[190] Graham BB, Mathisen DJ, Mark EJ, Takvorian RW. Primary pulmonary lymphoma. The Annals of Thoracic Surgery. 2005;**80**(4):1248-1253

[191] Yachoui R, Leon C, Sitwala K, Kreidy M. Pulmonary MALT lymphoma in patients with Sjogren's syndrome. Clinical Medicine & Research. 2017;**15**(1-2):6-12

[192] Milani P, Basset M, Russo F, Foli A, Palladini G, Merlini G. The lung in amyloidosis. European Respiratory Review: An Official Journal of the European Respiratory Society. 2017;**26**(145):170046-170054

[193] Baqir M, Kluka EM, Aubry MC, Hartman TE, Yi ES, Bauer PR, et al. Amyloid-associated cystic lung disease in primary Sjogren's syndrome. Respiratory Medicine. 2013;**107**(4): 616-621

[194] Simsek E, Caliskan A, Tutun U, Sahin S. Cause of a rare acute renal insufficiency: Rupture aortocaval fistula. Vascular. 2014;**22**(4):290-292

[195] Rajagopala S, Singh N, Gupta K, Gupta D. Pulmonary amyloidosis in Sjogren's syndrome: A case report and systematic review of the literature. Respirology. 2010;**15**(5):860-866

[196] Wong BC, Wong KL, Ip MS, Wang EP, Chan KW, Cheng LC. Sjogren's syndrome with amyloid a presenting as multiple pulmonary nodules. The Journal of Rheumatology. 1994;**21**(1):165-167

[197] Nakamura N, Yamada G, Itoh T, Suzuki A, Morita-Ichimura S, Teramoto S, et al. Pulmonary MALT lymphoma with amyloid production in a patient with primary Sjogren's syndrome. Internal medicine. 2002;**41**(4):309-311

[198] Polansky SM, Ravin CE. Nodular pulmonary infiltrate in a patient with Sjogren's syndrome. Chest. 1980;**77**(3): 411-412

[199] Carbone R, Cosso C, Cimmino MA. Pulmonary nodular amyloidosis in Sjogren syndrome. The Journal of Rheumatology. 2015;**42**(1):134

[200] Kobayashi H, Matsuoka R, Kitamura S, Tsunoda N, Saito K. Sjogren's syndrome with multiple bullae and pulmonary nodular amyloidosis. Chest. 1988;**94**(2):438-440

[201] Rodrigues K, Neves FS, Stoeterau KB, Werner Castro GR, Nobre LF, Zimmermann AF, et al. Pulmonary amyloidosis in Sjogren's syndrome: A rare diagnosis for nodular lung lesions. International Journal of Rheumatic Diseases. 2009;**12**(4): 358-360

[202] Kluka EM, Bauer PR, Aubry MC, Ryu JH. Enlarging lung nodules and cysts in a 53-year-old woman with primary Sjogren syndrome. Chest. 2013;**143**(1):258-261

[203] Seguchi T, Kyoraku Y, Saita K, Ihi T, Nagai M, Akiyama Y, et al. Human T-cell lymphotropic virus type I (HTLV-1) associated myelopathy and Sjogren's syndrome representing pulmonary nodular amyloidosis and multiple bullae: Report of an autopsy case. Virchows Archiv. 2006;**448**(6):874-876

[204] Jing ZC, Xu XQ, Han ZY, Wu Y, Deng KW, Wang H, et al. Registry and survival study in chinese patients with idiopathic and familial pulmonary arterial hypertension. Chest. 2007;**132**(2):373-379

[205] Teruuchi S, Bando M, Hironaka M, Ohno S, Sugiyama Y. Sjogren's syndrome with multiple bullae and pulmonary nodular amyloidosis. Nihon Kokyūki Gakkai Zasshi. 2000;**38**(12):918-922

[206] Liu Z, Yang X, Tian Z, Qian J, Wang Q, Zhao J, et al. The prognosis of pulmonary arterial hypertension associated with primary Sjogren's syndrome: A cohort study. Lupus. 2018;**27**(7):1072-1080

[207] Zhao Y, Wang H, Chen M, Zhang N, Yang ZW, Li D, et al. Primary Sjogren's syndrome associated pulmonary arterial hypertension: 20 new cases. Zhonghua Yi Xue Za Zhi. 2019;**99**(37):2921-2925

[208] Zuily S, Domingues V, Suty-Selton C, Eschwege V, Bertoletti L, Chaouat A, et al. Antiphospholipid antibodies can identify lupus patients at risk of pulmonary hypertension: A systematic review and meta-analysis. Autoimmunity Reviews. 2017;**16**(6):576-586

[209] Fox PC, Datiles M, Atkinson JC, Macynski AA, Scott J, Fletcher D, et al. Prednisone and piroxicam for treatment of primary Sjogren's syndrome. Clinical

and Experimental Rheumatology. 1993;**11**(2):149-156

[210] Fauci AS. Corticosteroids in autoimmune disease. Hospital Practice (Office ed.). 1983;**18**(10): 99-103, 7-18, 13-4

[211] Fox RI, Chan E, Benton L, Fong S, Friedlaender M, Howell FV. Treatment of primary Sjogren's syndrome with hydroxychloroquine. The American Journal of Medicine. 1988;**85**(4A):62-67

[212] Kruize AA, Hene RJ, Kallenberg CG, van Bijsterveld OP, van der Heide A, Kater L, et al. Hydroxychloroquine treatment for primary Sjogren's syndrome: A two year double blind crossover trial. Annals of the Rheumatic Diseases. 1993;**52**(5): 360-364

[213] Schnabel A, Reuter M, Gross WL. Intravenous pulse cyclophosphamide in the treatment of interstitial lung disease due to collagen vascular diseases. Arthritis and Rheumatism. 1998;**41**(7): 1215-1220

[214] Tsuzaka K, Akama H, Yamada H, Akizuki M, Tojo T, Homma M. Pulmonary pseudolymphoma presented with a mass lesion in a patient with primary Sjogren's syndrome: Beneficial effect of intermittent intravenous cyclophosphamide. Scandinavian Journal of Rheumatology. 1993;**22**(2): 90-93

[215] Yum HK, Kim ES, Ok KS, Lee HK, Choi SJ. Lymphocytic interstitial pneumonitis associated with Epstein-Barr virus in systemic lupus erythematosus and Sjogren's syndrome. Complete remission with corticosteriod and cyclophosphamide. The Korean Journal of Internal Medicine. 2002;**17**(3):198-203

[216] Oldham JM, Lee C, Valenzi E, Witt LJ, Adegunsoye A, Hsu S, et al. Azathioprine response in patients with

fibrotic connective tissue disease-associated interstitial lung disease. Respiratory Medicine. 2016;**121**:117-122

[217] Saketkoo LA, Espinoza LR. Experience of mycophenolate mofetil in 10 patients with autoimmune-related interstitial lung disease demonstrates promising effects. The American Journal of the Medical Sciences. 2009;**337**(5):329-335

[218] Swigris JJ, Olson AL, Fischer A, Lynch DA, Cosgrove GP, Frankel SK, et al. Mycophenolate mofetil is safe, well tolerated, and preserves lung function in patients with connective tissue disease-related interstitial lung disease. Chest. 2006;**130**(1):30-36

[219] Klinowski G, Gozzi F, Trentacosti F, Andrisani D, Sebastiani M, Clini EM. Rituximab for the treatment of acute onset interstitial lung disease in primary Sjogren's syndrome. Pulmonology. 2021;**27**(6):575-578

[220] Benad M, Koschel D, Herrmann K, Wiefel K, Kleymann A, Aringer M. Effects of cyclophosphamide and rituximab in patients with connective tissue diseases with severe interstitial lung disease. Clinical and Experimental Rheumatology. 2021. Epub ahead of print

[221] Chen MH, Chen CK, Chou HP, Chen MH, Tsai CY, Chang DM. Rituximab therapy in primary Sjogren's syndrome with interstitial lung disease: A retrospective cohort study. Clinical and Experimental Rheumatology. 2016;**34**(6):1077-1084

[222] Watanabe Y, Koyama S, Miwa C, Okuda S, Kanai Y, Tetsuka K, et al. Pulmonary mucosa-associated lymphoid tissue (MALT) lymphoma in Sjogren's syndrome showing only the LIP pattern radiologically. Internal Medicine. 2012;**51**(5):491-495

[223] Wise LM, Arkfeld DG. A patient with primary Sjogren's syndrome, cystic

lung disease, and MALT lymphoma treated successfully with rituximab: A case-based review. Clinical Rheumatology. 2020;**39**(4):1357-1362

[224] Blanco Perez JJ, Perez Gonzalez A, Guerra Vales JL, Melero Gonzalez R, Pego Reigosa JM. Shrinking lung in primary Sjogren syndrome successfully treated with rituximab. Archivos de Bronconeumología. 2015;**51**(9):475-476

[225] Justet A, Ottaviani S, Dieude P, Taille C. Tocilizumab for refractory organising pneumonia associated with Sjogren's disease. BML Case Reports. 2015;**2015**

[226] Thompson G, McLean-Tooke A, Wrobel J, Lavender M, Lucas M. Sjogren syndrome with associated lymphocytic interstitial pneumonia successfully treated with tacrolimus and Abatacept as an alternative to rituximab. Chest. 2018;**153**(3):e41-ee3

[227] Lee AS, Scofield RH, Hammitt KM, Gupta N, Thomas DE, Moua T, et al. Consensus guidelines for evaluation and management of pulmonary disease in Sjögren's. Chest. 2021;**159**(2):683-698

[228] Plemons JM, Al-Hashimi I, Marek CL. Managing xerostomia and salivary gland hypofunction: Executive summary of a report from the American Dental Association Council on Scientific Affairs. Journal of the American Dental Association (1939). 2014;**145**(8):867-873

[229] Furness S, Worthington HV, Bryan G, Birchenough S, McMillan R. Interventions for the management of dry mouth: Topical therapies. The Cochrane Database of Systematic Reviews. 2011;(12):Cd008934, 1-93

[230] Salum FG, Medella-Junior FAC, Figueiredo MAZ, Cherubini K. Salivary hypofunction: An update on therapeutic strategies. Gerodontology. 2018;**35**(4): 305-316

[231] Tan ECK, Lexomboon D, Sandborgh-Englund G, Haasum Y, Johnell K. Medications that cause dry mouth as an adverse effect in older people: A systematic review and Metaanalysis. Journal of the American Geriatrics Society. 2018;**66**(1):76-84

[232] Papas AS, Sherrer YS, Charney M, Golden HE, Medsger TA Jr, Walsh BT, et al. Successful treatment of dry mouth and dry eye symptoms in Sjögren's syndrome patients with oral pilocarpine: A randomized, placebo-controlled, dose-adjustment study. Journal of Clinical Rheumatology: Practical Reports on Rheumatic & Musculoskeletal Diseases. 2004;**10**(4): 169-177

[233] Wu CH, Hsieh SC, Lee KL, Li KJ, Lu MC, Yu CL. Pilocarpine hydrochloride for the treatment of xerostomia in patients with Sjögren's syndrome in Taiwan—A double-blind, placebo-controlled trial. Journal of the Formosan Medical Association. 2006;**105**(10):796-803

[234] Tsifetaki N, Kitsos G, Paschides CA, Alamanos Y, Eftaxias V, Voulgari PV, et al. Oral pilocarpine for the treatment of ocular symptoms in patients with Sjögren's syndrome: A randomised 12 week controlled study. Annals of the Rheumatic Diseases. 2003;**62**(12):1204-1207

[235] Rao RS, Akula R, Satyanarayana TSV, Indugu V. Recent advances of pacemakers in treatment of xerostomia: A systematic review. Journal of International Society of Preventive and Community Dentistry. 2019;**9**(4):311-315

[236] Ami S, Wolff A. Implant-supported electrostimulating device to treat xerostomia: A preliminary study. Clinical Implant Dentistry and Related Research. 2010;**12**(1):62-71

[237] Holland EJ, Whitley WO, Sall K, Lane SS, Raychaudhuri A, Zhang SY,

et al. Lifitegrast clinical efficacy for treatment of signs and symptoms of dry eye disease across three randomized controlled trials. Current Medical Research and Opinion. 2016;**32**(10): 1759-1765

[238] Foulks GN. Treatment of dry eye disease by the non-ophthalmologist. Rheumatic Diseases Clinics of North America. 2008;**34**(4):987-1000 x

[239] Sall K, Stevenson OD, Mundorf TK, Reis BL. Two multicenter, randomized studies of the efficacy and safety of cyclosporine ophthalmic emulsion in moderate to severe dry eye disease. CsA phase 3 study group. Ophthalmology. 2000;**107**(4):631-639

[240] Kim EC, Choi JS, Joo CK. A comparison of vitamin a and cyclosporine a 0.05% eye drops for treatment of dry eye syndrome. American Journal of Ophthalmology. 2009;**147**(2):206-13.e3

[241] Belafsky PC, Postma GN. The laryngeal and esophageal manifestations of Sjögren's syndrome. Current Rheumatology Reports. 2003;**5**(4): 297-303

[242] Fischer A, Brown KK, Du Bois RM, Frankel SK, Cosgrove GP, Fernandez-Perez ER, et al. Mycophenolate mofetil improves lung function in connective tissue disease-associated interstitial lung disease. The Journal of Rheumatology. 2013;**40**(5): 640-646

[243] Amlani B, Elsayed G, Barvalia U, Kanne JP, Meyer KC, Sandbo N, et al. Treatment of primary sjogren's syndrome-related interstitial lung disease: A retrospective cohort study. Sarcoidosis, Vasculitis, and Diffuse Lung Diseases: Official Journal of WASOG. 2020;**37**(2):136-147

[244] Isaksen K, Jonsson R, Omdal R. Anti-CD20 treatment in primary

Sjögren's syndrome. Scandinavian Journal of Immunology. 2008;**68**(6): 554-564

[245] Seror R, Sordet C, Guillevin L, Hachulla E, Masson C, Ittah M, et al. Tolerance and efficacy of rituximab and changes in serum B cell biomarkers in patients with systemic complications of primary Sjögren's syndrome. Annals of the Rheumatic Diseases. 2007;**66**(3): 351-357

[246] Daoussis D, Melissaropoulos K, Sakellaropoulos G, Antonopoulos I, Markatseli TE, Simopoulou T, et al. A multicenter, open-label, comparative study of B-cell depletion therapy with rituximab for systemic sclerosis-associated interstitial lung disease. Seminars in Arthritis and Rheumatism. 2017;**46**(5):625-631

[247] Narvaez J, Luch JL, Molina-Molina M, Vicens-Zygmunt V, Luburich P, Yanez MA, et al. Rituximab as a rescue treatment added on mycophenolate mofetil background therapy in progressive systemic sclerosis associated interstitial lung disease unresponsive to conventional immunosuppression. Seminars in Arthritis and Rheumatism. 2020;**50**(5):977-987

[248] Rimar D, Rosner I, Slobodin G. Upfront combination therapy with rituximab and mycophenolate Mofetil for progressive systemic sclerosis. The Journal of Rheumatology. 2021;**48**(2): 304-305

[249] Nadashkevich O, Davis P, Fritzler M, Kovalenko W. A randomized unblinded trial of cyclophosphamide versus azathioprine in the treatment of systemic sclerosis. Clinical Rheumatology. 2006;**25**(2):205-212

[250] Tashkin DP, Elashoff R, Clements PJ, Goldin J, Roth MD, Furst DE, et al. Cyclophosphamide versus placebo in scleroderma lung

disease. The New England Journal of Medicine. 2006;**354**(25):2655-2666

[251] Iudici M, Cuomo G, Vettori S, Bocchino M, Sanduzzi Zamparelli A, Cappabianca S, et al. Low-dose pulse cyclophosphamide in interstitial lung disease associated with systemic sclerosis (SSc-ILD): Efficacy of maintenance immunosuppression in responders and non-responders. Seminars in Arthritis and Rheumatism. 2015;**44**(4):437-444

[252] Tashkin DP, Roth MD, Clements PJ, Furst DE, Khanna D, Kleerup EC, et al. Mycophenolate mofetil versus oral cyclophosphamide in scleroderma-related interstitial lung disease (SLS II): A randomised controlled, double-blind, parallel group trial. The Lancet Respiratory Medicine. 2016;**4**(9): 708-719

[253] Khanna D, Denton CP, Jahreis A, van Laar JM, Frech TM, Anderson ME, et al. Safety and efficacy of subcutaneous tocilizumab in adults with systemic sclerosis (faSScinate): A phase 2, randomised, controlled trial. Lancet. 2016;**387**(10038):2630-2640

[254] Khanna D, Denton CP, Lin CJF, van Laar JM, Frech TM, Anderson ME, et al. Safety and efficacy of subcutaneous tocilizumab in systemic sclerosis: Results from the open-label period of a phase II randomised controlled trial (faSScinate). Annals of the Rheumatic Diseases. 2018;**77**(2):212-220

[255] Felten R, Meyer N, Duffaut P, Saadoun D, Hachulla E, Hatron P, et al. IL-6 receptor inhibition in primary sjögren syndrome: Results from a randomized multicenter academic double blind placebo-controlled trial of tocilizumab in 110 patients [abstract]. Arthritis and Rheumatism. 2019;71. Available from: https://acrabstracts.org/abstract/il-6-receptor-inhibition-in-primary-sjogren-syndrome-results-from-a-randomized-multicenter-academic-double-blind-placebo-controlled-trial-of-tocilizumab-in-110-patients/

[256] Sankar V, Brennan MT, Kok MR, Leakan RA, Smith JA, Manny J, et al. Etanercept in Sjogren's syndrome: A twelve-week randomized, double-blind, placebo-controlled pilot clinical trial. Arthritis and Rheumatism. 2004;**50**(7):2240-2245

[257] Moutsopoulos NM, Katsifis GE, Angelov N, Leakan RA, Sankar V, Pillemer S, et al. Lack of efficacy of etanercept in Sjogren syndrome correlates with failed suppression of tumour necrosis factor alpha and systemic immune activation. Annals of the Rheumatic Diseases. 2008;**67**(10):1437-1443

[258] Herrero-Beaumont G, Martinez Calatrava MJ, Castaneda S. Abatacept mechanism of action: Concordance with its clinical profile. Reumatologia Clinica. 2012;**8**(2):78-83

[259] Nakashita T, Ando K, Takahashi K, Motojima S. Possible effect of abatacept on the progression of interstitial lung disease in rheumatoid arthritis patients. Respiratory Investigation. 2016;**54**(5): 376-379

[260] Mochizuki T, Yano K, Ikari K, Hiroshima R, Takaoka H, Kawakami K, et al. The efficacy of abatacept in Japanese patients with rheumatoid arthritis: 104 weeks radiographic and clinical results in clinical practice. Modern Rheumatology. 2016;**26**(4):499-506

[261] Kurata I, Tsuboi H, Terasaki M, Shimizu M, Toko H, Honda F, et al. Effect of biological disease-modifying anti-rheumatic drugs on airway and interstitial lung disease in patients with rheumatoid arthritis. Internal Medicine. 2019;**58**(12):1703-1712

[262] Kang EH, Jin Y, Desai RJ, Liu J, Sparks JA, Kim SC. Risk of exacerbation

of pulmonary comorbidities in patients with rheumatoid arthritis after initiation of abatacept versus TNF inhibitors: A cohort study. Seminars in Arthritis and Rheumatism. 2020;**50**(3):401-408

[263] Cassone G, Manfredi A, Atzeni F, Venerito V, Vacchi C, Picerno V, et al. Safety of Abatacept in Italian patients with rheumatoid arthritis and interstitial lung disease: A Multicenter retrospective study. Journal of Clinical Medicine. 2020;**9**(1):277-287

[264] Mena-Vazquez N, Godoy-Navarrete FJ, Manrique-Arija S, Aguilar-Hurtado MC, Romero-Barco CM, Urena-Garnica I, et al. Non-anti-TNF biologic agents are associated with slower worsening of interstitial lung disease secondary to rheumatoid arthritis. Clinical Rheumatology. 2021;**40**(1):133-142

[265] Fernandez-Diaz C, Castaneda S, Melero-Gonzalez RB, Ortiz-Sanjuan F, Juan-Mas A, Carrasco-Cubero C, et al. Abatacept in interstitial lung disease associated with rheumatoid arthritis: National multicenter study of 263 patients. Rheumatology (Oxford, England). 2020;**59**(12):3906-3916

[266] Ferandez-Díaz C, Castaneda S, Melero R, Loricera J, Ortiz-Sanju'an F, Juan-Mas A, et al. Poster #SAT0035. Response to abatacept of different patterns of interstitial lung disease in rheumatoid arthritis: National multicenter study of 263 patients. Annals of the Rheumatic Diseases. 2020;**79**(Suppl. 1):943-944. DOI: 10.1136/annrheumdis-2020-eular.1741

[267] Mori S. Management of rheumatoid arthritis patients with interstitial lung disease: Safety of biological antirheumatic drugs and assessment of pulmonary fibrosis. Clinical Medicine Insights: Circulatory, Respiratory and Pulmonary Medicine. 2015;**9**(Suppl 1):41-49

[268] Tsuboi H, Matsumoto I, Hagiwara S, Hirota T, Takahashi H, Ebe H, et al. Effectiveness of abatacept for patients with Sjogren's syndrome associated with rheumatoid arthritis. An open label, multicenter, one-year, prospective study: ROSE (Rheumatoid Arthritis with Orencia Trial toward Sjogren's syndrome Endocrinopathy) trial. Modern Rheumatology. 2016;**26**(6):891-899

[269] Pontarini E, Fabris M, Quartuccio L, Cappelletti M, Calcaterra F, Roberto A, et al. Treatment with belimumab restores B cell subsets and their expression of B cell activating factor receptor in patients with primary Sjogren's syndrome. Rheumatology (Oxford, England). 2015;**54**(8):1429-1434

[270] Mariette X, Seror R, Quartuccio L, Baron G, Salvin S, Fabris M, et al. Efficacy and safety of belimumab in primary Sjogren's syndrome: Results of the BELISS open-label phase II study. Annals of the Rheumatic Diseases. 2015;**74**(3):526-531

[271] Gandolfo S, De Vita S. Double anti-B cell and anti-BAFF targeting for the treatment of primary Sjogren's syndrome. Clinical and Experimental Rheumatology. 2019;**118**(3):199-208

[272] Hall JC, Baer AN, Shah AA, Criswell LA, Shiboski CH, Rosen A, et al. Molecular subsetting of interferon pathways in Sjogren's syndrome. Arthritis & Rheumatology. 2015;**67**(9):2437-2446

[273] Nezos A, Gravani F, Tassidou A, Kapsogeorgou EK, Voulgarelis M, Koutsilieris M, et al. Type I and II interferon signatures in Sjogren's syndrome pathogenesis: Contributions in distinct clinical phenotypes and Sjogren's related lymphomagenesis. Journal of Autoimmunity. 2015;**63**:47-58

[274] Furie R, Khamashta M, Merrill JT, Werth VP, Kalunian K, Brohawn P, et al. Anifrolumab, an anti-interferon-alpha

receptor monoclonal antibody, in moderate-to-severe systemic lupus erythematosus. Arthritis Rheumatology. 2017;**69**(2):376-386

[275] Wells AU, Brown KK, Flaherty KR, Kolb M, Thannickal VJ, Group IPFCW. What's in a name? That which we call IPF, by any other name would act the same. The European Respiratory Journal. 2018;**51**(5):1800692-1800704

[276] Wollin L, Wex E, Pautsch A, Schnapp G, Hostettler KE, Stowasser S, et al. Mode of action of nintedanib in the treatment of idiopathic pulmonary fibrosis. The European Respiratory Journal. 2015;**45**(5):1434-1445

[277] Hilberg F, Roth GJ, Krssak M, Kautschitsch S, Sommergruber W, Tontsch-Grunt U, et al. BIBF 1120: Triple angiokinase inhibitor with sustained receptor blockade and good antitumor efficacy. Cancer Research. 2008;**68**(12):4774-4782

[278] Gurujeyalakshmi G, Hollinger MA, Giri SN. Pirfenidone inhibits PDGF isoforms in bleomycin hamster model of lung fibrosis at the translational level. The American Journal of Physiology. 1999;**276**(2):L311-L318

[279] Corbel M, Lanchou J, Germain N, Malledant Y, Boichot E, Lagente V. Modulation of airway remodeling-associated mediators by the antifibrotic compound, pirfenidone, and the matrix metalloproteinase inhibitor, batimastat, during acute lung injury in mice. European Journal of Pharmacology. 2001;**426**(1-2):113-121

[280] Ruwanpura SM, Thomas BJ, Bardin PG. Pirfenidone: Molecular mechanisms and potential clinical applications in lung disease. American Journal of Respiratory Cell and Molecular Biology. 2020;**62**(4):413-422

[281] Liu H, Drew P, Cheng Y, Visner GA. Pirfenidone inhibits inflammatory responses and ameliorates allograft injury in a rat lung transplant model. The Journal of Thoracic and Cardiovascular Surgery. 2005;**130**(3):852-858

[282] Flaherty KR, Wells AU, Brown KK. Nintedanib in progressive fibrosing interstitial lung diseases. Reply. The New England Journal of Medicine. 2020;**382**(8):781

[283] Wells AU, Flaherty KR, Brown KK, Inoue Y, Devaraj A, Richeldi L, et al. Nintedanib in patients with progressive fibrosing interstitial lung diseases-subgroup analyses by interstitial lung disease diagnosis in the INBUILD trial: A randomised, double-blind, placebo-controlled, parallel-group trial. The Lancet Respiratory Medicine. 2020;**8**(5):453-460

[284] Distler O, Highland KB, Gahlemann M, Azuma A, Fischer A, Mayes MD, et al. Nintedanib for systemic sclerosis-associated interstitial lung disease. The New England Journal of Medicine. 2019;**380**(26):2518-2528

[285] Khanna D, Albera C, Fischer A, Khalidi N, Raghu G, Chung L, et al. An open-label, phase II study of the safety and tolerability of Pirfenidone in patients with scleroderma-associated interstitial lung disease: The LOTUSS trial. The Journal of Rheumatology. 2016;**43**(9):1672-1679

[286] Enomoto Y, Nakamura Y, Colby TV, Inui N, Suda T. Pirfenidone for primary Sjogren's syndrome-related fibrotic interstitial pneumonia. Sarcoidosis, Vasculitis, and Diffuse Lung Diseases: Official Journal of WASOG. 2017;**34**(1): 91-96

[287] Fischer A, Distler J. Progressive fibrosing interstitial lung disease associated with systemic autoimmune diseases. Clinical Rheumatology. 2019;**38**(10):2673-2681

Section 6

Lung Transplant in IPF

Chapter 8

Lung Transplantation in Idiopathic Pulmonary Fibrosis

Ryan Goetz, Nitesh Kumar Jain, Humayun Anjum and Thomas S. Kaleekal

Abstract

Idiopathic pulmonary fibrosis (IPF) is a progressive lung disease associated with a high degree of morbidity and mortality in its more advanced stages. Antifibrotic therapies are generally effective in delaying the progression of disease; however, some patients continue to progress despite treatment. Lung transplantation is a surgical option for selected patients with advanced pulmonary fibrosis that increases their overall survival and quality of life. Changes in the Lung Allocation Score (LAS) in 2005 have resulted in increased transplants and decreased waitlist mortality in this population. Indications for transplant evaluation and listing include the clinical progression of the disease and related mortality risk ≥50% at 2 years without a transplant. Patients with clinically rapid deterioration or acute flares needing hospitalization can be bridged to transplant on extracorporeal support while remaining ambulatory and free from mechanical ventilation.

Keywords: Idiopathic lung fibrosis, IPF, Pulmonary fibrosis, Lung transplantation, Single lung transplantation, Double lung transplantation, anti-fibrotics, Interstitial lung disease, survival, GERD, Acute exacerbation of IPF, ECMO, Immunosuppression

1. Introduction

Lung transplantation is a therapeutic option for selected patients with end-stage lung disease that may improve their survival and provide a good quality of life [1].

IPF is a progressive form of interstitial lung disease with characteristic clinical features, imaging, and histologic findings. Clinical features include progressive dyspnea on exertion, chronic dry cough, and fatigue. Physical exam findings include bilateral Velcro-like crackles, clubbing and in late stages sequelae of secondary pulmonary hypertension. Pulmonary function tests demonstrate restriction in the form of decreased lung volumes and decreased diffusion capacity along with resting or exertional hypoxemia [2]. Though therapeutic medications have been approved for the treatment of IPF, a lung transplant is a surgical option in selected cases. Currently, about 4500 transplants or more are being done yearly across the world, mostly in the United States (US), Europe, and Japan. Of these transplants, nearly 33% have a diagnosis of IPF with a clinical, radiological, and pathological pattern consistent with Usual Interstitial Pneumonitis (UIP). Secondary pulmonary fibrosis from Non-Specific Interstitial Pneumonitis (NSIP) in connective tissue diseases, chronic hypersensitivity pneumonitis, post-inflammatory fibrosis (infections, drugs, toxins, inhalational injuries, radiation), sarcoidosis, and other rare interstitial lung diseases also account for 30–35% of lung transplants making fibrotic lung disease the predominant indication for lung transplantation at most centers in the US.

2. Diagnosis and medical therapies

Along with the clinical features described above, computed tomography (CT) of the chest, preferably high-resolution cuts (≤1.25 mm) with inspiratory and expiratory imaging, is the initial diagnostic choice. The radiological findings on CT are used in correlation with the histologic findings to diagnose IPF. The typical UIP pattern is defined by heterogenous para-septal fibrosis, architectural distortion, reticulation, and honeycombing with a peripheral and lower lobe predominance. These findings have a high positive predictive value for UIP and are diagnostic for IPF when autoimmune and hypersensitivity features are not present. There is no requirement to obtain a surgical lung biopsy due to the increased risk of complications like developing a bronchopleural fistula at the surgical site or setting off an IPF "flare." Current recommendations are to refer these patients to a transplant center at the time of diagnosis for consideration of the transplant evaluation. "Probable UIP" is the nomenclature used for bilateral reticulation with predominance in peripheral and lower lung fields with traction bronchiectasis but without honeycombing. This is also diagnostic for IPF in older adults and does not necessarily mandate a surgical lung biopsy or cryo-biopsy. In patients without these classic imaging findings or "atypical" cases, referral to an interstitial lung disease center is highly recommended for engaging a multi-disciplinary clinical, radiologic, and pathologic approach to diagnosis and management [2].

A full discussion of therapeutics in IPF is covered in other sections. Non-pharmacologic and pharmacologic therapies are essential in the pre-transplant patient. Non-pharmacologic therapies include supplemental oxygen where indicated, cardio-pulmonary rehabilitation, smoking cessation, and appropriate vaccinations (including influenza, pneumococcal, and now novel coronavirus-19 (COVID-19) [2].

Pharmacology therapy has revolutionized IPF care over the past decade. Nintedanib is a tyrosine kinase inhibitor inhibiting vascular endothelial growth factor (VEGF), fibroblast growth factor (FGF), and platelet-derived growth factor (PDGF). Pirfenidone is an anti-inflammatory/anti-fibrotic agent with various mechanisms, including inhibiting collagen synthesis with decreased fibroblast activity and decreasing tumor growth factor-beta and tumor necrosis factor-alpha activity. These drugs were initially approved with clinical trials demonstrating stabilization of forced vital capacity (FVC), a common marker of disease progression. More recently, meta-analyses have demonstrated mortality benefits with both agents [3].

3. The natural course of the disease

Before the availability of antifibrotic therapies, the median survival following IPF diagnosis was quite dismal at 3.8 years. While there was considerable variability in the clinical course, many patients experience a decline in their lung function with associated shortness of breath at rest, exertion, and supplemental oxygen dependency. The chronic hypoxic state induces secondary pulmonary hypertension and right ventricular strain, dysfunction, and eventually failure. Acute exacerbations of IPF (AE-IPF) are also a common etiology of morbidity with mortality varying from 50 to 85% with hospitalization [4].

4. Lung transplantation

Lung transplantation is the only curative modality for end-stage IPF with both survival and quality of life benefits. The first lung transplant in humans was performed by J.D. Hardy at the University of Mississippi in 1963 on a patient with lung cancer [5]. Dr. Joel Cooper performed the first successful single lung transplant in IPF in 1983 [6]. In 2019, a total of 4500 lung transplants were performed, and nearly 33% of these had a primary diagnosis of IPF (UIP pattern), making this one of the most common indications for a lung transplant [1]. Prior to 2005, patients with Chronic Obstructive Lung Disease (COPD) were the most common recipients of lung transplants as the transplant waitlist was based on a queue system with the time of the list as the primary determinant for allocation. Many IPF patients expired while awaiting potential donors on the waitlist. In the US, the Organ Procurement and Transplant Network (OPTN) is the organization entrusted with the responsibility to optimize organ allocation in line with the ethical principles of utility, justice, and respect for persons. In 2005, due to a recognition of high lung transplant waitlist mortality, the LAS system was implemented by the OPTN to optimize the allocation of donor's lungs with the intent to balance the urgency of transplant need with the post-transplant survival benefit. The clinical parameters, underlying diagnosis of the recipient, and statistical modeling determine the waitlist urgency and post-transplant benefit, thereby generating the LAS for the recipient and the subsequent allocation of available donor lungs. Additional changes in the allocation system were implemented by the Department of Health in November 2017 after a lawsuit in New York challenged the allocation system. The emergency action changed allocation priority from the local Donor Service Area (DSA) to regional priority resulting in patients with the highest LAS within a 250 nautical mile radius of the donor center being eligible for allocation. Before this change, the DSA would offer the donor lungs first to all listed local patients irrespective of their LAS before expanding offers to sicker patients outside the service area. As a result of this change, higher LAS patients in the region are receiving more access to donors' lungs, and listed IPF patients are benefiting from these changes with an increasing number of transplants [7].

5. Criteria for referral and transplantation in IPF

Conceptually, lung transplantation should be considered in patients with a high risk of death (quantified as >50%) within 2 years if lung transplantation is not performed. High (defined as >80%) likelihood of 5-year survival post-transplant from a general medical perspective (**Table 1**) [1, 8].

Indications for Referral
• At the time of diagnosis irrespective of starting antifibrotic therapies
• FVC ≤ 80% predicted or DLCO ≤40% predicted
• Decline in FVC ≥ 10% or decline in DLCO ≥15%
• Decline in FVC ≥ 5% with clinical or radiological progression
• Supplemental oxygen requirements at rest or with exertion
Indications for Listing
• Decline in FVC ≥ 10% or ≥ 5% with radiological progression or decline in DLCO ≥10% within a 6-month period
• Desaturation to ≤88% on the 6 Minute Walk Test (6 MWT)
• The decline of ≥50 m walk the distance on the 6MWT
• Diagnosis of secondary pulmonary hypertension
• Hospitalization for acute exacerbations or other respiratory complications

Table 1.
Indications for transplant referral and listing [8].

6. Contraindications to transplant

The International Society for Heart and Lung Transplantation (ISHLT) categorizes contraindications to transplantation as absolute, high risk, and standard risk factors. Absolute contraindications are factors that generally preclude successful lung transplantation. The ISHLT recommends that most transplant centers avoid transplantation in patients with these features, except under "very exceptional or extenuating circumstances." Importantly, these criteria include patients with severe extrapulmonary organ dysfunction who are not candidates for multi-organ transplants (**Table 2**) [1, 8].

Next are patients with risk factors associated with high or substantially increased risks. Patients with these features can be considered in centers with experience and expertise in addressing the underlying factors. Lung transplant centers with a higher volume of transplants per year (typically centers ≥40 lung transplants per year) may have better outcomes with these groups of patients. Modifiable risk factors like obesity, malnutrition, deconditioning, treatable infections, coronary disease amenable to stenting or percutaneous interventions, etc., need to be optimized as best possible before listing active for transplantation. If several of these factors are present, the risk factors are multiplicative for the poor post-transplantation outcome (**Table 3**).

Finally, standard risk factors may predispose patients to poor transplant outcomes in the short and long term. Again these factors are considered to be multiplicative (**Table 4**) [1, 8].

Social issues:

• Lack of patient willingness/acceptance of transplant

• Limited functional status (i.e., not ambulatory), the poor potential for rehabilitation

• Recurrent non-adherence

• Active substance use (tobacco, vaping, marijuana, IV drug use)

Systemic infections:

• Septic shock

• Active disseminated infection

• Active tuberculosis

• HIV with detectable viremia

Extra-pulmonary organ dysfunction (if not a candidate for multi-organ transplant):

• Renal dysfunction with glomerular filtration rate < 40 mL/min/1.73m^2

• Liver cirrhosis

• Acute liver failure

• Acute renal failure (with a low likelihood for recovery)

Other significant illnesses with resultant mortality risk/morbidity:

• Recent cerebrovascular accident

• Malignancy with a high risk of recurrence/death

• Progressive/severe cognitive impairment

• Other severe uncontrolled conditions in which patient is expected to have limited long term survival

---

Table 2.
Absolute contraindications for lung transplantation [1, 8].

Age > 70 years
Cardiac issues include:

- Severe coronary disease requiring coronary artery bypass grafting at transplant

- Reduced left ventricular ejection fraction <40%

Untreatable hematologic issues:

- Bleeding diathesis

- Thrombophilia

- Severe bone marrow suppression

Significant cerebrovascular disease
Severe esophageal issues, i.e., dysmotility
Re-transplant:

- <1 year following initial transplant

- For restrictive chronic lung allograft dysfunction (CLAD)

- For AMR as etiology of CLAD

Extra-corporeal support
Hepatitis B or C with detectable viral load and liver fibrosis
Infection:

- Mycobacterium abscessus

- Lomentospora prolificans

- Burkholderia cenocepacia or gladioli

Social issues:

- Lack of understanding of disease and/or transplant despite education

- Poor caregiving plan/social support

Weight: BMI <16 or > 35 kg/m^2
Functional limitations with potential for rehabilitation post-transplant

Table 3.
Relative contraindications or high-risk conditions for transplant.

Age 65–70 years
Non-pulmonary organ dysfunction:

- Chronic kidney disease with a Glomerular filtration rate of 40–60 mL/min/1.73 m^2

- Mild to moderate coronary artery disease

- Severe coronary artery disease amenable to percutaneous intervention prior to transplant

- LVEF 40–50%

- Peripheral vascular disease

- Severe gastroesophageal reflux disease

- Esophageal dysmotility

- Poorly controlled diabetes

- Bone marrow suppression with thrombocytopenia, anemia, or leukopenia

- Hypoalbuminemia

Connective tissue disease (scleroderma, lupus, inflammatory myopathy)
Retransplant >1 year for obstructive chronic lung allograft dysfunction (CLAD)
Mechanical ventilation pre-transplant
Surgical issues:

- Prior pleurodesis

- Previous thoracic surgery

Infections:

- HIV with undetectable viral load

- Scedosporium apiospermum

Frailty
Weight: BMI 30–34.9 or BMI 16–17 kg/m^2

Table 4.
Other general risk factors for poor post-transplant outcomes.

7. Listing considerations

7.1 Age

The issue of candidacy for patients with advanced age is controversial in lung transplantation. Historically older patients had worsened outcomes, with multiple case-control studies showing worsened long and short-term mortality in patients over 60 years of age [9]. However, more recently, an increasing number of lung transplants are being performed on older patients, with a database showing that 11.1% of patients being above age 70 from 2006 to 2013. In this study, survival at 1 year was similar in patients in 60s vs. 70s. However, 3 and 5-year survival was worsened in the group in 70s [10]. Successful transplantation has even been reported in an 80-year-old patient [11]. UNOS registry showed similar outcomes up to age 74, but worsened survival between ages 75 and 79. Various complications are more common in patients over 65, including infections, rejection, venous thrombo-emboli, malignancy, and drug toxicity [12].

7.2 Obesity

Overweight and obese patients (defined as body mass index >25 kg^*m^{-2} and > 30 kg^*m^{-2} respectively) had a higher risk of death post-transplant (15 and 22% higher respectively on the multi-variate analysis) [13]. Weight loss both improves pre-transplant symptoms and post-transplant survival with dose-response improvements [14]. We refer these patients for nutritional counseling and pulmonary rehabilitation. We use a threshold of BMI >35 as an absolute contraindication to transplant.

7.3 Medical frailty

Medical Frailty can be characterized as declining physiologic and functional reserve leading to a general susceptibility to physiologic insults, leading to potentially deleterious outcomes. The prevalence of frailty increases with age. The decline in lean body mass, strength, endurance, balance, walking performance, and low activity are markers of medical frailty [15].

Multiple tools have been developed to assess and quantify medical frailty. Previous work in IPF has utilized the Fried Frailty Phenotype (FFP) score. This score includes 5 components: Unintentional weight loss, exhaustion, slowness, physical activity, and weakness. **Table 5** further describes these features. Each component is scored 0 or 1. A score of zero represents the absence of frailty, a score of 1–2 represents pre-frailty status, score ≥ 3 indications frailty.

28% of lung transplant candidates meet the criteria for frailty by FFP. Higher FFP is associated with increased risk of delisting, mortality before lung transplant, and mortality within 1-year post-transplantation. Cardiopulmonary rehabilitation can be helpful to preserve or even improve functional status in patients with end-stage lung disease [16]. It is our practice to refer patients with medical frailty to cardiopulmonary rehabilitation in addition to nutrition evaluation very early in the evaluation process.

7.4 Telomeropathy

Chromosomal telomeres protect against the loss of genetic information in normal cell division. Mutations in telomerase can lead to the shortening of the telomeres. This further leads to cell cycle arrest with associated bone marrow failure,

Component	Criteria
Unintentional weight loss	>10 lbs. self-reported or 5% measured total body weight over 1 year
Exhaustion	How many days over the past week have you:
	• Felt that everything you did was an effort
	• Felt as though you could not get going
	Meets criteria if >3 days
Slowness	Self-report of slow walking pace (or difficulty walking across the room)
Physical activity	Self-reported decreased activity compared to the average person
Weakness	Handgrip strength measured by dynamometer
Adapted from [15].	

Table 5.
Fried frailty phenotype score.

malignancy, hepatic failure, and IPF. Pre-transplant telomere shortening is associated with earlier age of presentation and progressive phenotype [17]. Leukocyte telomere length < 10th percentile is seen in 25% of sporadic IPF cases and 37% of familial IPF cases [18]. Patients with short telomere length (coined short telomere syndrome) also have been seen to have worsened lung transplantation outcomes with worse survival, shorter time interval to CLAD, and higher incidence of grade 3 PGD [19]. These patients also have a high incidence of cytopenias, especially given that many medications given in the post-transplant period are associated with further bone marrow toxicity (such as mycophenolate, valganciclovir) [20]. Several studies have also demonstrated increased renal impairment and calcineurin toxicity [21, 22]. The current recommendation is that all patients with possible familial IPF be evaluated for signs of telomeropathy with attention to hematologic abnormalities and liver cirrhosis. Our center tests all IPF patients with a strong family history undergoing transplant work-up for telomere length studies based on significant complications encountered in patients with short telomere syndrome. In patients diagnosed with short telomere syndrome, pre-transplant evaluation with hematology to assess baseline bone marrow function, including bone marrow biopsy, liver function assessment, and cirrhosis evaluation with ultrasound elastography, MRI, or even MRI trans-jugular liver biopsy may be required in some patients. Post-transplant therapy modifications in this group, including strategies to preserve bone marrow function by avoiding cell cycle inhibitor-based immunosuppression may be helpful in ensuring long-term success in this group of patients.

8. Cardiac issues

8.1 Coronary artery disease

Coronary artery disease is common in patients with IPF, being common comorbidity in the age group affected by this disease, inflammation, lipid abnormalities, and the impact of disease-specific therapies. Incidence as high as 65.8% has been described in cohorts with left heart catheterization data pre-transplant [23]. Optimization pre-transplant is recommended by cardiologists and cardiovascular surgeons experienced with the transplant process. Percutaneous interventions, particularly in IPF patients, should be discussed in a multidisciplinary manner depending on the understanding of illness related to the IPF, severity of the coronary lesions, and type of intervention, especially the placement of drug-eluting stents, which may require prolonged dual antiplatelet regimens for several months and complicate the listing or transplant of the patient. There is increasing literature that patients can safely undergo coronary artery bypass grafting and still undergo lung transplantation with equivalent outcomes, although there may be technical limitations. Most of these patients may be eligible only for a single lung transplant (typically right single lung transplant) secondary to the prior sternotomy status, disruption of the left pleural space, and danger of disrupting the bypass grafts [24].

8.2 Left ventricular diastolic dysfunction

In patients with intact LV systolic function by ejection fraction, it is important to evaluate LV diastolic dysfunction. This is defined by evaluating early mitral inflow velocity (E) to early diastolic mitral annular velocity (e prime). In patients with poor echocardiographic visualization, an elevated pulmonary capillary wedge pressure on right heart catheterization or a directly measured elevated left ventricular end diastolic pressure (LVEDP) can also be suggestive. Diastolic dysfunction greatly increases the risk of primary graft dysfunction in the immediate post-operative period and increases the duration of mechanical ventilation post-transplant [25]. Optimization of volume status is essential in these patients.

8.3 Pulmonary hypertension

Secondary Pulmonary hypertension (PH) is common in patients with end-stage IPF. Pulmonary hypertension is defined as a mean pulmonary artery pressure of more than 20 mmHg (decreased from 25 mmHg in most recent guidelines) [26]. One prior study of IPF patients undergoing transplant evaluation found that 49% demonstrated PH (utilizing 25 mmHg as cutoff). PH is associated with lower FVC and a greater need for supplemental oxygen pre-transplant. However, a prior study of UNOS data in IPF showed no difference in mortality post-transplant [27].

9. Gastro-esophageal issues

Gastro-esophageal issues have long been associated with lung disease. There is a strong association between gastroesophageal reflux disease as a major independent risk factor with IPF. In a 2005 study 78 consecutive patients referred for lung transplantation found 63% of patients had GERD symptoms, 72% had a hypotensive lower esophageal sphincter, 44% had prolonged gastric emptying, and 38% at abnormal pH testing [28]. These issues are not limited to patients with symptoms, and testing is recommended in all patients being evaluated for transplant. Post-transplant gastro-esophageal reflux, including intra-esophageal reflux from esophageal dysmotility and potential for micro-aspiration or frank oropharyngeal aspiration, is a major factor in poor outcomes post-transplant with early allograft dysfunction, development of donor-specific antibodies and chronic lung allograft dysfunction (CLAD) [29].

Post-transplant gastro-esophageal issues are associated with worsened outcomes. Patients with GERD post-transplant has been shown to have diminished recovery of FEV1 [30]. Aspiration is closely associated with both chronic and acute rejection, with an increased rate of bronchiolitis obliterans syndrome [31]. Patients with significant reflux should be considered for anti-reflux surgery. Pre-transplant surgery (where tolerated) is associated with trend toward fewer IPF exacerbations [32]. In patients unable to undergo pre-transplant anti-reflux surgery, early post-transplant surgery is associated with preserved lung function in addition to decreased bronchiolitis obliterans and a signal toward improved mortality [33, 34].

10. Pre-transplant work-up

Once a patient is referred for consideration of lung transplantation, further evaluation is undertaken to uncover risk factors and/or contraindications for transplantation.

11. Cardiovascular evaluation

An echocardiogram is obtained with a bubble study to identify structural heart issues, including ventricular dysfunction, valvulopathy, and cardiac/pulmonary shunts. Right heart catheterization is performed, evaluating for pulmonary hypertension, and filling pressures, and cardiac output. Left heart catheterization is performed to evaluate for coronary arterial disease. A baseline ECG is obtained. A peripheral arterial disease evaluation includes carotid ultrasound and ankle-brachial index.

12. Gastro-intestinal evaluation

Given the association of gastro-esophageal reflux with IPF and its association with poor transplant outcomes, a gastro-esophageal workup is pursued even in the asymptomatic patient with IPF. We typically order a modified barium swallow to assess oral pharyngeal function and aspiration risk, a barium esophagram to assess dysmotility, intra-esophageal reflux, hiatal hernias, or esophageal strictures, and a gastric emptying study to assess gastric motility. Further testing based on this initial screen includes formal esophageal manometry and pH probe monitoring. We do not recommend surgical intervention prior to the transplant in these IPF patients. However, protocol-based reassessment of these tests is done 3 months post-transplant for potential early surgical intervention, including fundoplication and hiatal hernia repair.

13. Malignancy evaluation

Age-appropriate cancer screening is ensured, including prostate, breast, cervical, and colorectal. If eligible, lung cancer screening with a low dose CT chest is performed. Patients are counseled regarding skin lesions and referred to dermatology if concerning. Apart from malignant melanoma, other skin cancers are not considered a contraindication to proceeding with lung transplantation. However, depending on the sun exposure a patient may have had during their lifetime and the burden of pre-existing cancers, this can cause major post-transplant morbidity. Transplant immunosuppression clearly predisposes to increased incidence of new and recurrent skin cancers, rapid rate of growth or doubling time, and higher than expected rate of metastasis compared to the general population [35]. There is also increasing evidence that the use of voricoazole as anti-fungal prophylaxis may be independently associated with skin cancers in the predisposed population [36].

14. Criteria/timing for listing

A decision to list a patient for lung transplantation is a multi-disciplinary effort that should only be undertaken after careful workup and counseling the patient extensively on the risks and benefits. A multi-disciplinary committee should make this decision with input from both transplant pulmonology, transplant surgery, consultants, social work, physical therapy, and nutrition.

15. Impact of anti-fibrotic therapy on listing

Anti-fibrotic therapy has improved the outcomes for patients with IPF, with initial studies showing a decreased decline in FVC and more recent meta-analyses demonstrating improved mortality [3]. Patients should be starting on these therapies immediately, and they may delay the need for transplantation. Early in their use, there were concerns regarding the impact of anti-fibrotic on wound healing. However, observational studies have demonstrated no impaired wound or anastomotic healing [37, 38]. While the efficacy of anti-fibrotic agents in late IPF with FVC < 30% is not clear, there is no contraindication to continue these drugs through to the transplant if the patient is already on the same. Anti-fibrotic combination therapies with different mechanisms of action for IPF are undergoing clinical trials. There is no current literature evidence outside of anecdotal case reports to justify the use of anti-fibrotic agents routinely after the lung transplant, even in single lung transplant recipients with a native IPF lung. A clinical trial is currently investigating the continuation of Nintedanib following single lung transplantation in IPF (NCT 03562416).

16. Single vs. double lung transplant

The modern growth in lung transplant volume has been largely that of a double lung transplant. In general, double lung transplantation is preferred over single lung with superior long-term outcomes (7.8 years versus 4.8 years) [1]. However, short-term outcomes may favor offering single lung transplantation in elderly and frail patients, as there is typically less ischemic time to the allograft, a shorter ICU stay, hospitalization, and less overall perioperative morbidity [39]. In patients who are candidates for both single and double lung transplants, the current recommendation is to list for both, as there is decreased waiting list mortality, increased transplantation rate, and no difference in 1- or 5-year mortality [40, 41].

17. Management of acute exacerbations of IPF (AE-IPF) in transplant candidates

AE-IPF (colloquially referred to as flares) are frequently observed in patients with IPF and can result in rapidly progressive respiratory failure and death within days. AE-IPF is categorized by increasing hypoxia and dyspnea with bilateral ground-glass opacities and negative infectious evaluation [2]. The in-hospital mortality is above 50–85% for these episodes. Standard empiric therapy for AE-IPF includes corticosteroids, empiric antimicrobials, and supplemental oxygen. However, no therapeutic modality has demonstrated effectiveness in randomized controlled trials. These exacerbations' exact pathophysiology and mechanisms have yet to be fully elucidated. However, infections, post-operative, drug toxicity, and aspiration have been identified as triggers. More recently, autoantibodies have been identified as a possible trigger of IPF flares. A randomized controlled clinical trial for consisting of plasmapheresis, rituximab, and intra-venous immunoglobulin (IVIG) to reduce auto-antibody burden is currently ongoing [42]. Notably, treatment outcomes are much worse in patients who require mechanical ventilation, with studies reporting 87–96% mortality [43]. The American Thoracic Society guidelines recommend having a value-based goal of care discussion prior to instituting mechanical ventilation [44]. Notably, mechanical ventilation is a significant barrier to lung transplantation as it predisposes patients to immobility, over-sedation, deconditioning, and ventilator induced lung injury (VILI) [45]. In patients who are listed (preferably) or undergoing evaluation for lung transplantation, the use of veno-venous extracorporeal membrane oxygenation (VV-ECMO) is an attractive therapeutic modality for patients with refractory hypoxemia to avoid mechanical ventilation as a bridge to lung transplantation. Our center has a large amount of experience with ambulatory ECMO to help improve patient conditioning while an acceptable donor organ is found.

18. Mechanical ventilation in the pre-transplant period

Mechanical ventilation is a relative contraindication to transplant. It is associated with several deleterious effects, including sedation and immobility, leading to rapid deconditioning and ventilatory induced lung injury. Additionally, given the high incidence of pulmonary hypertension in this population, the induction period can be associated with high morbidity and even mortality. For these reasons, our center avoids mechanical ventilation where possible in lung transplantation candidates with IPF in an acute flare with high oxygen needs that would typically need mechanical ventilatory support. Instead, we prefer to use a strategy of elective veno-venous ECMO cannulation and maintenance once oxygen needs exceed a FiO2 of 80% on a high flow nasal cannula or non-invasive ventilatory support. This enables us to provide adequate oxygenation and ventilation to the patient while allowing ambulation to avoid deconditioning, nutrition via oral means and lets the patient maintain communication.

19. ECMO as a bridge to transplant

Despite early cohorts showing poor outcomes, ambulatory ECMO has emerged as an attractive option to bridge candidates with poor native lung function to transplant. A recent cohort study demonstrated 59% survival to transplant in those bridged with ECMO and excellent long-term outcomes in those surviving to discharge with 88% 1 year and 83% 3 year survival [46]. Ambulation is one of the greatest benefits of ECMO in the pre-transplant period. The improved oxygenation and physiologic reserve provided by ECMO allow these patients to ambulate to a greater extent. In fact, the above cohort found that ambulation was the only independent predictor of survival to transplantation. A dual lumen right internal jugular cannula is often preferred over femoral cannulation strategies for ease of ambulation. Bi- femoral venous cannulation is not a contraindication to ambulation, and we routinely ambulate patients with femoral cannulas in our center with specific practical safety measures to avoid accidental decannulation or adverse events.

20. Immunosuppression

In the immediate peri-transplant therapy, induction immunosuppression is achieved with high dose corticosteroids and traditionally thymoglobulin; however, basiliximab, an IL-2r monoclonal antibody, is being utilized with increased frequency. Following the transplant, standard immunosuppression is continued with calcineurin inhibitor (typically tacrolimus), a cell-cycle antagonist (typically mycophenolate mofetil or mycophenolic acid), and low dose prednisone.

21. Post-transplant infections and prophylaxis

Bacterial infections are common peri-transplant, and our practice is to cover prophylactically for 48–72 hours with vancomycin and cefepime. This addressed both gram positives (especially methicillin resistant staph aureus) and more resistant gram negatives (most prototypically pseudomonas).

Pneumocystis is a life-long concern post-transplant. Trimethoprim-sulfamethoxazole (TMP/SMX) is the preferred prophylaxis, given that it also has activity against Strep pneumoniae, staphylococcus, Enterobacteriaceae, Listeria, and Nocardia. Other agents, including dapsone and atovaquone can be utilized in the event TMP/SMX is not tolerated.

Cytomegalovirus (CMV) infection can be devastating following lung transplantation, and prophylaxis has been demonstrated to improve outcomes. Valganciclovir is the preferred option, however IV ganciclovir can be utilized if the patient does not have enteral access or is not absorbing medications. Donor-recipient CMV status informs the duration of treatment. In donor positive-recipient negative (D+/R-), the highest risk group, 12 months of prophylaxis is recommended. In D+/R+ and D−/R+ a minimum of 6 months of prophylaxis is recommended [47]. Prophylaxis is re-initiated if the patient undergoes additional immunosuppression and CMV viral PCR titers are followed regularly. Routine prophylaxis is not recommended in D−/R- subgroup; however, blood products administered to this group must be CMV negative.

Fungal infections are also common post-lung transplantation. This may be of particular importance in patients with IPF undergoing a single lung transplant as their native lungs may harbor or be colonized with fungal organisms. Some patients may develop aspergilloma cavities or progress to invasive fungal disease with the enhanced immunosuppression with invasive pulmonary aspergillosis and ulcerative tracheobronchitis being the most feared variants. The two most common approaches to prophylaxis are systemic azole therapy to cover aspergillus, and some centers will use nebulized liposomal amphotericin B to prevent aspergillus colonization at the anastomotic site.

22. Monitoring protocol post-transplantation

Most transplant centers have post-transplant protocols that address post-transplant follow-up in terms of clinic visits, post-transplant diagnostics, and laboratory tests. IPF patients undergoing transplants will typically follow the same protocol similar to other patients. Patients typically are encouraged to monitor and log their vitals, spirometry, blood glucose, activity levels, nutritional intake, participation in cardiopulmonary rehab and to call the transplant center for any medical problems. Frequent clinic visits in the first one to 3 months after transplant helps ensure frequent clinical assessment for medical or social and financial issues, compliance, establishing rapport and confidence with the transplant team.

23. Outcomes

Return of pulmonary function is dependent on graft characteristics, recipient thoracic cage, and post-operative complications. A value of 80% of predictive value can be achieved 3 months postoperatively in both FVC and FEV_1, and patients may reach 100% by 6–12 months. Lung function typically stabilizes more rapidly in single lung transplants; at 3 months, some patients achieve FVC and FEV1 over 80% predicted [48]. Since 2010, 1 year and 5-year survival have been 85% and 59%, respectively, with some variation with regards to pre-transplant risk factors and post-transplant complications. Younger patients with lesser comorbidities tend to have better survival overall [1, 49].

Furthermore, a lung transplant has been shown to improve health-related quality of life in a clinically meaningful way. Most of this change occurs in the first 6–7 months post-transplant. This is despite the systemic effects of immunosuppression and the development of often serious co-morbid conditions [50].

24. Conclusion

Overall, a lung transplant is a therapeutic option for patients with advanced IPF that continue to progress despite being on medical therapies. It has the potential to increase their survival and provide a quality of life. It is important to refer these patients with typical or probable UIP early to a lung transplant center due to the risk of rapid progression of disease or deterioration from AE-IPF. Acute decompensation can potentially make a transplant evaluation difficult to complete due to clinical instability. Transplant centers will typically list only patients with evidence of clinical deterioration and can help co-manage patients that may be stable on medical therapies. Access to resources at transplant centers may impact patients beyond the immediate medical needs, including referral or evaluations for cardiopulmonary rehab, nutrition, or weight loss, other medically indicated consultations, and clinical trials, and help introduce patients to other social forums like patient support groups.

Author details

Ryan Goetz[1], Nitesh Kumar Jain[2], Humayun Anjum[3] and Thomas S. Kaleekal[4*]

1 Department of Internal Medicine, University of Alabama at Birmingham, Birmingham, Alabama, USA

2 Department of Critical Care Medicine, Mayo Clinic Health System, Mankato, Minnesota, USA

3 Department of Medicine, University of North Texas, Denton, Texas, USA

4 Division of Pulmonary, Allergy and Critical Care Medicine, University of Alabama at Birmingham, Alabama, USA

*Address all correspondence to: kaleekal@uab.edu

IntechOpen

References

[1] Chambers DC, Cherikh WS, Harhay MO, Hayes D Jr, Hsich E, Khush KK, et al. The international thoracic organ transplant registry of the International Society for Heart and Lung Transplantation: Thirty-sixth adult lung and heart & lung transplantation report & 2019; focus theme: Donor and recipient size match. The Journal of Heart and Lung Transplantation. 2019;**38**(10):1042-1055

[2] Lederer DJ, Martinez FJ. Idiopathic pulmonary fibrosis. New England Journal of Medicine. 2018;**378**(19): 1811-1823

[3] Petnak T, Lertjitbanjong P, Thongprayoon C, Moua T. Impact of Antifibrotic therapy on mortality and acute exacerbation in idiopathic pulmonary fibrosis: A systematic review and meta-analysis. Chest. 2021;**160**(5):1751-1763

[4] Juarez MM, Chan AL, Norris AG, Morrissey BM, Albertson TE. Acute exacerbation of idiopathic pulmonary fibrosis-a review of current and novel pharmacotherapies. Journal of Thoracic Disease. 2015;7(3):499-519

[5] Hardy JD. The first lung transplant in man (1963) and the first heart transplant in man (1964). Transplantation Proceedings. 1999;**31**(1-2):25-29

[6] Toronto Lung Transplant Group. Unilateral lung transplantation for pulmonary fibrosis. The New England Journal of Medicine. May 1986;**314**(18):1140-1145. DOI: 10.1056/nejm198605013141802. PMID: 3515192

[7] Drolen C, Cantu E, Goldberg HJ, Diamond JM, Courtwright A. Impact of the elimination of the donation service area on United States lung transplant practices and outcomes at high and low competition centers. American Journal of Transplantation. 2020;**20**(12): 3631-3638

[8] Leard LE, Holm AM, Valapour M, Glanville AR, Attawar S, Aversa M, et al. Consensus document for the selection of lung transplant candidates: An update from the International Society for Heart and Lung Transplantation. The Journal of Heart and Lung Transplantation. 2021;**40**(11):1349-1379

[9] Gutierrez C, Al-Faifi S, Chaparro C, Waddell T, Hadjiliadis D, Singer L, et al. The effect of recipient's age on lung transplant outcome. American Journal of Transplantation. 2007;7(5):1271-1277

[10] Hayanga AJ, Aboagye JK, Hayanga HE, Morrell M, Huffman L, Shigemura N, et al. Contemporary analysis of early outcomes after lung transplantation in the elderly using a national registry. The Journal of Heart and Lung Transplantation. 2015;**34**(2):182-188

[11] Shigemura N, Brann S, Wasson S, Bhama J, Bermudez C, Hattler BG, et al. Successful lung transplantation in an octogenarian. The Journal of Thoracic and Cardiovascular Surgery. 2010;**139**(3):e47-ee8

[12] Biswas Roy S, Alarcon D, Walia R, Chapple KM, Bremner RM, Smith MA. Is there an age limit to lung transplantation? The Annals of Thoracic Surgery. 2015;**100**(2):443-451

[13] Lederer DJ, Wilt JS, D'Ovidio F, Bacchetta MD, Shah L, Ravichandran S, et al. Obesity and underweight are associated with an increased risk of death after lung transplantation. American Journal of Respiratory and Critical Care Medicine. 2009;**180**(9):887-895

[14] Chandrashekaran S, Keller CA, Kremers WK, Peters SG, Hathcock MA, Kennedy CC. Weight loss prior to lung transplantation is associated with improved survival. The Journal of Heart and Lung Transplantation. 2015;**34**(5): 651-657

[15] Sheth JS, Xia M, Murray S, Martinez CH, Meldrum CA, Belloli EA, et al. Frailty and geriatric conditions in older patients with idiopathic pulmonary fibrosis. Respiratory Medicine. 2019;**148**:6-12

[16] Singer JP, Diamond JM, Gries CJ, McDonnough J, Blanc PD, Shah R, et al. Frailty phenotypes, disability, and outcomes in adult candidates for lung transplantation. American Journal of Respiratory and Critical Care Medicine. 2015;**192**(11):1325-1334

[17] Armanios M. Telomeres and age-related disease: How telomere biology informs clinical paradigms. The Journal of Clinical Investigation. 2013;**123**(3): 996-1002

[18] Cronkhite JT, Xing C, Raghu G, Chin KM, Torres F, Rosenblatt RL, et al. Telomere shortening in familial and sporadic pulmonary fibrosis. American Journal of Respiratory and Critical Care Medicine. 2008;**178**(7):729-737

[19] Newton CA, Kozlitina J, Lines JR, Kaza V, Torres F, Garcia CK. Telomere length in patients with pulmonary fibrosis associated with chronic lung allograft dysfunction and post & lung transplantation survival. The Journal of Heart and Lung Transplantation. 2017;**36**(8):845-853

[20] Tokman S, Singer JP, Devine MS, Westall GP, Aubert JD, Tamm M, et al. Clinical outcomes of lung transplant recipients with telomerase mutations. The Journal of Heart and Lung Transplantation. 2015;**34**(10):1318-1324

[21] Borie R, Kannengiesser C, Hirschi S, Le Pavec J, Mal H, Bergot E, et al. Severe hematologic complications after lung transplantation in patients with telomerase complex mutations. The Journal of Heart and Lung Transplantation. 2015;**34**(4):538-546

[22] Silhan LL, Shah PD, Chambers DC, Snyder LD, Riise GC, Wagner CL, et al. Lung transplantation in telomerase mutation carriers with pulmonary fibrosis. European Respiratory Journal. 2014;**44**(1):178-187

[23] Nathan SD, Basavaraj A, Reichner C, Shlobin OA, Ahmad S, Kiernan J, et al. Prevalence and impact of coronary artery disease in idiopathic pulmonary fibrosis. Respiratory Medicine. 2010;**104**(7):1035-1041

[24] McKellar SH, Bowen ME, Baird BC, Raman S, Cahill BC, Selzman CH. Lung transplantation following coronary artery bypass surgery & improved outcomes following single-lung transplant. The Journal of Heart and Lung Transplantation. 2016;**35**(11): 1289-1294

[25] Li D, Weinkauf J, Hirji A, Kapasi A, Lien D, Nagendran J, et al. Elevated pre-transplant left ventricular end-diastolic pressure increases primary graft dysfunction risk in double lung transplant recipients. The Journal of Heart and Lung Transplantation. 2019;**38**(7):710-718

[26] Hoeper MM, Humbert M. The new haemodynamic definition of pulmonary hypertension: Evidence prevails, finally! European Respiratory Journal. 2019;**53**(3):1900038

[27] Hayes D Jr, Higgins RS, Black SM, Wehr AM, Lehman AM, Kirkby S, et al. Effect of pulmonary hypertension on survival in patients with idiopathic pulmonary fibrosis after lung transplantation: An analysis of the united network of organ sharing registry. The Journal of Heart and Lung Transplantation. 2015;**34**(3):430-437

[28] D'Ovidio F, Singer LG, Hadjiliadis D, Pierre A, Waddell TK, de Perrot M, et al. Prevalence of gastroesophageal reflux in end-stage lung disease candidates for lung transplant. The Annals of Thoracic Surgery. 2005;**80**(4):1254-1260

[29] Tangaroonsanti A, Lee AS, Crowell MD, Vela MF, Jones DR, Erasmus D, et al. Impaired esophageal motility and clearance post-lung transplant: Risk for chronic allograft failure. Clinical and Translational Gastroenterology. 2017;**8**(6):e102

[30] Posner S, Finn RT, Shimpi RA, Wood RK, Fisher D, Hartwig MG, et al. Esophageal contractility increases and gastroesophageal reflux does not worsen after lung transplantation. Diseases of the Esophagus. 2019;**32**(10):1-8

[31] Shepherd KL, Chambers DC, Gabbay E, Hillman DR, Eastwood PR. Obstructive sleep apnoea and nocturnal gastroesophageal reflux are common in lung transplant patients. Respirology. 2008;**13**(7):1045-1052

[32] Raghu G, Pellegrini CA, Yow E, Flaherty KR, Meyer K, Noth I, et al. Laparoscopic anti-reflux surgery for the treatment of idiopathic pulmonary fibrosis (WRAP-IPF): A multicentre, randomised, controlled phase 2 trial. The Lancet Respiratory Medicine. 2018;**6**(9):707-714

[33] Robertson AG, Krishnan A, Ward C, Pearson JP, Small T, Corris PA, et al. Anti-reflux surgery in lung transplant recipients: Outcomes and effects on quality of life. The European Respiratory Journal. 2012;**39**(3):691-697

[34] Davis RD Jr, Lau CL, Eubanks S, Messier RH, Hadjiliadis D, Steele MP, et al. Improved lung allograft function after fundoplication in patients with gastroesophageal reflux disease undergoing lung transplantation. The Journal of Thoracic and Cardiovascular Surgery. 2003;**125**(3):533-542

[35] Howard MD, Su JC, Chong AH. Skin cancer following solid organ transplantation: A review of risk factors and models of care. American Journal of Clinical Dermatology. 2018;**19**(4): 585-597

[36] Kuklinski LF, Li S, Karagas MR, Weng WK, Kwong BY. Effect of voriconazole on risk of nonmelanoma skin cancer after hematopoietic cell transplantation. Journal of the American Academy of Dermatology. 2017;**77**(4):706-712

[37] Delanote I, Wuyts WA, Yserbyt J, Verbeken EK, Verleden GM, Vos R. Safety and efficacy of bridging to lung transplantation with antifibrotic drugs in idiopathic pulmonary fibrosis: A case series. BMC Pulmonary Medicine. 2016;**16**(1):156

[38] Leuschner G, Stocker F, Veit T, Kneidinger N, Winter H, Schramm R, et al. Outcome of lung transplantation in idiopathic pulmonary fibrosis with previous anti-fibrotic therapy. The Journal of Heart and Lung Transplantation. 2018;**37**(2):268-274

[39] De Oliveira NC, Osaki S, Maloney J, Cornwell RD, Meyer KC. Lung transplant for interstitial lung disease: Outcomes for single versus bilateral lung transplantation. Interactive Cardiovascular and Thoracic Surgery. 2012;**14**(3):263-267

[40] Chauhan D, Karanam AB, Merlo A, Tom Bozzay PA, Zucker MJ, Seethamraju H, et al. Post-transplant survival in idiopathic pulmonary fibrosis patients concurrently listed for single and double lung transplantation. The Journal of Heart and Lung Transplantation. 2016;**35**(5):657-660

[41] Nathan SD, Shlobin OA, Ahmad S, Burton NA, Barnett SD, Edwards E. Comparison of wait times and mortality for idiopathic pulmonary fibrosis patients listed for single or bilateral lung transplantation. The Journal of Heart and Lung Transplantation. 2010;**29**(10): 1165-1171

[42] Donahoe M, Valentine VG, Chien N, Gibson KF, Raval JS, Saul M, et al. Autoantibody-targeted treatments for

acute exacerbations of idiopathic
pulmonary fibrosis. PLoS One.
2015;**10**(6):e0127771

[43] Mallick S. Outcome of patients with
idiopathic pulmonary fibrosis (IPF)
ventilated in intensive care unit.
Respiratory Medicine. 2008;**102**(10):
1355-1359

[44] Raghu G, Rochwerg B, Zhang Y,
Garcia CA, Azuma A, Behr J, et al. An
official ATS/ERS/JRS/ALAT clinical
practice guideline: Treatment of
idiopathic pulmonary fibrosis. An
update of the 2011 clinical practice
guideline. American Journal of
Respiratory and Critical Care Medicine.
2015;**192**(2):e3-e19

[45] Singer JP, Blanc PD, Hoopes C,
Golden JA, Koff JL, Leard LE, et al. The
impact of pretransplant mechanical
ventilation on short- and long-term
survival after lung transplantation.
American Journal of Transplantation.
2011;**11**(10):2197-2204

[46] Tipograf Y, Salna M, Minko E,
Grogan EL, Agerstrand C, Sonett J, et al.
Outcomes of extracorporeal membrane
oxygenation as a bridge to lung
transplantation. The Annals of Thoracic
Surgery. 2019;**107**(5):1456-1463

[47] Patel N, Snyder LD, Finlen-
Copeland A, Palmer SM. Is prevention
the best treatment? CMV after lung
transplantation. American Journal of
Transplantation. 2012;**12**(3):539-544

[48] Pêgo-Fernandes PM, Abrão FC,
Fernandes FL, Caramori ML,
Samano MN, Jatene FB. Spirometric
assessment of lung transplant patients:
One year follow-up. Clinics (São Paulo,
Brazil). 2009;**64**(6):519-525

[49] Bos S, Vos R, Van Raemdonck DE,
Verleden GM. Survival in adult lung
transplantation: Where are we in
2020? Current Opinion in Organ
Transplantation. 2020;**25**(3):268-273

[50] Singer JP, Singer LG. Quality of life
in lung transplantation. Seminars in
Respiratory and Critical Care Medicine.
2013;**34**(3):421-430